The concept of tumor immunogenicity has been around for almost as long as the study of immunology itself, and recent years have seen significant advances in the field of human tumor immunology. The purpose of this volume is to review these advances, particularly in relation to the potential for immune intervention in preventing or treating tumors.

The editors and contributors, all leading workers in the field, survey advances in the understanding of the relationship between cancer cell and the immune response. Chapters review in depth the function of immune surveillance and mechanisms of tumor immunity, the role of T lymphocytes and oncogenes in the immune response to cancer, and the potential for immunotherapy of cancer. New areas of tumor immunology are presented, including recent progress in the development of tumor vaccines with particular reference to melanoma.

Up-to-date and authoritative, volumes in this series are intended for a wide audience of clinicians and researchers with an interest in the applications of biomedical science to the understanding and management of cancer.

# TUMOR IMMUNOLOGY

## Immunotherapy and cancer vaccines

# ■ CANCER: CLINICAL SCIENCE IN PRACTICE

*General Editor*

Professor Karol Sikora
*Department of Clinical Oncology*
*Royal Postgraduate Medical School*
*Hammersmith Hospital, London*

A series of authoritative review volumes intended for a wide audience of clinicians and researchers with an interest in the application of biomedical science to the understanding and management of cancer.

Also in this series:
Molecular Endocrinology of Cancer
ISBN 0 521 460 670
Edited by Jonathan Waxman

Cell Therapy
ISBN 0 521 473 152
Edited by George Morstyn and William Sheridan

# ■TUMOR IMMUNOLOGY

## Immunotherapy and cancer vaccines

*Edited by*

### A. G. Dalgleish
*St. George's Hospital Medical School*
*London, UK*

### M. J. Browning
*University of Leicester*
*Leicester, UK*

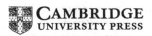

CAMBRIDGE UNIVERSITY PRESS
Cambridge, New York, Melbourne, Madrid, Cape Town, Singapore,
São Paulo, Delhi, Dubai, Tokyo, Mexico City

Cambridge University Press
The Edinburgh Building, Cambridge CB2 8RU, UK

Published in the United States of America by Cambridge University Press, New York

www.cambridge.org
Information on this title: www.cambridge.org/9780521159470

First published 1996
First paperback edition 2010

*A catalogue record for this publication is available from the British Library*

*Library of Congress Cataloguing in Publication Data*

Tumor immunology/edited by A. G. Dalgleish, M. J. Browning.
      p.   cm.–(Cancer, clinical science in practice)
   Includes bibliographical references
   ISBN 0-521-47237-7 (hardback)
   1. Tumors-Immunological aspects.  I. Dalgleish, A. G. (Angus G.)
II. Browning, M. J. (Michael J.) III. Series.
   [DNLM: 1. Neoplasms–therapy.  2. Immunotherapy.  3. Neoplasms–
immunology.  QZ 266 T924 1995]
   AR188.6.T862 1995
   616.99'2079–dc20
   DNLM/DLC                              95-36486
   for Library of Congress                      CIP

ISBN 978-0-521-47237-1 Hardback
ISBN 978-0-521-15947-0 Paperback

# Contents

# Contributors

Michael Browning
*University of Leicester School of Medicine, Leicester, England*

Kerry A. Chester
*MRC Centre, Cambridge, England*

Heung Chong
*Imperial Cancer Research Fund, Rayne Institute, London, England*

Pierre G. Coulie
*Ludwig Institute for Cancer Research, Brussels, Belgium*

A. Maria Dahl
*Courtauld Institute, London, England*

A. G. Dalgleish
*St. George's Hospital Medical School, London, England*

Sina Dorudi
*The Royal London Hospital, London, England*

Dr Richard Essner
*John Wayne Cancer Institute, Santa Monica, California*

Mariet C. W. Feltkamp
*Department of Immunohematology, University Hospital, Leiden, The Netherlands*

Robin Foa
*Centro di Immunogenetica ed Istocompacibilica, Torino, Italy*

Guido Forni
*Centro di Immunogenetica ed Istocompacibilica, Torino, Italy*

Bernard A. Fox
*Earle A. Chiles Research Institute, Portland, Oregon, USA*

Rosalind A. Graham
*Imperial Cancer Research Fund, London, England*

Robert E. Hawkins
*MRC Centre, Cambridge, England*

Dave S. B. Hoon
*John Wayne Cancer Institute, Santa Monica, California, USA*

W. Martin Kast
*Department of Immunohematology, University Hospital, Leiden, The Netherlands*

Cornelis J. M. Melief
*Department of Immunohematology, University Hospital, Leiden, The Netherlands*

Takashi Morisaki
*John Wayne Cancer Institute, Santa Monica, California, USA*

Donald L. Morton
*John Wayne Cancer Institute, Santa Monica, California, USA*

Gary J. Nabel
*Earle A. Chiles Research Institute, Portland, Oregon, USA*

Mepur H. Ravindranath
*John Wayne Cancer Institute, Santa Monica, California, USA*

Nicholas P. Restifo
*Department of Surgery, National Cancer Institute, Bethesda, Maryland, USA*

Pramod K. Srivastava
*Department of Biological Sciences, Fordham University, The Bronx, New York, USA*

Hans J. Stauss
*Courtauld Institute, London, England*

Ryuichiro Suto
*Department of Biological Sciences, Fordham University, The Bronx, New York, USA*

Joyce Taylor-Papadimitriou
*Imperial Cancer Research Fund, London, England*

Richard G. Vile
*Imperial Cancer Research Fund, Rayne Institute, London, England*

Michael Wang
*Department of Surgery National Cancer Institute, Bethesda, Maryland, USA*

# Series Editor's Preface

The immune response to cancer is an elusive topic. We know that tumor cells can be recognized but are not sure how important this recognition is in modifying the course of the disease. Like much in cancer research, its relative importance is dictated by fashion. Beginning with very crude transplantation experiments long before the ground rules of xenogeneic and alogeneic rejection were understood, through the development of syngeneic animal strains, and the immunological and subsequently structural understanding of histocompatibility proteins, we are now entering a remarkable era.

Recent advances in the dissection of both the cellular and humoral arms of the immune system have allowed a much clearer understanding of antigen recognition at a molecular level. Sophisticated tools are now available to analyse the effector side of the immune response effectively. Furthermore, a host of novel reagents are now available to tease apart the basic mechanisms of specific recognition, the generation of diversity, and the destructive mechanisms involved in tumor cell killing.

Tumor immunology is yet again in its ascendency. This volume, truly international in its authorship, puts together a compelling tribute to the power of molecular immunology. From the concept of immunosurveillance, through the molecular mechanisms of tumor antigen recognition to the involvement of cytokines in the inhibition of cancer cell growth, this book provides an excellent and timely summary. It concludes by examining the potential of gene therapy to modify the immune response to cancer in patients – an area of growing clinical investigation.

The next decade is likely to produce novel concepts in both our understanding and in the application of immunology to cancer. Cancer vaccines will almost certainly become available for routine use for the treatment and prevention of cancer. Here is an excellent source book to guide us on the journey through these exciting times.

Karol Sikora

# Abbreviations

| | |
|---|---|
| AAV | adeno-associated virus |
| ABC | ATP-binding cassette |
| Ad | human adenovirus |
| ADCC | antibody-dependent cellular cytoxicity |
| AJCC | American Joint Committee on Cancer |
| ALL | acute lymphoblastic leukemia |
| AML | acute myeloblastic leukemia |
| anti-ids | antidiotypic antibodies |
| APC | antigen presenting cell |
| | |
| BCG | bacille Calmette–Guerin |
| | |
| CD | cluster determinant |
| CEA | carcinoembryonic antigen |
| CML | chronic myeloid leukemia |
| CMV | cytomegalovirus |
| CNTF | ciliary neurotrophic factor |
| CTL | cytolytic T lymphocytes |
| CTL-P | precursors of CTL |
| | |
| DETOX | a combination of mycobacterial cell wall with trehalose dimycolate and monophosphoryl lipid A derived from *Salmonella* |
| DFS | disease-free survival |
| DNFB | dinitrofluorobenzene |
| DNP | dinitrophenol |
| DOPA | dihydroxyphenylanaline |
| DTH | delayed-type hypersensitivity |
| | |
| EBNA | Epstein–Barr virus nuclear antigens |
| EBV | Epstein–Barr virus |
| EGF | epidermal growth factor |

| | |
|---|---|
| EGFr | epidermal growth factor receptor |
| ELISA | enzyme-linked immunosorbent assay |
| EPO | erythropoietin |
| ER | endoplasmic reticulum |
| | |
| 5-FC | 5-fluorocytosine |
| Friend MuLV | Friend's murine leukemia virus |
| | |
| GalNac | N-acetylgalactosamine |
| G-CSF | granulocyte colony-stimulating factor |
| GD3 | ganglioside |
| GH | growth hormone |
| $GM_2$<br>$GM_3$ | gangliosides |
| GM-CSF | granolocyte–macrophage colony-stimulating factor |
| GVH | graft-versus-host |
| GVHD | graft-versus-host disease |
| | |
| HBV | hepatitis B virus |
| HCL | hairy cell leukemia |
| HEL | hen egg lysozyme |
| HGF | hepatocyte growth factor |
| HIV | human immunodeficiency virus |
| HLA | human leukocyte antigen |
| HMW | high molecular weight |
| HPLC | high-performance liquid chromatography |
| HPV | human papilloma virus |
| HSP<br>hsp | heat shock proteins |
| HSV | herpes simplex virus |
| HSVtk | herpes simplex virus thymidine kinase |
| HTLV-1 | human T lymphotrophic virus type-1 |
| | |
| IFA | incomplete Freund's adjuvant |
| IFN | interferon |
| IFN-$\alpha$ | interferon-$\alpha$ |
| Ig | immunoglobulin |
| Ii | invariant chain polypeptide |
| IL | interleukin |
| IL-1RI | interleukin-1 type I receptor |
| IL-1RII | interleukin-1 type II receptor |
| rIL-2 | recombinant interleukin-2 |
| Ir | immune response |

| | |
|---|---|
| IRS-1 | insulin receptor substrate-1 |
| i.v. | intravenous |
| | |
| kb | kilobase |
| KLH | keyhole limpet hemocyanin |
| | |
| LAK | lymphocyte activated killer |
| LDA | limiting dilution analysis |
| LMP | latent membrane protein |
| | |
| $\beta_2$m | $\beta_2$-microglobin |
| MAA | melanoma-associated antigens |
| Mab | monoclonal antibody |
| MAGE | melanoma antigen E |
| MART | melanoma antigen recognized by T cells |
| MCP | monocyte chemoattractant protein |
| MCV | melanoma cell vaccine |
| M-CSF | macrophage colony-stimulating factor |
| cMET | hepatocyte growth factor receptor |
| MHC | major histocompatibility complex |
| MLTC | mixed lymphocyte–tumor cell cultures |
| MLTR | mixed lymphocyte tumor reaction |
| MMTV | mouse mammary tumor virus |
| MPyV | mouse polyomavirus |
| MT | middle T (tumor antigen) |
| MTP | MHC-linked transporter protein |
| MUC1 | mucin gene |
| MUC1-S | secreted MUC1 |
| MUC1-T | transmembrane MUC1 |
| | |
| NeuGc | $N$-glycolyl neuraminic acid |
| NK | natural killer |
| | |
| OSM | oncostatin M |
| OSM | ovine submaxillary mucin |
| | |
| PBL | peripheral blood lymphocytes |
| PCR | polymerase chain reaction |
| PEM | polymorphic epithelial mucin |
| PKC | protein kinase C |
| PLC | phospholipase C |
| PRL | prolactin |
| PSF | peptide supply factor |

| | |
|---|---|
| PTK | protein tyrosine kinase |
| Rbp | retinoblastoma protein |
| RT-PCR | reverse transcriptase polymerase chain reaction |
| SAg | microbial superantigens |
| s.c. | subcutaneous |
| SCCHN | squamous cell carcinoma of the head and neck |
| SEG | a staphylococcal superantigen |
| sFv | intracellular chain antibodies |
| SV40 | simian virus 40 |
| T | large tumor antigen |
| t | small tumor antigen |
| TAA | tumor-associated antigens |
| TAL | tumor-associated lymphocytes |
| TAM | tumor-associated macrophages |
| TAP | transporter associated with antigen processing |
| TATA | tumor-associated transplantation agents |
| $TCID_{50}$ | 50% tissue culture infectious dose |
| TCR | T cell receptor |
| TDLN | tumor-draining lymph node |
| TGF-$\beta$ | tumor growth factor-$\beta$ |
| $T_{H1}$, $T_{H2}$ | T helper cells |
| TIL | tumor-infiltrating lymphocytes |
| TNF | tumor necrosis factor |
| TNF-$\alpha$ | tumor necrosis factor-$\alpha$ |
| TSTA | tumor-specific transplantation antigen |
| TS/A | spontaneous mammary adenocarcinoma of Balb/c mice |
| UV | ultraviolet |
| VMO | vital melanoma oncolysate |
| VV | vaccinia virus |

# 1

# Introduction and Historical Perspective

MICHAEL BROWNING AND A. G. DALGLEISH

The concept of tumour immunogenicity has been around for almost as long as the study of immunology itself, and it has remained one of the most controversial areas in immunology throughout this time. It is over one hundred years since William Coley observed that tumour regression could be induced by stimulating the immune system with bacterial toxins. However, the use of immunotherapy in the treatment of cancer has advanced relatively little since then. In spite of many peaks and troughs of enthusiasm along the way, the concept of a role for the immune response in the control and elimination of malignant cells survived, giving rise in the later 1960s to the 'immune surveillance' theory of cancer (Burnet, 1970), whereby cells of the immune system continuously patrol the body, seeking out and eliminating cells in the process of malignant transformation. The extent to which this actually occurs in vivo remains a topic of debate to this day. Direct evidence of a role for the immune response in the elimination of cancer cells has come from a number of animal models of tumour immunity. The extent to which these mechanisms apply to the majority of human cancers remains unclear, although the last few years have seen significant advances in the field of human tumor immunology.

In the first half of this century, a number of experimental systems showed the rejection of tumours following transplantation within outbred species or across species. In effect, these experiments only demonstrated the strength of the allogeneic and xenogeneic immune response, and with hindsight told us little of the tumour-specific immune response. The introduction of inbred laboratory animal strains allowed similar experiments to be carried out using spontaneously arising tumour transplants in syngeneic recipients. In general, these tumours grew progressively, with little or no evidence of rejection of the tumours or of induction of tumour-specific immunity, leading to the opinion that tumours were largely nonimmunogenic in the hosts in which they arose. The balance of opinion swung in favour of tumour immunogenicity

1

again with the advent of animal models of virally, chemically or irradiation-induced tumours in inbred laboratory strains. In these models, whilst the primary tumour grew progressively in the host, it was shown that an animal, which had been exposed to a tumour and then been surgically cured of that tumour, was capable of rejecting a secondary challenge of cells derived from the same tumour. These experiments showed that the tumours induced immune responses, which exhibited two of the key features of the cognitive immune response, namely specificity and memory. In general, however, prior exposure to the tumour was required in order to observe the protective effects of the immune response in eliminating a tumour cell challenge. In the case of virally induced tumours, the immune response conferred a degree of protection against other syngeneic tumours induced by the same causative agent. In the case of chemically or irradiation-induced tumours, however, this cross reactivity was not observed.

Buy the end of the 1960s, a number of 'paradigms' of tumour immunity were established, in experimental systems at least. Firstly, that most virally induced tumours were immunogenic, and that a degree of protection could be induced in a syngeneic host by prior exposure to the tumour, or to another (syngeneic) tumour caused by the same virus, or in some cases to cell free virus. Secondly, that chemically or irradiation-induced tumours could also, in certain cases, induce a protective immune response capable of rejecting a secondary tumour cell challenge. In these cases, however, the response was specific for the immunizing tumour and showed no cross reactivity for other tumours, even when induced by the same oncogenic process. Thirdly, that most 'spontaneous' tumours were either non- or poorly immunogenic in the host. However, if such tumours were infected with a transforming virus, then they could become immunogenic and then followed the same rules as described above for virally induced tumours.

More recently, the mechanisms that operate in the recognition and elimination of tumour cells in these model systems have been worked out (reviewed by Greenberg, 1991), and have shown a key role for T lymphocytes in conferring the specificity of tumour rejection. In particular, CD8+ cytotoxic T lymphocytes (CTL) were identified as an important effector population in the elimination of tumour cells. In many cases, whilst these responses were mediated by CD8+ CTL, the induction of the response were dependent also on the presence of CD4+ T cells. In addition to these antigen-specific effectors, roles have been identified in tumour rejection for natural killer (NK) cells, and for nonspecific effector cells such as macrophages and eosinophils. It should be noted, however, that a strict delineation between specific and nonspecific effector mechanisms is somewhat arbitrary, as the elimination of tumours in vivo is likely to involve both effector arms acting in concert, rather than one or other acting in isolation. Also, through cytokine signalling pathways, specific effectors may play a major role in the induction and activation of nonspecific effector cells and vice versa.

In humans, direct evidence for a role of the immune response in immunity to tumours was lacking for many years. The occurrence of spontaneous regressions of a number of tumours, the presence of mononuclear cellular infiltrates in many tumour types, and the response of certain tumours to immunotherapy all provided circumstantial evidence of the presence of an immune response to the tumour in a proportion of patients at least, and kept alive the hopes that immune intervention might provide a therapeutic strategy for human cancer. In the last twenty years, there have been very significant advances in our understanding of the molecular mechanisms involved both in the immune response and in the process of cellular transformation resulting in tumours. From the immunological aspect, the identification of the role of molecules encoded by the major histocompatibility complex (MHC) in 'restricting' T cell responses (Zinkernagel & Doherty, 1979) and presenting antigenic peptides to the T cell antigen receptor (Bjorkman et al., 1987) has enabled us to understand how T lymphocytes 'see' antigens. The demonstration by Townsend and colleagues that intracellular proteins encode antigens for CTL and that these can be substituted by exogenous short synthetic peptides corresponding to the antigenic epitope (Townsend et al., 1985, 1986) greatly expanded the range of potential tumour antigens to include virtually any cellular protein expressed in the tumour as long as it was recognized by the immune system as 'nonself' (this would include mutated cellular proteins, and differentiation and tissue specific antigens not expressed in the thymus during T cell ontogeny). The recognition that malignant transformation represents a multi-step process, with mutations occurring in proto-oncogenes and tumour suppressor genes, as well as mutations and aberrant expression of other cellular proteins (reviewed by Fearon & Vogelstein, 1990) gave new insights into the processes by which tumours develop. Together these advances in immunology and in oncology allowed a more rational approach to be taken to the study of human tumour immunity, and the potential for tumour vaccination and immunotherapy, and have led to spectacular advances in the field of tumour immunology in the last few years.

The purpose of this volume is to review these advances, particularly in relation to the role of immune intervention in the prevention or treatment of human cancers. In selecting the topics for inclusion in the volume, we have invited contributions from experts in a variety of fields of tumour immunology in which the greatest advances have been made in the last few years. This approach has inevitably led to some overlap between the subject matter in certain chapters in the book. This overlap, we feel, adds to rather than detracts from the book, in that certain key areas of current research interest are addressed by several authorities, each bringing a slightly different perspective to the data that are emerging in that area. (From the editors' point of view, it has been reassuring that these opinions have not given rise to areas of conflict between authors, but rather that a concensus view of the directions that future work should take and of the potential for immune intervention in cancer therapy appears to be emerging.)

The context is set by Vile and colleagues (Chapter 2), who provide an overview of the role of immune surveillance against cancer, the range of antigens that have been associated with immune recognition of tumours, and the mechanisms, both specific and nonspecific, which operate in tumour immunity.

This is followed by several chapters that address different aspects of the role of T lymphocytes in the immune response to cancer, and their importance as effector cells in the prevention and treatment of cancers. In Chapter 3, Restifo and Wang describe the pathways of antigen processing and presentation via MHC class I and class II molecules to CD8+ and CD4+ T cells respectively, and the role of antigen processing and presentation in malignancy. These pathways provide the basis for the recognition of all antigens by T lymophocytes and are therefore central to our understanding of the specific immune response to tumours. Browning (Chapter 4) describes the role of MHC class I molecules in tumour immunity in general and focuses specifically on the effects of the frequently observed loss of MHC class I expression on tumour cells, the mechanisms that underlie it, and its significance for tumour immunity and immunotherapy. One of the key areas of research in tumour immunology at present is the search for a vaccine or vaccines that can be used to prevent the development of cancers in high-risk groups, or as therapeutic agents in the treatment of established malignancies. Central to this is the need to identify relevant tumour-specific antigens that can be used to induce or augment the immune response. In Chapter 5, Coulie describes the identification and characterization of a number of human tumour antigens that are recognized by tumour-specific cytotoxic T lymphocytes. Another approach to cancer vaccination is the definition of tumour-specific peptides which bind to MHC class I molecules and stimulate the induction of CTL, that are capable of recognizing and lysing tumour cells, which express the antigen from which the peptide sequences were derived (described by Feltkamp, Melief and Kast in Chapter 6). The authors describe this work within a context of the induction of CTL directed against viral oncogene products, and so Chapter 6 also describes the basis of the immune response to virally induced tumours and to viral oncogene products. The role of oncogene products in tumour immunity is elaborated on in Chapter 7, in which Stauss and Dahl describe how cellular oncogene products may act as targets for immune responses in tumour immunity and immunotherapy.

Whilst the potenital for effector T cells as agents in tumour prevention and treatment is now apparent, it is clear also that many tumours are poor stimulators of the immune response, and that there is a disparity between a tumour cell's antigenicity (that is, its ability to present antigen and be recognized by a primed effector cell) and its immunogenicity (that is, its ability to stimulate *de novo* an immune response in the host). This disparity has been addressed recently and methods for enhancing a tumour's immunogenicity have been explored. Two principal approaches have emerged, and these are described in Chapters 8 and 9. Recent studies have indicated that, for an antigen to be immunogenic it must not only be presented in an appropriate way to the immune system (for example, MHC/peptide complex–TcR interaction), but that there is a requirement also for additional 'co-stimulatory' signals delivered to the T lymphocyte to induce activation. In Chapter 8, Dalgleish describes the role of T cell co-stimulatory molecules and their ligands in the induction of tumour-specific immune responses, and in Chapter 9, Forni and Foa describe the role that cytokines play in immune induction and in tumour rejection. These latter studies have implicated a range of effector mechanisms, both specific and nonspecific, in the rejection of tumours. Hoon, Morisaki and Essner, in Chapter 10, further explore the role of cytokines in tumour immunity, by addressing the regulatory effects of interleukin-4 and related cytokines, not on the cells of the immune system, but on non-haematopoietic cancer cells themselves.

The preceding chapters relate largely to the role of the immune response in tumour immunity, and its potential for immunotherapy of cancer. In fact, therapeutic cancer vaccine studies are already in hand, and in Chapter 11, Morton and Ravindranath describe the current concepts concerning melanoma vaccines, and the results obtained using predominantly a mixed allogeneic whole cell melanoma vaccine.

Several new areas of tumour immunology have emerged in the last few years. In Chapter 12, Graham and Taylor-Papadimitriou review the family of epithelial mucins, and their role in immunity to cancers involving glandular epithielium. Chapter 13, by Suto and Srivastava, describes the heat shock proteins, and how heat shock protein–peptide complexes interact with the immune system to provide a novel strategy for vaccination against cancer and infectious disease. A number of the strategies that are being employed to develop cancer vaccines or to enhance the immunogenicity involve the use of recombinant genetic techniques, and in Chapter 14, Fox and Nabel look forward to the potential role of gene transfer and gene therapy in the treatment of malignant disease. Finally, the emphasis is shifted back to the humoral arm of the immune response and its possible role in the treatment of cancer by Hawkins and Chester, in Chapter 15, who describe the application of gene technology to the production of antibodies for use in cancer therapy.

At the time of writing, the manipulation of the immune response to provide strategies for the treatment of human tumours is based largely on potential. The spectacular advances that have been made in our understanding of the relationship between the cancer cell and the immune response in the last few years now need to be translated into practical therapies for this potential to be realized. That is likely to be the main challenge for tumour immunologists for the next few years. The results already obtained with vaccination in late-stage malignant disease, in melanoma at least, are encouraging. The range of approaches that could be taken are legion, however, and it is of paramount importance that properly controlled studies of the safety and efficacy of these potential immunotherapies are carried out in order to develop rational approaches to cancer immunotherapy. Whilst the overall goal of immunotherapy remains the eradication of cancer, it should be remembered that a therapeutic effect that prolongs or improves quality of life, whether achieved by immunotherapy alone or by adjuvant immunotherapy, would be of substantial benefit. The prospects at present are bright.

## REFERENCES

Bjorkman P., Saper M. A., Samraoui B., Bennet W. S., Strominger J. L & Wiley D. C. (1987) The foreign antigen binding site and T cell recognition regions of class I histocompatibility antigens. *Nature*, 329, 512–18.

Burnet F. M. (1970) *Immunological surveillance*. Oxford, Pergamon Press.

Fearon E. R. & Vogelstein B. (1990) A genetic model for colorectal tumorigenesis. *Cell*, 61, 759–67.

Greenberg P. D. (1991) Adoptive T cell therapy of tumors: mechanisms operative in the recognition and elimination of tumor cells. *Advances in Immunology*, 49, 281–355.

Townsend A. R. M., Gotch F. M. & Davey J. (1985) Cytotoxic T cells recognize fragments of influenza nucleoprotein. *Cell*, 42, 457–67.

Townsend A. R. M., Rothbard J., Gotch F., Bahadur G., Wraith D. & McMichael A. J. (1986) The epitopes of influenza nucleoproteins recognized by cytotoxic T lymphocytes can be defined with short synthetic peptides. *Cell*, 44, 959–68.

Zinkernagel R. M. & Doherty P. C. (1979) MHC restricted cytotoxic T cells: studies on the biological role of polymorphic major transplantation antigens determining T cell restriction specificity, function and responsiveness. *Advances in Immunology*, 26, 51–177.

# 2

## The Immunosurveillance of Cancer: Specific and Nonspecific Mechanisms

RICHARD G. VILE, HEUNG CHONG AND SINA DORUDI

## ■ DOES THE IMMUNE SYSTEM PLAY A PART IN THE CONTROL OF TUMOUR GROWTH?

### Antigenicity and Immunogenicity

The role of immune modulation upon the growth of human tumours is a topic of intense interest because it offers the potential for immune-mediated treatments for cancer. Unfortunately, despite many years of high optimism oscillating with great sceptism, the outlook for the use of immunotherapy in the control of tumour growth still remains fraught with uncertainty.

The role of the immune system in modulating the growth of tumour cells in animal model systems in vivo is studied by considering the immunogenicity of a tumour. An immunogenic tumour is one that induces resistance to the growth of a secondary challenge of that tumour following immunization of syngeneic animals with the tumour cells. Experiments in rodents showed that some tumour cell lines, especially those which were induced in vivo by strong chemical carcinogens, when transplanted to syngeneic hosts, demonstrate clear immunogenicity (Globerson & Feldman, 1964; Baldwin, 1973). Moreover, under these circumstances, this immunogenicity was highly tumour specific (Globerson & Feldman, 1964). The conclusion from such studies was that the immunogenic rodent tumours must express determinants, which can be recognized specifically by the immune system and against which an effective immune response can be mounted following appro-priate presentation. These determinants were initially known as tumour-associated transplantation antigens (TATA). From these studies has arisen the concept of tumour antigens, which we will define as determinants on

7

tumour cells, which, under appropriate circumstances, can be recognized by components of the immune system.

The first paradox that arises from these types of studies is why the primary tumour, induced in the animal by chemical carcinogenesis or irradiation, is not itself rejected in vivo, whereas cells from the same tumour can be used to vaccinate naive animals against subsequent challenges with tumorigenic doses of the cells. Presumably, in the rodent models, the antigens that are created by the transformation process can be recognized by the immune system only following a previous exposure, although the immune mechanisms which are involved are unclear (Prehn, 1994). Importantly, however, studies on many spontaneously arising tumours showed that these are only poorly, if at all, immunogenic (Hewitt, Blake & Walder, 1976).

It is not possible to test the immunogenicity of spontaneously arising human tumours in the same way as with animal models. Hence, the definition of immunogenicity, as applied to human tumours, must necessarily be reconsidered. For the purposes of this discussion we will make a functional definition for tumour immunogenicity as the ability of the tumour cells to express determinants: (1) that can be recognized by components of the immune system; and (2) against which an effective immune response can be mounted.

Initially, it would seem that, given this operating definition, any tumour that develops in an immunocompetent patient could be considered to be nonimmunogenic since, if it was not, the immune system would presumably have already mounted an effective (clearative) immune response. However, this may not necessarily be the case; tumour cells may still be immunogenic but the rate of growth of the transformed cells in vivo may be faster than the ability of the immune system to clear them. Therefore, the rate of growth of human tumours in vivo is dependent upon both its immunogenicity (expression of relevant immune-activating antigens) and its rate of growth (determined by the nature of the mutations that have led to the growth transformation of the cells).

## Human Tumours Can be Antigenic but Not Immunogenic

What now seems clear is that at least some tumour cells express tumour antigens that are apparently recognizable by components of the immune system (Boon et al., 1994; Houghton, 1994), that is, they are antigenic. The molecular characterization of these of these antigens is discussed in more detail in the section on Are Tumours Antigenic? and in later chapters. However, these antigens may not be sufficient, per se, to stimulate an effective antitumour immune response, so that many tumours are only poorly, if at all, immunogenic (Pardoll, 1992). Indeed, in patients in which tumours develop, which are known to express such antigens, this must be the case (Boon et al., 1992) (see below). It follows, therefore, that the aim of the range of molecular immunotherapies that are currently being developed for the treatment of cancer (see elsewhere in this volume) is to increase the immunogenicity of tumour cells to above the threshold over which effective immune reactions are generated (Pardoll, 1993).

## Immune Surveillance

The demonstration of tumour/transplantation antigens on tumour cells led to the proposal that tumour growth in vivo might be controlled by the immune system (Burnet, 1970): if a clone of tumour cells evolves which expresses antigens that are truly immunogenic, an intact immune system would, by definition, recognize and clear those clones (Doherty, Knowles & Weittstein, 1984). The failure of spontaneous tumours to be rejected in the same way as tumours generated by highly mutagenic, immunosuppressive methods was used as an argument that an immune screening of emerging tumour cells takes place in vivo to eliminate any tumour cells expressing immunogenic determinants. Thus, the concept of immune surveillance arose in which the immune system was seen as a frontline active protection against the development of cancer (Burnet, 1970; Doherty et al., 1984; Kripke, 1988). This surveillance could only be circumvented if the immune system was depressed by immuno-suppressive treatments (Malmgren, Benneson & McKinley, 1952) or by increased aggressiveness with which tumour cells grow in vivo.

The immune surveillance hypothesis has many intrinsic attractions and can be used to explain several clinical observations. For instance, many human tumours take several years to develop from the time of the initiating molecular mutations in the parental cell. In part, this may be due to the time required for a cell to accumulate sufficient growth-transforming mutations (to oncogenes and tumour suppresor genes) for it to become freed of the constraints of normal growth controls (Vogelstein & Kinzler, 1993). In addition, it may be that this lag period is also due to the time required for the evolution of a population of growth-transformed cells that have lost the expression of immunogenic determi-nants (Kripke, 1988). The population of tumour cells that finally emerges would, therefore, be both fully growth transformed and nonimmuno-genic. Years of growth in situ in the presence of an intact immune system would indeed provide a powerful selection against the emergence of immunogenic tumour cells, using immune surveillance mechanisms to remove immunogenic progeny along the way (Figure 2.1).

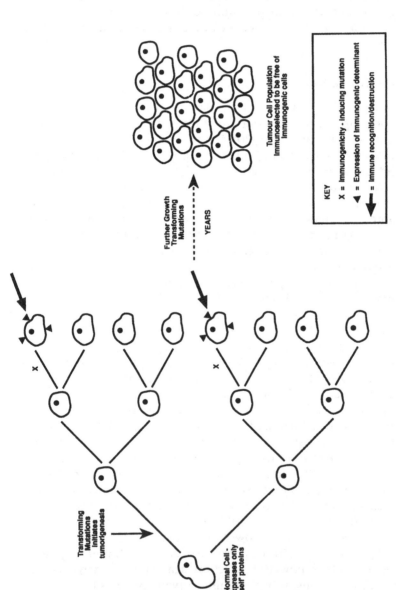

**Figure 2.1** Immune surveillance may not be the primary defence against the development of most tumours but it may contribute to the selection of nonimmunogenic tumour populations. Tumours derive initially from mutations to genes of growth differentiation (proto-oncogens and tumour suppressor genes) and so may not be overtly immunogenic. However, genetic instability during the subsequent multiple cell divisions may generate expression of immunogenic determinants on the cell surface of specific daughter clones and immune surveillance by T cells and NK cells may act to 'mop up' these cells.

Tumour Cell Population
Immunoselected to be free of
immunogenic cells

Further Growth
Transforming
Mutations

YEARS

Transforming
Mutations
Initiates tumorigenesis

Normal Cell -
expresses only
'self' proteins

KEY

X = Immunogenicity - inducing mutation

▲ = Expression of immunogenic determinant

→ = Immune recognition/destruction

Other clinical evidence also suggests a role for the immune system in an antitumour protective role. For example, some tumours undergo spontaneous regressions, albeit vary rarely, associated with detectable immune activity (Rosenberg, 1991). In addition, prognosis of certain tumour types is favourably associated with the histological identification of plentiful infiltrates of immune cells into the tumour site (Oliver & Nouri, 1992). These observations would argue that immune surveillance of tumour populations may be a dynamic process in which subpopulations of immunogenic tumour cells are continually emerging and being recognized by immune cells.

However, recent advances in the understanding of the immune system, more clinical correlations between immune status and tumour incidence, and the application of molecular techniques to the identification of tumour antigens have led to necessary modifications to, but not complete abandonment of, the immune surveillance hypothesis.

If immunosurveillance were truly an important guardian of the body's defence against tumour development, impairing the functioning of the immune system should lead to an increase in the number of tumours that develop. There are, undoubtedly, a few cases where immunosuppression does appear to lead to an increased incidence of a few extremely immunogenic tumour types (Kripke, 1988; Ioachim, 1990). However, a review of the available data from both human and animal models suggests that, at least for most of the common human cancers, this phenomenon is not repeated (Stutman, 1975; Penn, 1988). Similarly, experiments using mice in which the T cell component of the immune system has been eradicated (such as athymic nude mice) have not demonstrated convincing evidence that the absence of an immune system automatically leads to increased incidence of spontaneous tumours (Rygard & Poulson, 1974).

Patients who have not obviously experienced conditions of major immune deficiency do still develop tumours, which must have developed in the presence of intact immune systems, often over a period of years. It would seem likely then that, if tumour clones emerge that do express strongly immunogenic determinants, they would indeed be cleared by the immune system. To this degree, it seems that immune surveillance may well operate in humans, perhaps to 'mop up' any tumours that emerge through gross mutagenic processes, which generate overtly immunogenic cells (Figure 2.1). However, removing the constraints of a functioning immune system does not appear to have a significant effect on the incidence of most common cancers. Therefore, it seems probable that immune surveillance, at least in the form proposed initially, does not act as the primary defence against tumour development in the way that the immune system is the frontline against infectious agents.

Hence, the final tumour population that grows aggressively in vivo and represents the clinically relevant problem:

1. Contains immunogenic cells that cannot be cleared fast enough by the immune system because of the emergence of a particular clone with a very high intrinsic rate of growth (Figure 2.2A), in which case the immune response is arising too late to be of value;
2. Contains cells that are neither antigenic nor immunogenic (Figures 2.1 and 2.2B); or
3. Contains cells that are antigenic but are only poorly immunogenic (Figure 2.2C), in which case these cells are able to ellicit an immune response but this is insufficient for rejection to occur; or
4. Contains a heterogeneous mixture of cells with the properties of any of (1), (2) and (3).

## Therapeutic Implications

If the population of tumour cells is immunogenic but simply outgrows the immune response, returning the patient to a state of minimal residual disease by surgery/chemotherapy/radiation therapy might swing the therapeutic balance in favour of the immune system (although many chemotherapy regimens are also immunosuppressive) (Situation 1). However, if the tumour cells are completely nonantigenic, immunotherapy will be largely futile against such tumours (Situation 2). It is, however, Situation 3 that offers the most hope for effective intervention with immunotherapy. If tumour cells really are antigenic but not yet sufficiently immunogenic for immune clearance due to defects in the pathways of antigen presentation, then modifications of tumour cells or immune cells with immunomodulatory genes/proteins may be able to swing the balance in favour of immune-mediated control of tumour growth (Pardoll, 1993; Rosenberg et al., 1993; Colombo & Forni, 1994; Culver & Blaese, 1994; Tepper & Mule, 1994). This option is particularly attractive because it offers the hope of a new generation of biologically-based therapies, which may be significantly less toxic than the current range of chemotherapeutic drugs. Situation 4 may also be favourable, since infiltrating specific T cells successfully activated by the antigenic cells may be able to release cytokines which are cytotoxic to the adjacent nonantigenic tumour cells, or which activate NK cells (see below in section on Immune Mechanisms of Tumour Recognition and Clearance), which do not depend upon the presence of antigen for killing.

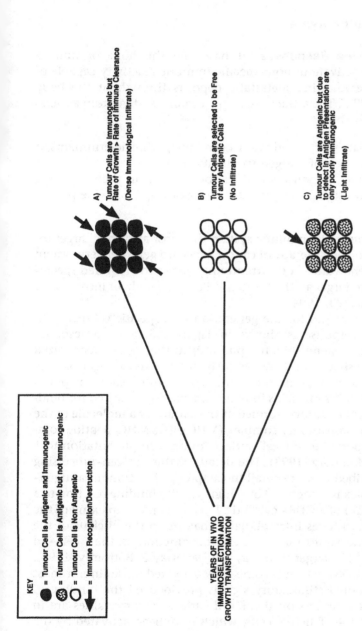

**KEY**

● = Tumour Cell is Antigenic and Immunogenic

◉ = Tumour Cell is Antigenic but not Immunogenic

○ = Tumour Cell is Non Antigenic

↓ = Immune Recognition/Destruction

**YEARS OF IN VIVO
IMMUNOSELECTION AND
GROWTH TRANSFORMATION**

A)
Tumour Cells are Immunogenic but
Rate of Growth > Rate of Immune Clearance

(Dense Immunological Infiltrate)

B)
Tumour Cells are selected to be Free
of any Antigenic Cells

(No Infiltrate)

C)
Tumour Cells are Antigenic but due
to defect in Antigen Presentation are
only poorly Immunogenic

(Light Infiltrate)

**Figure 2.2** Tumours may develop in vivo because of a variety of possible interactions between tumour cells and the immune system – the correlation between in vivo growth of tumour cells, antigenicity, immunogenicity and clinically observable immune infiltrates. (A) The tumour consists of immunogenic cells, which cannot be cleared fast enough by the immune system because of the emergence of a particular clone with a very high intrinsic rate of growth. (B) In the opposite extreme, the tumour contains cells that are neither antigenic nor immunogenic, and so is invisible to the immune system. (C) In the intermediate situation, the tumour contains cells that are antigenic but, because of defects in the antigen presentation pathway, are only poorly immunogenic. Human tumours probably simultaneously contain a heterogeneous mixture of cells that have the properties of (A), (B) and (C).

# ■ IMMUNE MECHANISMS OF TUMOUR RECOGNITION AND CLEARANCE

## Specific Mechanisms

**Cellular Immune Responses** It has been the hope of tumour immunologists to activate tumour-specific immune reactivity capable of recognizing and eradicating metastatic deposits throughout the body (Kedar & Klein, 1992). The attraction of the immune system from a therapeutic viewpoint is that:

1. Once appropriately activated against tumour-specific determinants, it has very high levels of antigen specificity; and
2. It has an in-built response amplification so that, in theory, only a small activation signal can produce a long-lasting bodywide protection.

These properties make the immune system the most attractive target for current attempts at gene therapy of cancer, since no gene delivery system or even chemotherapeutic drug currently has either the required specificity or efficiency to target all the tumour cells in the body of most cancer patients (Vile & Russell, 1994).

The best-case scenario for the generation of a specific cellular antitumour immune response is shown in Figure 2.3. Such a response depends upon the existence of a tumour antigen that can be recognized by the immune system. The endogenously synthesized antigen is processed intracellularly within the proteasome into short peptides (typically about nine amino acids in length), which are selected for binding into the molecular 'groove' formed at the surface of a molecule of the class I major histocompatibility complex (MHC). The MHC–peptide complex is then transported to the cell surface for antigen presentation to T cells (Neefjes & Momburg, 1993). The details of this antigen–processing pathway are described in more detail in Chapter 9. The tumour antigen–MHC class I complex is recognized by a high-affinity binding reaction to a T cell receptor (TCR) of a CD8+ cytolytic T cell (CTL). Complexing of the TCR with antigen initiates intracellular signalling to the nucleus of the CTL stimulating the expression of the effector functions of the T cell – in this case killing of the target (tumour) cell (Janeway & Bottomly, 1994). However, for the CD8+ cell to become fully activated for killing, it must also receive additional stimulatory signals provided by the binding of cytokines to their receptors on the T cell surface. The cytokines are in turn secreted by CD4+ T helper cells, which have been activated by the presentation of the tumour antigen by a professional antigen presenting

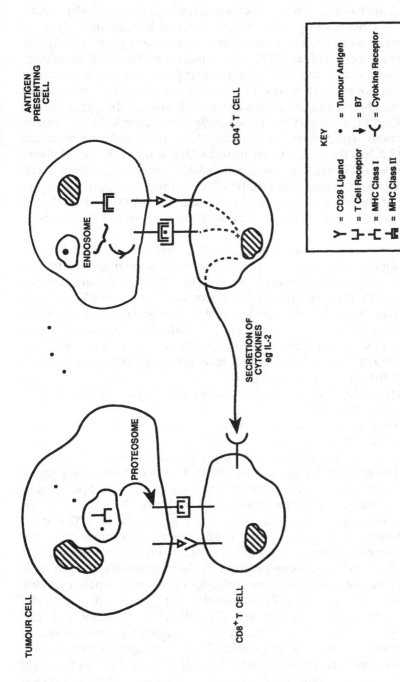

**Figure 2.3** The cellular interactions involved in antigen presentation leading to antigen-specific recognition of tumour cells by cytolytic CD8+ T cells (see text for details).

cell (APC), such as a dendritic cell or a macrophage (Paul & Seder, 1994). These APCs must take up shed antigen, process it proteolyticaly via a separate endosomal antigen processing pathway, and present antigenic peptides complexed with an MHC class II molecule (Neefjes & Momburg, 1993). In addition to the MHC–antigen complexes on the tumour and APC cell surface binding to the TCR on the T cells, full activation also requires the complexing of other surface molecules at the opposing cell surfaces. One such interaction, increasingly recognized as being important in tumour rejection, is the binding of the co-stimulatory molecule B7.1 or B7.2 (on the APC), to its ligand CD28 (on the T cell) (Allison, 1994; June et al., 1994). Therefore, for an MHC-restricted cytolytic T cell response to be generated to a specific tumour antigen requires both presentation of the antigenic peptide by the tumour cell (MHC class I) and cytokine 'help' produced by presentation of the antigen to CD4+ helper T cells (Figure 2.3).

Following successful activation, the CTL will divide so that many daughter clones are produced, all with identical antigen specificity (the same TCR). In addition, certain types of helper T cells will persist in the periphery with the capacity to recognize any future challenge with tumour cells expressing the same antigen. Ideally, this will provide a pool of effector CD8+ T cells that can circulate through the body and are able to destroy any tumour cells that have metastasised as well as a pool of memory cells, which can in future initiate an attack on any cells expressing the same tumour antigen.

Unfortunately, this system clearly does not operate optimally, if at all, in patients who develop cancer. This failure could be for a variety of reasons, some of which will be discussed later in this chapter. For example, many tumour cells down-regulate or lose expression of MHC class I molecules so that antigens cannot be presented (Browning & Bodmer, 1992; Restifo et al., 1993; Vegh et al., 1993). The lack of immunogenicity of tumour cells may also be due to the absence of effective operation of the CD4+ T helper arm of the presentation pathway (Pardoll, 1992). For instance, shedding of tumour antigens and their uptake by APC may be very ineffective in the patient so that full activation of tumour-specific CD4+ helper cells is prevented and complete activation of the CTL fails due to a lack of cytokine secretion from the helper cells (Figure 2.3). This has led to the suggestion that gene transfer of the appropriate cytokine genes directly into tumour cells may be able to bypass the defects in the helper arm of the immune response (Pardoll, 1992; Colombo & Forni, 1994; Tepper & Mule, 1994). Tumour cells modified by gene transfer to express cytokines, such as interleukin-2 (IL-2) or granulocyte–macrophage colony-stimulating factor (GM-CSF), may then act more effectively as antigen presenting cells, fulfilling the functions both of direct antigen presentation to CD8+ cells and cytokine activation of the same cells by local secretion of the cytokine genes (Dranoff et al., 1993) (Figure 2.4) (see Chapter 9). Similarly, gene transfer of accessory molecules such as MHC genes (Tanaka et al., 1988) or co-stimulatory molecules such as B7 (Townsend & Allison, 1993; Ramarathinam et al., 1994), may also enhance the antigen presenting nature of the tumour cells and generate tumour specific CTL responses (Figure 2.4).

The best demonstration that specific, T cell-mediated reactivity to tumour antigens exists, comes from the recovery of MHC-restricted

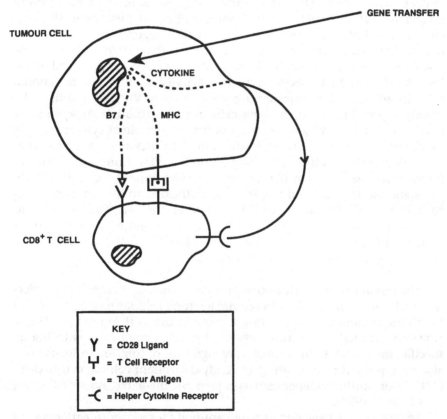

**Figure 2.4** Molecular immunotherapy using gene transfer into tumour cells. Gene transfer into tumour cells, using genes encoding MHC (Tanaka et al, 1988), B7 (Allison, 1994), or cytokines (Tepper and Mule, 1994), for example, might be used to overcome defects in the antigen presenting pathways in vivo. Such molecular therapies aim to make the tumour cell itself into as effective an antigen presenting cell as possible.

CD8+ T cells, which have infiltrated the tumour (Ioannides & Whiteside, 1993). These T cells, called tumour infiltrating lymphocytes (TIL), can be grown in vitro and can subsequently lyse autologous tumour cells from the same patient as well as some tumour cells of the same histological type as long as they are MHC matched (Kawakami et al., 1992). Several workers have tried to exploit the in vivo generation of TIL for therapeutic purposes using adoptive immunotherapy protocols principally in human melanoma patients (Rosenberg et al., 1988; Economou et al., 1992; Lotze et al., 1992). TIL are expanded in vitro in the presence of high levels of IL-2 and returned to the patient in the hope that they will traffic specifically to tumour deposits, which are expressing the tumour antigens against which the TIL were raised (Figure 2.5). A recent study (Mackensen et al., 1994) of TIL from a malignant melanoma showing clinical and histological signs of spontaneous regression demonstrated that a particular clone of T cells, expressing the $V(\beta)16$ variable gene segment of the TCR, was predominant in situ. When purified these $V(\beta)16+$ T cells had specific cytolytic activity against the melanoma cells. In addition, immunostaining showed these $V(\beta)16+$ T cells to be closely apposed to the melanoma cells in situ. Although these data are only derived from a single patient, it points to the role of cytolytic T cells in the specific recognition and destruction of a regressing human tumour.

Unfortunately, although tumour preferential homing of TIL to tumours has been shown (Griffith et al., 1989; Rosenberg et al., 1990), there are also large amounts of residual trafficking to liver and spleen in patients treated with their own TIL. As is often the case, the use of TIL to produce regressions in animal models has been more successful so far than in human patients (Kedar & Klein, 1992) and the routine use of TIL still remains some distance in the future.

**Humoral Immune Responses**    It is generally believed that effective antitumour immunity will require a strong cellular response in order to kill the tumour cells expressing tumour antigens (Knuth et al., 1991). However, antibody responses, deriving from B lymphocytes with highly specific immunoglobulin-mediated recognition of tumour antigens, may also be important in generating antibody-dependent cellular cytotoxicity (ADCC) or antibody-dependent complement-mediated lysis of tumour cells (Lloyd, 1991).

Several groups have documented antibody responses in patients with certain types of tumour (Disis et al., 1994) and in patients treated with cancer vaccines that have been reported to show some clinical efficacy (Kwak et al., 1992; Hoover et al., 1993; Barth et al., 1994; Mittelman et al., 1994). However, there is a paucity of evidence that antibody responses have a significant role on controlling tumour cell growth in patients and

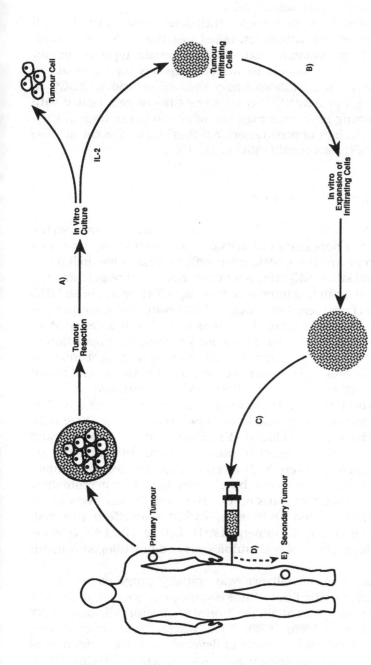

**Figure 2.5** Adoptive immunotherapy with tumour infiltrating immune cells. CD8+, MHC-restricted T lymphocytes infiltrating the tumour can be recovered from the tumour and grown in vitro (A), expanded in the presence of added IL-2 (B), and replaced in vivo (C). Since these cells are believed to recognize specific antigens expressed by the tumour cells, the hope is that, once returned to the patient, their natural tumour-homing specificity will allow them to traffic to tumour deposits throughout the body (D) and lyse the tumour cells (E). Similar experimental treatments have been tried using nonspecific effectors of tumour immunity including NK cells, LAK cells, and TAM.

the majority of current research effort is directed at generating powerful cell-mediated immunity to tumour cells.

Perhaps the most important role for antibodies in cancer therapy will be the use of monoclonal antibodies, raised specifically to tumour antigens known to be preferentially expressed on certain types of tumour cells, to target cytotoxic agents to tumour deposits (Eccles et al., in press). In addition, such antibodies may themselves lead to ADCC in which macrophages or natural killer cells lyse tumour cells coated with antibody. A recurring problem for the use of antibodies in tumour therapy is, however, the lack of penetration that these molecules can achieve into the tumour deposits (Reithmuller et al., 1993).

## Non-specific Mechanisms

**Natural Killer Cells**  As well as antigen-specific T lymphocytes, there are also other populations of activated leukocytes that have been shown to be potent effectors of defence against tumours. One such population, the natural killer (NK) cells, is a non-B, non-T cell population of T lymphocytes, which can lyse tumour cells nonspecifically and in an MHC unrestricted way (Trinchieri, 1989; Klein & Mantovani, 1993; Kurosawa et al., 1993). NK cells lack TCR but do express other T cell differentiation markers. Experiments in mice have previously identified a population of peripheral blood lymphocytes from tumour-bearing hosts that infiltrate tumours to high levels, and can be removed from the tumour and grown in high levels of IL-2 (Lotze et al., 1981). When transferred back to a tumour-bearing host, the cells traffic to tumour deposits and can mediate significant regressions (Yashumura et al., 1994) (Figure 2.5). These cells, named lymphokine activated killer (LAK) cells are a subset of NK cells and have been used for the treatment of human patients (Rosenberg et al., 1985). Unfortunately, the very high levels of IL-2 required to maintain adequate LAK cell activation in vivo have proved to be largely prohibitive because of the associated toxicities of IL-2. However, the discovery of TIL showed that MHC-restricted T cells were fiftyfold more effective in mediating tumour cell killing (Rosenberg, 1991). Unlike TIL, LAK cells are effective in mediating lysis of both autologous and heterologous tumour cells.

Although immune surveillance was initially proposed to be the domain of antigen-specific T cells, there is some evidence that, if immune surveillance does take place at all, the frontline effector cells may be NK cells (Herberman & Holden, 1978). Thus, whereas nude mice lacking functional CD8+ T cells do not tend to develop increased incidences of spontaneous tumours, beige mice which lack NK cells do (Prehn, 1994).

No immunological priming is required to activate antitumour NK activity, although T cell induced activation of NK cells can occur (Herberman & Holden, 1978).

Although the mechanism of NK recognition of the tumour cells is unknown it is not dependent upon the presence of specific tumour antigens (described below).

## Tumour-associated Macrophages

Tumour-associated macrophages (TAM) represent a major component of the lymphoreticular infiltrates of several human tumours (Mantovani et al., 1992; Van Ravenswaay Classen et al., 1992; Klein & Mantovani, 1993). TAM express very high levels of MHC class II antigens, which allow them to present tumour antigens to CD4+ T helper cells at the site of tumour development (see section on Specific Mechanisms of Tumour Recognition and Clearance). This class II-mediated presentation pathway is very important to promote the secretion of helper cytokines by antigen-specific CD4+ cells to complete the antigen-specific activation of CTL. In addition, several groups have shown that eradication of CD8+ CTL does not necessarily prevent tumour rejection. In these circumstances, CD4+ cells are required to secrete cytokines, which recruit nonspecific effectors directly to sites of tumour growth. There is also evidence for a direct role of bone marrow-derived APC in MHC class I-restricted antigen presentation of tumour antigens (Huang et al., 1994).

In addition to antigen presentation, TAM also have tumour cytotoxic capacities themselves but only when activated by cytokines, such as interferon (IFN), secreted from activated CD4+ T cells, or at sites of inflammation (Mantovani et al., 1992). Tumoricidal properties of TAM have been demonstrated extensively in vitro. The mechanisms of cell killing include the release of tumour necrosis factor (TNF), interleukin-1 (IL-1) free radicals, proteases and nitric oxide. The cytokines released by TAM will, in turn, recruit secondary immune cells to the tumour site to amplify the nonspecific tumoricidal effects. In general, the tumoricidal properties of TAM from tumours that are regressing is greater than that from tumours that are actively growing, suggesting that the properties of TAM documented in vitro correlate well with their in vivo functions (Klein & Mantovani, 1993).

In addition, TAM can also kill antibody-sensitized tumour cells as the nonspecific effector of the antibody-dependent, antigen-specific cellular cytotoxicity pathway (ADCC, see section on humoral immune responses).

Therefore, TAM appear to play a central role in the pathways of both specific antitumour immunity (via activation of the CD4+ helper pathway) and of nonspecific antitumour immunity (via their own tumor-icidal properties and their cytokine-secreting functions). For these reasons, TAM have been proposed as good candidates for adoptive transfer to patients for therapy (Bartholeyns, 1993). Clinical trials are currently underway using adoptive transfer of $10^8$ to $10^9$ TAM recovered (and amplified) from patients' tumours and re-infused systemically. Preliminary results have demonstrated accumulation of re-infused macrophages at the necrotic periphery of melanoma and carcinoma biopsies, but efficacy data are still awaited. In addition, TAM may be candidates in the future as vehicles for delivery of cytotoxic drugs, immunomodulators or therapeutic genes to tumour deposits in vivo (Bartholeyns, 1993). In this respect, the longevity of macrophages in the circulation (up to several years) makes them attractive delivery vehicles for cancer gene therapy.

Finally, it is also important that several reports have also documented an apparently synergistic interaction of TAM with tumour cells in which the macrophages appear to secrete growth factors that may enhance tumour cell growth and/or metastasis (Mantovani et al., 1992). Therefore, the use of TAM in tumour immunotherapy may be a double-edged sword that can be exploited, but only with care.

### Other Cell Types Mediating Nonspecific Immunity

A variety of other immune cells have been implicated in mediating tumour regression, including eosinophils, mast cells and neutrophils. These cell types are typically recruited to sites of inflammation, often in response to cytokine secretion by activated CD4+ helper cells and TAM. The efficacy of eosinophils in mediating rejection of rodent tumours has been demonstrated clearly by experiments in which tumour cells engineered to express interleukin-4 (IL-4) were shown to be rejected in vivo (Golumbek et al., 1991; Tepper, Coffman & Leder, 1992). The rejection was accompanied by distinctive infiltration of the regressing tumour by eosinophils and macrophages, and, under certain circumstances, short-lived immunological memory was produced, which conferred some resistance to subsequent challenge with unmodified tumour cells.

## ■ ARE TUMOURS ANTIGENIC?

For immune control of tumours to be possible, in whatever form, the cells must express determinants that are, at least potentially, capable of being recognized by components of the immune system. In addition, these determinants must be qualitatively or quantitatively sufficiently different from normal cellular determinants to ensure that any subsequent immunity raised against them does not lead to autoimmune destruction of normal cells (Golumbek et al., 1993).

The early work on transplantation of tumours between syngeneic hosts demonstrated the existence of transplantation antigens on tumour cells. As already discussed, these antigens, when seen as a vaccinating challenge, lead to the stimulation of immune responses, which mediate rejection of secondary challenges of immunogenic tumour cells. Such animal data led to, and continue to provoke, hopes that tumour cell preparations might be used as cancer vaccines to stimulate antitumour immunity in patients with established disease (Bystryn, 1990; Oettgen & Old, 1991; Morton et al., 1993). Recently, however, molecular techniques have been used to identify and clone individual genes that fulfil some of the criteria of tumour antigens, but only so far from a limited range of human tumours (Boon et al., 1992; Houghton, 1994). This has led to a new era of tumour vaccination trials. However, as well as generating new hopes for the use of 'molecular vaccines' in cancer therapy, these results have also raised complex apparent paradoxes, which must also be confronted even in the light of the new enthusiasm.

### Classes of Tumour Antigens

Several classes of molecules have now been identified at a molecular level, which might act as tumour antigens and even perhaps as tumour immunogens. These are described in detail elsewhere (Boon et al., 1994; Houghton, 1994; Pardoll, 1994) and are listed by type in Table 2.1.

**Nonself Tumour Antigens**  The most obvious types of determinants, which could act as rejection antigens on tumour cells, are viral proteins that derive from an oncogenic virus. These proteins may be those derived directly from the transforming proteins themselves, such as the human papilloma virus E6 or E7 proteins (Chen, et al., 1991), or they may be other viral antigens, which are not directly involved in the process by which the virus transforms the cell – for instance, the viral structural proteins. In fact, only between 15 and 25% of human cancers are thought to have a viral aetiology (Schulz & Vile, 1992) and even then there is good evidence that viral-induced tumour cells have very often down-regulated expression of the most immunogenic viral proteins (such as envelope proteins) (Klein & Boon, 1993). This probably represents a form of immunosurveillance, since virally infected cells expressing foreign antigens will be rapidly selected out; only infected cells which lose, or down-regulate expression of these proteins will survive immune clearance long enough to become transformed by the action of the viral transforming proteins. Nonetheless, this still leaves the transforming proteins as potential targets for T cell and humoral immune responses and considerable research effort is currently being directed to determining the most immunogenic parts of proteins, such as the papilloma virus E6 and E7 proteins, which are known to be maintained in transformed cells in cervical neoplasia (Chen et al., 1991).

The other class of 'nonself' antigens that might be available to signal the emergence of a tumour population to the immune system is the mutated cellular proteins whose mutation is integral to the transformation process (Table 2.1). Mutations to proto-oncogenes and mutated tumour suppressor genes produce protein products that differ from the normal proteins by one or a few amino acid residues. There is growing evidence that cytotoxic T cells can be detected from both animal models and patient populations, which have reactivity against mutated regions of oncoproteins, such as RAS and tumour suppressor proteins such as p53, whilst having minimal reactivity against the normal proteins (Jung & Schluesener, 1991; Chen et al., 1992; Schlichtholz et al., 1992; Skipper & Stauss, 1993; Nijman et al., 1994) (see Chapter 7). Therefore, even though these 'antigens' are derived from host cell-encoded, self genes (as opposed to virally encoded, 'foreign' genes), they may serve as immunogenic targets for the immune system – provided the appropriate peptides can pass successfully through the proteasome processing pathway and be presented by class I MHC molecules on the surface of tumour cells.

**Self Tumour Antigens**   Within the last few years, molecular biology has been used to clone a new set of potential human tumour antigens. These studies have revealed that proteins, which are neither foreign (nonself) nor mutated versions of normal cellular proteins, can serve as targets for cytotoxic T cell responses against tumour cells (Table 2.1).

The first class of such genes was cloned from human melanomas using a biological assay in which CTL clones derived from a patient were used to identify a specific molecule expressed by the melanoma cells from the same patient (Van der Bruggen et al., 1991; Gaugler et al., 1994). The MAGE family of genes have been shown to be unmutated versions of a cellular gene that is normally only expressed in early ontogeny but not normally on mature tissues other than in the testes. In addition, screening of other tumour types show that MAGE is expressed on a variety of tumour cells (Brasseur et al., 1992) but not on their corresponding normal cellular counterparts (see Chapter 5). Similar biological assays based on the use of patient CTL have also been used to clone other antigens, including the melanocyte-specific enzyme, tyrosinase (Brichard et al., 1993), and MART protein (Kawakami et al., 1994a), which differ from the MAGE family of antigens in that they are normally expressed on

**Table 2.1** The Spectrum of Antigens that the Immune System is likely to Encounter and their Relationship to Known Classes of Tumour Antigens to which T and B Cell Responses have been shown

| Self | | Altered self | | Nonself |
|---|---|---|---|---|
| 'Dangerous self' | 'Nondangerous self' | | Mutated version of self | Foreign |
| Important for development – against which autoimmunity would be greatly deleterious | Abnormal levels of expression on normal tissues | Abnormal levels of expression and inappropriate timing | | Viral antigens |
| e.g. Normal RAS, normal p53 | HER-2/neu Tyrosinase MART | MAGE family | Oncogenic RAS* Mutated p53* Translocation bcr-abl | Papilloma:- E6, E7 EBV:- EBNA HBV: x antigen HTLV-1: tax; env |
| | | **Immunological reaction** | | |
| All reactive T/B cells negatively selected in thymus | *Either* low affinity immune cells sneak through tolerization process because of low levels of expression of antigen in thymus *Or* high-affinity immune cells in periphery because of absence of antigen in thymus *Or* low affinity (?) cells raised against only 'cryptic' or 'subdominant' epitopes of antigen | | CTL/antibodies raised against mutated peptides but not (?) against the corresponding normal peptide | Antiviral CTL raised, provided the antigens which are not down-regulated in the infected cell are still immunogenic (can be presented by MHC class I in tumour cells) |

melanocytes but are expressed in greater quantities in patients with melanoma, partly because of the large numbers of cells expressing the proteins.

The CTL response to these antigens appears to be specific as judged by two related observations:

1. Melanoma cells not expressing the antigens are not killed by the respective patient CTL (Brichard et al., 1993; Boon et al., 1994);
2. The antigenic peptides must be presented in the context of specific MHC molecules (Kawakami et al., 1994b) (melanoma cells expressing the antigen but lacking the appropriate MHC class I molecule are not lysed by the patient CTL).

This property of the presentation of tumour antigens has recently been used to identify a tumour antigenic epitope in human melanoma (Cox et al., 1994). Peptides were eluted from MHC class I molecules on tumour cells, fractionated by chromatography and analysed using tandem mass spectrometry. A peptide epitope was identified, which, when complexed with the appropriate MHC class I molecule, was recognized by CTLs derived from the same patient as well as from five other melanoma patients. This peptide forms part of a previously unidentified protein, which is specific to melanocyte and melanoma cells.

These classes of antigens have the hallmarks of being able to be recognized in specific, MHC-restricted, T cell-mediated immune responses. This has been used to argue that such antigens could be used as vaccines in patients with tumours, which are known to express the antigen and who have the correct MHC haplotype, to ensure that the antigen will be correctly presented to the immune system (Traversari et al., 1992; Marchand et al., 1993) (see Chapter 4).

In contrast, a population of T lymphocytes has also been identified that resembles NK cells in that they lyse their targets in an MHC unrestricted fashion but resemble CTL in that they appear to be specific for the target antigen encoded by the *MUC*-1 gene, which is expressed on the surface of breast and pancreatic tumours (Barnd et al., 1989; Taylor-Papadimitriou et al., 1993). MUC-1 does not have to be processed via the proteasome pathway typical of MHC class I presentation but is recognized by virtue of its cell surface expression by a mechanism that is still unclear.

## ■ PARADOXES OF T CELL-MEDIATED TUMOUR IMMUNE SURVEILLANCE

Despite the great attraction and elegance of these types of studies, there would seem to be two conceptual paradoxes which have, as yet, to be fully resolved.

## Tumour Surveillance Requires the Breaking of Tolerance to Self Antigens

The first is that the use of genes such as MAGE, tyrosinase and MART as vaccines requires the breaking of immunological tolerance to what are, after all, normal self antigens (Golumbek et al., 1993; Parmiani, 1993; Houghton, 1994). As such, it might be expected that all reactive T cells against these self antigens would already have been negatively selected in the thymus. However, the means by which these antigens were cloned clearly demonstrate the existence in melanoma patients of self antigen-reactive T cells, which are precursors of the CTL induced in vitro, suggesting that tolerance can be broken to these antigens. This conflict might be explained by postulating one of the following:

1. There is a population of T cells, which have already encountered the antigens in the thymus but were not eliminated because their TCR interaction with the antigenic peptide is only of low affinity.
2. The T cell population selected by the experiments used to clone the antigens never actually encountered the antigen during thymic development, perhaps because of the low expression of the antigen in the thymus. This situation is possible only if (inadvertant) elimination of the normal cells, which express the antigen by an auto-immune response, would not pose an acute threat to normal development. Alternatively, it may be that the same normal cells are sequestered away from contact with immune cells.
3. The CTL derived from these patients have been raised against 'subdominant' or 'cryptic' determinants on the self antigens, rather than against the 'dominant' determinants, which are processed from the native molecule and are efficiently presented by MHC molecules. In contrast, subdominant determinants are only poorly presented to T cells – such clones are thus not negatively selected and tolerance is not induced to these determinants.

Therefore, the study of antitumour immune responses has shown that the distinction between 'self' and 'nonself' is not a sharply defined one (Table 2.1). Indeed, it has been suggested that certain antigens might be recognized not as 'self' or 'nonself' but as 'dangerous' or 'nondangerous' (Moudgil & Sercarz, 1994). Dangerous antigens would be those that are widely expressed on important tissues and, if they formed the focus of an autoimmune reaction, would pose a threat to development. In contrast, nondangerous antigens would be ones that, if weakly reactive T cells are raised against them or cryptic determinants within them, will not cause an acute threat to the development of the organism. It may be significant in this respect that the majority of T cell-mediated tumour antigens have been cloned only from melanoma and that loss of melanocytes (vitiligo) during certain pathological conditions does not not lead to any serious, acutely life-threatening condition. In addition, many patients who show positive responses to immunotherapy in melanoma also develop vitiligo (Richards, 1991). This suggests that it is possible (and even beneficial in melanoma patients) to stimulate immunity to components of normal melanocytes and, furthermore, loss of melanocyte function, although cosmetically undesirable, does not seem to be especially deleterious to the patient.

Whatever the mechanism by which potentially self-reactive T cells are maintained in the periphery, they seem to be unresponsive (anergic) until a perturbation in the system occurs. This perturbation could be produced by the emergence of a tumour population in which suprathreshold levels of the antigen are expressed. This may be sufficient to break anergy and allow interaction of either low-affinity T cells with the antigen [(1) in list above] or interaction of normal affinity T cells with a self antigen against which they have never learned tolerance [(2) in list above]. Hence, immune recognition of self tumour antigens may use a similar mechanism to that seen in autoimmunity where the reactive T cells have a limited repertoire of TCRs (otherwise they would not have escaped thymus selection).

If the scenario described in (1) above is actually the case, it remains to be seen if the normally anergic T cells with only low-affinity TCR for the antigen will, when activated to become CTLs, be able to clear tumours in vivo.

## Are Self Antigens Relevant to Tumour Immunity?

These considerations lead to the second dilemma presented by the identification of these self proteins as potential tumour antigens and highlights a danger of producing what may be essentially circular arguments in the justification of the importance of these genes in antitumour immunity. The argument goes that, because CTLs derived from precursor T cells in the patient's peripheral blood have been used to identify these antigens, they might potentially be good targets for use in vaccines. For self antigens, such as MAGE, the point has been made that these antigens can be presented to the immune system in a specific, MHC-restricted fashion (Kawakami et al., 1992) and effectively enough to activate a CTL response in vitro (Van der Bruggen & Van den Eynde, 1992). Therefore, the following questions arise:

1. Why, in the presence of such an antigen, an effective immune response is not elicited leading to tumour rejection,

2. Is the immune reactivity, which has been selected out by these experiments, really relevant to a clearative antitumour immune response in vivo; and, therefore,
3. Are these antigens really appropriate targets for vaccination?

Several theoretical arguments can be offered as reconciliation. The most optimistic one is that the CTL identified in the experiments of Boon (Van der Bruggen et al., 1991; Brichard et al., 1993) and others (Kawakami et al., 1994) exist in the periphery as precursor T cells with the potential to recognize tumour antigens (correct TCRs) but lack the functional signals in vivo that complete the circle of T cell activation (Figures 2.3 and 2.4) (such as appropriate T cell help, via cytokine secretion, or co-stimulatory signals). The in vitro experiments, in which the antigens are identified using what are clearly fully activated CTL, are all carried out after incubation of the precursor T cells for several weeks in the presence of added IL-2, irradiated cells derived from the autologous tumour as well as feeder cells (for example, Brichard et al., 1993), that is, under conditions in which adequate T cell 'help' is already artificially supplied by the investigator. If such help can be provided to the tumour cell–T cell recognition reaction in vivo, for instance using gene transfer of cytokine (Tepper & Mule, 1994) or B7 (Allison, 1994) genes, it might be possible to replicate the in vitro situation of effective recognition and killing of tumour cells in an MHC-restricted, antigen-specific manner (Figure 2.4).

There are also other possible explanations for the failure of the antitumour immune response despite the existence of defined tumour antigens and potentially reactive CTL. For example, an immunological 'sneak through' mechanism may allow the development of tumours that express tumour antigens, but at low levels and for long periods. Indeed, animal experiments have demonstrated what may be a similar phenomenon whereby a large inoculum of tumour cells (Humphreys et al., 1962), or *Taenia taeniaformis* (Mitchell, Rajasekariah & Richard, 1980), can be rejected by naive mice but a small inoculum is not. Therefore, induction of tolerance, rather than immunity, by a nascent tumour or infection may occur in a patient over a long period of time despite the presence of potentially antigenic and immunogenic targets. Other explanations have also been proposed for the absence of effective immune clearance of tumours despite the presence of immunogens, including the possibility that the orthotopic site in which the tumour develops may be a poor site for immunization and that vascularization of small tumours may be delayed so that the immune system cannot 'see' a tumour that grows from a small inoculum.

Finally, Prehn has suggested that the interaction between an immunogenic tumour and the immune system may be a complex one such that many tumours may actually be stimulated by cytokines and antibodies resulting from a weak immune reaction raised against itself (Prehn, 1994). The theoretical arguments of Prehn suggest that immunotherapy may even lead to an increased growth of human tumours if the increment of the antitumour immune response that is produced by the therapy is not large enough and even that tumour inhibition may be more effectively brought about by immunosuppression. Indeed, this author even suggests that the immunodepression seen in many cancer patients, possibly as a result of chemotherapy, may be a protective response to take away any stimulatory effects on the growth of the tumour produced by a weak immune response against it (Prehn, 1994). It thus appears that the interaction of a tumour expressing putative immunogens with the immune system is likely to be much more complex than might appear at first inspection.

## ◼ IN VIVO TUMOUR CELL KILLING MAY ENHANCE GENERATION OF ANTITUMOUR

We have recently shown that multiple intravenous (i.v.) injections of high titre retroviral supernatant encoding the herpes simplex virus thymidine kinase (*HSVtk*) cytotoxic gene produced significant reductions in the number of lung metastases in mice treated with ganciclovir compared to saline-treated controls (Vile et al., 1994). When DNA was prepared from a variety of tissues, proviral integration was detected only in the tumour-bearing lungs of mice subsequently treated with saline (four of six) but not ganciclovir. It seems probable that these PCR signals represent infection of the dividing tumour cells in the lungs of saline-treated mice, whereas they are not detected in the ganciclovir-treated animals because expression of the *HSVtk* gene leads to eradication of the infected cells in this group. Although expression of the *HSVtk* gene leads to a considerable bystander killing effect in vitro (Vile & Hart, 1993), it seemed unlikely that the substantial in vivo reduction in the number of disseminated lung metastases could be explained by this localized bystander killing, which is effective over only a short distance (Bi et al., 1993; Freeman et al., 1993). It also seemed unlikely that efficiency of viral infection alone could account for the observed effects, since the delivery of viral particles to such a high proportion of lung nodules would be hindered by adsorption to endothelial cells on the passage through the heart into the lungs. When we repeated our experiments in athymic mice, the results suggested that a T cell-dependent immune-mediated mechanism may be amplifying the therapeutic effect of direct killing of a few tumour cells in the lungs, a result which is consistent with two other recently published reports (Barba et al., 1994; Mullen et al., 1994).

Therefore, although the *HSVtk*-expressing B16 tumour cells, which were used in these studies, are normally only very poorly immunogenic (Hock et al., 1993), when B16 cells express the *HSVtk* gene, they are killed in situ by ganciclovir treatment and the treated mice become partially protected against subsequent challenge with parental, B16 tumour cells. Two other similar reports have been published showing the development of a similar antitumour immunity following in vivo killing of tumour cells using either the cytosine deaminase (Mullen et al., 1994) or *HSVtk* gene (Barba et al., 1994), the latter effect being associated with infiltrates of CD8+ T cells and macrophages (Barba et al., 1994). The mechanisms by which the killing of B16 tumour cells in vivo by ganciclovir but not by in vitro lethal irradiation confers a protective immunity to challenge by parental cells is of great potential interest for the development of better approaches to antitumour vaccination protocols. It is possible that these effects may be mediated in part by the release of inhibitory factors from the dying tumour that inhibit the growth of tumour cells growing at distant sites (O'Reilly et al., 1994). However, the importance of a functional immune system suggests that immune-based mechanisms are also involved. One possibility is that the killing of a large number of cells in vivo, which have already formed established tumours, leads to the release of a massive load of dead tumour cells debris, and the efficient uptake and presentation of their tumour antigens by cells of the immune system (such as macrophages and dendritic cells) (Cavallo et al., 1993; Raychaudhuri & Morrow, 1993; Colombo & Forni, 1994; Udono et al., 1994). This may involve some novel mechanisms of antigen presenting (Huang et al., 1994), in a manner different from that which occurs when lethally irradiated cells die in vivo. If so, such effects might be enhanced by the use of vectors, which, as well as encoding cytotoxic genes such as *HSVtk*, also encode cytokines, such as GM-CSF, which promote differentiation of antigen presenting cells and are effective in generating protective antitumour immunity (Dranoff et al., 1993; Levitsky et al., 1994).

# ■ SUMMARY

It is now clear that, despite being a disease of immunologically speaking 'self' cells, some tumours can be recognized by both specific and nonspecific effector arms of the immune system. Clearly, however, the interconnecting network of immune cells that are responsible for antitumour reactivity will act in concert rather than in isolation. Therefore, the distinction between specific and nonspecific mechanisms may be somewhat arbitrary. For example, there is accumulating evidence suggesting specificity in NK cell recognition of targets (Trinchieri, 1994); antigen nonspecific macrophages may mediate the ADCC clearance of tumour cells coated with highly antigen-specific antibody, and secretion of cytokines by CD4+ helper cells may activate both antigen-specific CTL and nonspecific effectors of tumour cell killing.

The last few years have seen major developments in the understanding of how tumours may be antigenic and/or immunogenic. Molecular characterization of viral antigens and mutated cellular proteins intimately associated with the transformation process, have highlighted potential sequences that tumour cells might express, leading to classical rejection reactions directed at immunologically 'foreign' immunogens. Identification of proteins that are expressed on human tumour cells and against which MHC-restricted CTLs have been raised by the patient have also recently provided a new set of targets for antitumour vaccination. However, it is important not to ignore the theoretical problems and apparent contradictions that these findings have posed for the understanding of the immunological reaction to tumour cells. Whilst it is hoped that such proteins will genuinely provide novel, effective therapeutic targets for tumour immunotherapy, an open mind must also be kept to the possibility that such proteins are decoys against which, at best, only weak and nonclearative immunity can be raised. After all, these are self antigens against which immunological tolerance must be broken (if it exists) and which have already been proven to be able to coexist, at high levels of expression, with the immune system in patients who develop tumours. Although much has still to be learned about the basic immunological mechanisms by which tumour cells are recognized or ignored by the immune system, the possibility of augmenting responses against these tumour-associated antigens gives real hope that molecular immunotherapies may soon make a clinical impact on tumour control.

# ■ DEDICATION

This chapter is dedicated to Sandy Jaffe, who died of cancer whilst it was being prepared, and to her family.

## REFERENCES

Allison J.P. (1994) CD28-B7 interactions in T-cell activation. *Current Opinion in Immunology*, 6, 414–19.

Baldwin R.W. (1973) Immunological aspects of chemical carcinogenesis. *Advances in Cancer Research*, 18, 1–75.

Barba D., Hardin J., Sadelain M. & Gage F.H. (1994) Development of anti tumour immunity following thymidine kinase-mediated killing of experimental brain tumours. *Proceedings of the National Academy of Sciences USA*, 91, 4348–52.

Barnd D.L., Lan M.S., Metzgar R.S. & Finn O.J. (1989) Specific tumor histocompatibility complex – unrestricted recognition of tumor-associated mucins by human cytotoxic T cells. *Proceedings of the National Academy of Sciences USA*, **86**, 7159–63.

Barth A., Hoon D.S.B., Foshag L.J. et al. (1994) Polyvalent melanoma cell vaccine induces delayed-type hypersensitivity and in vitro cellular immune response. *Cancer Research*, **54**, 3342–5.

Bartholeyns J. (1993) Monocytes and macrophages in cancer immunotherapy. *Research in Immunology*, **144**, 288–91.

Bi W.L., Parysek L.M., Warnick R. & Stambrook P.J. (1993) In vitro evidence that metabolic co-operation is responsible for the bystander effect observed with HSG tk retroviral gene therapy. *Human Gene Therapy*, **4**, 725–31.

Boon T., Cerottini J.C., Van den Eynde B., van der Bruggen P. & Van Pel A. (1994) Tumor antigens recognised by T lymphocytes. *Annual Review of Immunology*, **12**, 337–65.

Boon T., De Plaen E., Lurquin C., Van Den Eynde B., Van Der Bruggen P. et al. (1992) Identification of tumour rejection antigens recognised by T lymphocytes. *Cancer Surveys*, **13**, 23–37.

Brasseur F., Marchand M., Vanwijck R. et al. (1992) Human gene MAGE-1, which codes for a tumor-rejection antigen, is expressed by some breast tumors. *International Journal of Cancer*, **52**, 839–41.

Brichard V., Van Pel A., Wolfel T. et al. (1993) The tyrosinase gene encodes for an antigen recognised by autologous cytolytic T lymphocytes on HLA-A2 melanomas. *Journal of Experimental Medicine*, **178**, 489–95.

Browning M.J. & Bodmer W.F. (1992) MHC antigens and cancer: implications for T-cell surveillance. *Current Opinion in Immunology*, **4**, 613–18.

Burnet F.M. (1970a) The concept of immunological surveillance. *Progress in Experimental Tumour Research*, **13**, 1–27.

Burnet F.M. (1970b) *Immunological surveillance*. Oxford, Pergamon Press.

Bystryn J.C. (1990) Tumour vaccines. *Cancer and Metastasis Reviews*, **9**, 81–91.

Cavallo F., Di Pierro F., Giovarrelli M. et al. (1993) Protective and curative potential of vaccination with interleukin-2-gene transfected cells from a spontaneous mouse mammary adenocarcinoma. *Cancer Research*, **53**, 5067–70.

Chen I., Thomas E.K., Hu S.L., Hellstrom I. & Hellstrom K.E. (1991) Human papilloma virus type 16 nucleoprotein E7 is a tumor rejection antigen. *Proceedings of the National Academy of Sciences USA*, **88**, 110–14.

Chen W., Peace D.J., Rovira D.K. et al. (1992) T cell immunity to the joining region of p210-bcr-abl protein. *Proceedings of the National Academy of Science USA*, **89**, 1468–72.

Colombo M.P. & Forni G. (1994) Cytokine gene transfer in tumor inhibition and tumor therapy: where are we now? *Immunology Today*, **15**, 48–51.

Cox A.L., Skipper J., Chen Y. et al. (1994) Identification of a peptide recognised by five melanoma-specific human cytotoxic T cell lines. *Science*, **264**, 716.

Culver K.W. & Blaese R.M. (1994) Gene therapy for cancer. *Trends in Genetics*, **10**, 174–8.

Disis M.L., Calenoff E., McLaughlin G. et al. (1994) Existent T cell and antibody immunity to HER2/neu protein in pateints with breast cancer. *Cancer Research*, **54**, 16–19.

Doherty P.C., Knowles B.B. & Wettstein P.J. (1984) Immunological surveillance of tumors in the context of major histocompatibility complex restriction of T cell function. *Advances in Cancer Research*, **42**, 1–65.

Dranoff G., Jaffee E., Lazenby A. et al. (1993) Vaccination with irradiated tumor cells engineered to secrete murine granulocyte macrophage colony stimulating factor stimulates potent, specific, and long lasting anti-tumor immunity. *Proceedings of the National Academy of Sciences USA*, **90**, 3539–43.

Eccles S.A., Court W.J., Box G.A., Dean C.J., Melton R.G. & Springer C.J. (in press) Regression of established breast carcinoma xenografts with antibody-directed enzyme prodrug therapy against c-erbB2 p185. *Cancer Research*, **54**.

Economou J.S., Figlin R.A., Jacobs E. et al. (1992) The treatment of patients with metastatic melanoma and renal cell cancer using in vitro expanded and genetically engineered (neomycin phosphotransferase) bulk, CD8+ and/or CD4(+) tumor infiltrating lymphocytes and bulk, CD8(+) and/or CD4(+) peripheral blood leukocytes in combination with recombinant interleukin-2 alone, or with recombinant interleukin-2 and recombinant alpha interferon. *Human Gene Therapy*, **3**, 411–30.

Freeman S.M., Abboud C.N., Whartenby K.A. et al. (1993) The 'bystander effect' tumour regression when a fraction of the tumour mass is genetically modified. *Cancer Research*, **53**, 5274–83.

Gaugler B.B., Van den Eynde B., van der Bruggen P. et al. (1994) Human gene MAGE-3 codes for an antigen recognised on a human melanoma by autologous cytolytic T lymphocytes. *Journal of Experimental Medicine*, **179**, 921.

Globerson A. & Feldman M. (1964) Antigenic specificity of benzo(a)pyrene-induced sarcomas. *Journal of the National Cancer Institute*, **32**, 1229–43.

Golumbek P., Levitsky H., Jaffee E. & Pardoll D.M. (1993) The antitumor immune response as a problem of self–nonself discrimination: implications for immunotherapy. *Immunological Research*, **12**, 183–92.

Golumbek P.T., Lazenby A.J., Levitsky H.I. et al. (1991) Treatment of established renal cancer by tumor cells engineered to secrete interleukin-4. *Science*, **254**, 713–16.

Griffith K.D., Read E.J., Carrasquillo J.A. et al. (1989) In vivo distribution of adoptively transferred indium-111-labeled tumor infiltrating lymphocytes and peripheral blood lympocyes in patients with metastatic melanoma. *Journal of the National Cancer Institute*, **81**, 1709–17.

Herberman R.B. & Holden H.T. (1978) Natural cell mediated immunity. *Advances in Cancer Research*, **27**, 305–77.

Hewitt H.B., Blake E.R. & Walder A.S. (1976) A critique of the evidence for active host defence against cancer, based on personal studies of 27 murine tumours of spontaneous origin. *British Journal of Cancer*, **33**, 241–59.

Hock I.I., Dorsch M., Kunzendorf U. et al. (1993) Vaccinations with tumour cells genetically engineered to produce different cytokines: effectivity not superior to a classical adjuvant. *Cancer Research*, **53**, 714–16.

Hoover H.C., Brandhorst J.S., Peters L.C. et al. (1993) Adjuvant active specific immunotherapy for human colorectal cancer: 6.5-year median follow up of a phase III prospectively randomised trial. *Journal of Clinical Oncology*, **11**, 390–99.

Houghton A.N. (1994) Cancer antigens: immune recognition of self and altered self. *Journal of Experimental Medicine*, **180**, 1–4.

Huang A.Y.C., Golumbek P., Ahmadzadeh M., Jaffee E., Pardoll D. & Levitsky H. (1994) Role of bone marrow derived cells in presenting MHC class I-restricted tumor antigens. *Science*, **264**, 961–5.

Humphreys S.R., Glynn J.P., Chirigos M.A. & Goldin A. (1962) Further studies on the homograft response in BALB/c mice with L1210 leukaemia and a resistant subline. *Journal of the National Cancer Institute*, **28**, 1053–63.

Ioachim H.L. (1990) The opportunistic tumors of immune deficiency. *Advances in Cancer Research*, **54**, 301–17.

Ioannides C.G. & Whiteside T.L. (1993) T cell recognition of human tumors: implications for molecular immunotherapy of cancer. *Clinical Immunology and Immunopathology*, 66, 91–106.

Janeway C.A. & Bottomly K. (1994) Signals and signs for lymphocyte responses. *Cell*, 76, 275–85.

June C.H., Bluestone J.A., Nadler L.M. & Thompson C.B. (1994) The B7 and CD28 receptor families. *Immunology Today*, 15, 321–31.

Jung S. & Schluesener H.J. (1991) Human T lymphocytes recognise a peptide of a single point mutated, oncogenic ras protein. *Journal of Experimental Medicine*, 173, 273–6.

Kawakami Y., Eliyahu S., Delgado C.H. et al. (1994b) Cloning of the gene coding for a shared human melanoma antigen recognised by autologous T cells infiltrating into tumor. *Proceedings of the National Academy of Sciences USA*, 91, 3515–19.

Kawakami Y., Eliyahu S., Sakaguchi K. et al. (1994a) Identification of the immunodominant peptides of the MART-1 human melanoma antigen recognised by the majority of HLA-A2-restricted tumor infiltrating lymphocytes. *Journal of Experimental Medicine*, 180, 347–52.

Kawakami Y., Zakut R., Topalian S.L., Stotter H. & Rosenberg S.A. (1992) Shared human melanoma antigens. Recognition by tumor infiltrating lymphocytes in HLA-A2.1-transfected melanomas. *Journal of Immunology*, 148, 638–43.

Kedar E. & Klein E. (1992) Cancer immunotherapy: Are the results discouraging? Can they be improved? *Advances in Cancer Research*, 59, 245–322.

Klein E. & Mantovani A. (1993) Action of natural killer cells and macrophages in cancer. *Current Opinion in Immunology*, 5, 714–18.

Klein G. & Boon T. (1993) Tumor immunology: present perspectives. *Current Opinion in Immunology*, 5, 687–92.

Knuth A., Wolfel T. & Meyer zum Buschenfelde K.-H. (1991) Cellular and humoral immune responses against cancer: implications for cancer vaccines. *Current Opinion in Immunology*, 3, 659–64.

Kripke M.L. (1988) Immunoregulation of carcinogenesis: past present and future. *Journal of the National Cancer Institute*, 80, 722–7.

Kurosawa S., Matsuzaki G., Harada M., Ando T. & Nomoto K. (1993) Early appearance and activation of natural killer cells in tumor-infiltrating lymphoid cells during tumor development. *European Journal of Immunology*, 23, 1029–33.

Kwak L.W., Campbell M.J., Czerwinski D.K., Hart S., Miller R.A. & Levy R. (1992) Induction of immune responses in patients with B-cell lymphoma against the surface immunoglobulin idiotype expressed by their tumors. *New England Journal of Medicine*, 327, 1209–15.

Levitsky H.I., Lazenby A., Hayashi R.J. & Pardoll D. (1994) In vivo priming of two distinct anti-tumour effector populations: the role of MHc Class I expression. *Journal of Experimental Medicine*, 179, 1215–24.

Lloyd K.O. (1991) Humoral immune responses to tumor-associated carbohydrate antigens. *Seminars in Cancer Biology*, 2, 421–5.

Lotze M.T., Grimm D.A., Mazumder A., Strausser J.L. & Rosenberg S.A. (1981) Lysis of fresh and cultured autologous tumour by human lymphocytes cultured in T-cell growth factor. *Cancer Research*, 41, 4420–5.

Lotze M.T., Rubin J.T., Edington H.D., Posner M.G., Wolmark N. et al. (1992) The treatment of patients with melanoma using interleukin-2, interleukin-4 and tumor infiltrating lymphocytes. *Human Gene Therapy*, 3, 167–77.

Mackensen A., Carcelain G., Viel S. et al. (1994) Direct evidence to support the immunosurveillance concept in a human regressive melanoma. *Journal of Clinical Investigation*, 93, 1397–402.

Malmgren R.A., Benneson B.E. & McKinley T.W. (1952) Reduced antibody titres in mice treated with carcinogenic and chemotherapeutic agents. *Proceedings of the Society for Experimental Biology and Medicine*, 79, 484–8.

Mantovani A., Bottazzi B., Colotta F., Sozzani S. & Ruco L. (1992) The origin and function of tumor-associated macrophages. *Immunology Today*, 13, 265–70.

Marchand M., Brasseur F., Van der Bruggen P., Coulie P. & Boon T. (1993) Perspectives for immunisation of HLA-A1 patients carrying a malignant melanoma expressing gene MAGE-1. *Dermatology*, 186, 278–80.

Mitchell G.F., Rajasekariah G.R. & Richard M.D. (1980) A mechanism to account for the mouse strain variation in resistance to the larval cestode, *Teania taeniaeformis*. *Immunology*, 39, 481–9.

Mittelman A., Chen Z.J., Liu C.C., Hirai S. & Ferrone S. (1994) Kinetics of the immune response and regression of metastatic lesions following development of humoral anti-high molecular weight-melanoma associated antigen immunity in three patients with advanced malignant melanoma immunised with mouse antiidiotypic monoclonal antibody MK2-23. *Cancer Research*, 54, 415–21.

Morton D.L., Foshag L.J., Hoon D.S.B. et al. (1993) Prolongation of survival in metastatic melanoma after active specific immunotherapy with a new polyvalent melanoma vaccine. *Annals of Surgery*, 216, 463–82.

Moudgil K.D. & Sercarz E.E. (1994) Can antitumor immune responses discriminate between self and nonself? *Immunology Today*, 15, 353–5.

Mullen C.A., Coale M.M., Lowe R. & Blaese R.M. (1994) Tumors expressing the cytosine deaminase suicide gene can be eliminated in vivo with 5-fluorocytosine and induce protective immunity to wild type tumor. *Cancer Research*, 54, 1503–6.

Neefjes J.J. & Momburg F. (1993) Cell biology of antigen presentation. *Current Opinion in Immunology*, 5, 27–34.

Nijman H.W., Van der Burg S.H., Vierboom M.P.M., Houbiers J.G.A., Kast W.M. & Melief, C.J.M. (1994) p53, a potential target for tumor-directed T cells. *Immunology Letters*, 40, 171–8.

O'Reilly M.S., Holmgren L., Shing Y. et al. (1994) Angiostatin: a novel angiogenesis inhibitor that mediates the suppression of metastases by a Lewis lung carcinoma. *Cell*, 79, 315–28.

Oettgen H.F. & Old L.J. (1991) The history of cancer immunotherapy. In *Biologic therapy of cancer*, V.T. Devita, S. Hellman & S.A. Rosenburg (eds) pp. 87–119. Philadelphia, J.B. Lippincott Company.

Oliver R.T.D. & Nouri A.M.E. (1992) T cell immune response to cancer in humans and its relevance for immunodiagnosis and therapy. *Cancer Surveys*, 13, 173–204.

Pardoll D. (1992) New strategies for active immunotherapy with genetically engineered tumor cells. *Current Opinion in Immunology*, 4, 619–23.

Pardoll D.M. (1993) Cancer vaccines. *Immunology Today*, 14, 310–16.

Pardoll D.M. (1994) Tumour antigens: a new look for the 1990s. *Nature*, 369, 357–8.

Parmiani G. (1993) Tumor immunity as autoimmunity: tumor antigens include normal self proteins which stimulate anergic peripheral T cells. *Immunology Today*, 14, 536–8.

Paul W.E. & Seder R.A. (1994) Lymphocyte responses and cytokines. *Cell*, 76, 241–51.

Penn I. (1988) Tumors of the immunocompromised patient. *Annual Review of Medicine*, 39, 63–73.

Prehn R.T. (1994) Stimulatory effects of immune reactions upon the growths of untransplanted tumors. *Cancer Research*, 54, 908–14.

Ramarathinam L., Castle M., Wu Y. & Liu Y. (1994) T cell co-stimulation by B7/BB1 induces CD8 T cell-dependent tumor rejection: an important role of B7/BB1 in the induction, recruitment, and effector function of antitumor T cells. *Journal of Experimental Medicine*, **179**, 1205–14.

Raychaudhuri S. & Morrow W.J.W. (1993) Can soluble antigens induce CD8+ cytotoxic T-cell response? A paradox revisited. *Immunology Today*, **14**, 344–8.

Reithmuller G., Schneider-Gadicke E. & Johnson J.P. (1993) Monoclonal antibodies in cancer therapy. *Current Opinion in Oncology*, **5**, 732–9.

Restifo N.P., Esquivel F., Kawakami Y. et al. (1993) Identification of human cancers deficient in antigen processing. *Journal of Experimental Medicine*, **177**, 265–72.

Richards J.M. (1991) Sequential chemoimmunotherapy for metastatic melanoma. *Seminars in Oncology*, **18** (Suppl. 7), 91–5.

Rosenberg S.A. (1991) Immunotherapy and gene therapy of cancer. *Cancer Research*, **51** (Suppl.), 5074s–5079s.

Rosenberg S.A., Aebersold P., Cornetta K. et al. (1990) Gene transfer into humans – immunotherapy of patients with advanced melanoma using tumor-infiltrating lymphocytes modified by retroviral gene transduction. *New England Journal of Medicine*, **323**, 570–8.

Rosenberg S.A., French Anderson W., Blaese M. et al. (1993) The development of gene therapy for the treatment of cancer. *Annals of Surgery*, **218**, 455–64.

Rosenberg S.A., Lotze M.T., Muul L.M. et al. (1985) Observations on the systemic administration of autologous lymphokine-activated killer cells and recombinant interleukin-2 to patients with metastatic cancer. *New England Journal of Medicine*, **313**: 1485–92.

Rosenberg S.A., Packard B.S., Aebersold P.M. et al. (1988) Use of tumor-infiltrating lymphocytes and interleukin-2 in the immunotherapy of patients with metastatic melanoma, special report. *New England Journal of Medicine*, **319**, 1676–80.

Rygard J. & Poulson C.O. (1974) The mutant nude mouse does not develop spontaneous tumours. *Acta Pathologica Microbiologica et Immunologica Scandinavica*, **82**, 99–107.

Schlichtholz B., Legros Y., Gillet D. et al. (1992) The immune response to p53 in breast cancer patients is directed against immunodominant epitopes unrelated to the mutationsl hot spot. *Cancer Research*, **52**, 6380–4.

Schulz T.F. & Vile R.G. (1992) Viruses in human cancer. In *Introduction to the molecular genetics of cancer*, R.G. Vile (ed.) pp. 137–76. Chichester, UK, John Wiley & Sons.

Skipper J. & Stauss H.J. (1993) Identification of two cytotoxic T lymphocyte-recognised epitopes in the ras protein. *Journal of Experimental Medicine*, **177**, 1493–9.

Stutman O. (1975) Immunodepression and malignancy. *Advances in Cancer Research*, **22**, 261–422.

Tanaka K., Gorelik E., Watanabe M., Hozumi N. & Jay G. (1988) Rejection of B16 melanoma induced by expression of a transfected major histocompatibility complex class I gene. *Molecular and Cellular Biology*, **8**, 1857–61.

Taylor-Papadimitriou J., Stewart L., Burchell J. & Beverley P. (1993) The polymorphic epithelial mucin as a target for immunotherapy. *Annals of the New York Academy of Sciences*, **5**, 69–79.

Tepper R.I., Coffman R.L. & Leder P. (1992) An eosinophil-dependent mechanism for the antitumor effect of interleukin-4. *Science*, **257**, 548–51.

Tepper R.I. & Mule J.J. (1994) Experimental and clinical studies of cytokine gene-modified tumor cells. *Human Gene Therapy*, **5**, 153–64.

Townsend S.E. & Allison J.P. (1993) Tumour rejection after direct co-stimulation of CD8+ T cells by B7-transfected melanoma cells. *Science*, **259**, 368–70.

Traversari T., Van der Bruggen P., Luescher I.F. et al. (1992) A nonapeptide encoded by haman gene MAGE-1 is recognized on HLA-A1 by cytolytic T lymphocytes directed against tumor antigen MZ2-E. *Journal of Experimental Medicine*, **176**, 1453–7.

Trinchieri G. (1989) Biology of natural killer cells. *Advances in Immunology*, **47**, 187.

Trinchieri G. (1994) Recognition of major histocompatibility complex Class I antigens by natural killer cells. *Journal of Experimental Medicine*, **180**, 417–21.

Udono H., Levery D.L. & Srivastava P.K. (1994) Cellular requirements for tumor-specific immunity elicited by heat shock proteins: tumor rejection antigen gp96 primers CD8+ T-cells in vivo. *Proceedings of the National Academy of Sciences USA*, **91**, 3077–81.

Van der Bruggen P., Traversari C., Chomez P. et al. (1991) A gene encoding an antigen recognised by cytolytic T lymphocytes on a human melanoma. *Science*, **254**, 1643–7.

Van der Bruggen P. & Van den Eynde B. (1992) Molecular definition of tumor antigens recognised by T-lymphocytes. *Current Opinion in Immunology*, **4**, 608–12.

Van Ravenswaay Claasen H.H., Kluin P.M. & Fleuren G.J. (1992) Tumor infiltrating cells in human cancer. *Laboratory Investigation*, **67**, 166–74.

Vegh Z., Wang P., Vanky F. & Klein E. (1993) Selectively down regulated expression of major histocompatibility complex class I alleles in human solid tumors. *Cancer Research*, **53**, 2416–20.

Vile R.G. & Hart I.R. (1993) Use of tissue specific expression of the Herpes Simplex Virus thymidine kinase gene to inhibit growth of established murine melanomas following direct intratumoral injection of DNA. *Cancer Research*, **53**, 3860–4.

Vile R.G., Nelson J.A., Castleden S.C., Chong H. & Hart I.R. (1994) Systemic gene therapy of murine melanoma using tissue specific expression of the KSVtk gene involves an immune component. *Cancer Research*, **54**, 6228–34.

Vile R.G. & Russell S.J. (1994) Gene transfer technologies for the gene therapy of cancer. *Gene Therapy*, **1**, 88–98.

Vogelstein B. & Kinzler K.W. (1993) The multistep nature of cancer. *Trends in Genetics*, **9**, 138–41.

Yashumura S., Lin W.C., Hirabayashi H., Vujanovic N.L., Herberman R.B. & Whiteside T. (1994) Immunotherapy of liver metastases of human gastric carcinoma with interleukin 2-activated natural killer cells. *Cancer Research*, **54**, 3808–16.

# 3

# Antigen Processing and Presentation

## NICHOLAS P. RESTIFO AND MICHAEL WANG

## ■ INTRODUCTION

Specificity is the hallmark of immune responses mediated by lymphocytes. T lymphocytes provide this specificity to the cellular branch of the immune system, while B lymphocytes produce antibodies which are the essence of recognition by the humoral immune system. There are fundamental differences in the ways that the cellular and the humoral immune systems recognize antigens (Table 3.1). T cells recognize only antigens composed of protein or glycoprotein, while B cells are capable of recognizing such substances as polysaccharides and nucleic acids in addition to protein and glycoprotein antigens. B cells can recognize antigens not presented in the context of other molecules. T cells, on the other hand, have a restricted antigen world in that they generally recognize antigens in the context of a 'self' major histocompatibility complex (MHC) molecule on the surface of a cell. T cells utilize structures on their surfaces called T cell receptors (TCR) to recognize antigen/MHC molecule com-

Table 3.1. Towards a Molecular Understanding of Immune Recognition of Antigens

|  | Humoral | Cellular |
|---|---|---|
| Recognizing cell | B lymphocyte | T lymphocyte |
| Recognizing molecule | Immunoglobulin | T cell receptor |
| 'Self' molecules required? | No | Yes |
| Chemical identity of antigen | Protein, nucleic acid, polysaccharide, other | Protein |
| Phase of antigen | Fluid or solid | Solid |
| State of antigen | Native or denatured | 'Processed' |

plexes; B cells use immunoglobulin (Ig) molecules to react specifically to antigenic stimuli. While Ig is secreted, sometimes in extremely large quantities, little if any TCR is shed by T cells. Underlying the differences in the molecules used for recognition is an important difference in the types of antigens recognized: B cells can recognize antigen in its native conformation, whereas T cells generally recognize antigen that has been 'processed', then presented by MHC molecules. More specifically, antigen is denatured, cleaved within the cell, and transported into specific subcellular compartments where it is bound by MHC molecules. After a complex of antigen and MHC completes its journey to the cell surface, it is potentially recognizable by a T cell. It is the molecular and cell biology of the processing and presentation of antigens that forms the basis of this chapter.

The importance, for tumor immunologists, of how antigens are recognized by T cells (that is, what T cells 'see') is linked largely to the establishment of new immunotherapies based on T cells. These new therapies have ushered in a new set of challenges having to do with how T cells recognize, or may fail to recognize tumor-associated antigens (TAA). Early experiments showed that the growth of a syngeneic tumor in a mouse could be prevented by prior immunization with that same tumor (Prehn and Main, 1957; Klein et al., 1960). Since then, the mechanisms involved in the antitumor immune response have been partially elucidated (Schreiber et al., 1988; Greenberg, 1991) and T cells have been shown to play a critical role (Shimizu & Shen, 1979; Greenberg et al., 1981; Rosenberg, Spiess & Lafreniere, 1986). Guided by results from animal model studies, human T cells that accumulate within the mass of a tumor have been shown in some cases to specifically lyse autologous tumor cells in vitro (Itoh et al., 1988; Topalian, Solomon & Rosenberg, 1989). The T cells can also specifically secrete cytokines, such as interleukin-2 (IL-2), interferon-$\gamma$ (IFN-$\gamma$), granulocyte–macrophage colony stimulating factor (GM-CSF) and tumor necrosis factor-$\alpha$ (TNF-$\alpha$), and proliferate in response to stimulation with autologous tumor cells (Barth et al., 1991). Antitumor T cells can be grown to large numbers in vitro, and transferred adoptively to treat even substantial tumor burdens in both humans and mice (Rosenberg et al., 1988). Finally, TAA recognized by autologous human T cells have been identified by the use of molecular cloning techniques. Taken together, these findings provide strong evidence that a T cell immune response can occur against an autologous tumor.

# ■ THE MOLECULAR BASIS OF THE SPECIFICITY OF T CELLS

T cell responses were found by early investigators to be controlled by the presence of particular genes encoded in the MHC. Polymorphisms at this genetic region were observed to control the ability of an animal to mount a T cell response. Early attempts to demonstrate direct binding of antigen to T cells failed while attempts succeeded in the case of B cells. While a relatively straightforward and still useful model of the recognition of antigen by humoral factors was promulgated before the turn of the century, it took nearly another hundred years for a similar event to occur for T cells.

T cells express molecules of exquisite sensitivity on their cell surfaces that are very much like the antibody molecules found on the surfaces of B cells. These molecules, called T cell receptors, recognize peptide fragments of antigens that are noncovalently complexed with MHC molecules. The MHC-bound peptide recognized by the TCR is often referred to as an 'epitope.' An antigenic molecule frequently contains several different antigenic epitopes, the consequences of which are considered below in the context of antigen processing.

There are two major types of MHC molecules, class I and class II, which are integral membrane glycoproteins that are ultimately expressed on the surfaces of cells. These two types of MHC molecules, noncovalently complexed with antigenic peptides, constitute ligands for two different types of cells. Class I molecules serve as antigen receptors for $CD8^+$ lymphocytes, while class II molecules perform the same function for $CD4^+$ lymphocytes. While some of their functions overlap, there exists a very definite division of labor between $CD8^+$ and $CD4^+$ lymphocytes. $CD8^+$ cells are sometimes termed cytotoxic T lymphocytes (CTL) because they are generally capable of directly killing target cells through the release of lytic granules as well as cytokines. $CD4^+$ cells, while also capable in some cases of cytotoxic activity, are also called helper T cells, since they enhance antibody responses by activating B cells, promote other T cell responses, and activate a variety of other immune effector cells, for example, macrophages.

# ■ MHC MOLECULES AS ANTIGEN RECEPTORS

MHC molecules have been associated with diverse immunological phenomena (Hansen, Correno & Sachs, 1993). Amongst the earliest descriptions of these phenomena are the observations that mixing lymphocytes from MHC distinct strains of mice can cause proliferation (Bach et al., 1972) and that immune responses are 'restricted,' that is, a T lymphocyte can specifically recognize a target cell only if it bears not only the antigen but also the appropriate MHC molecule (Zinkernagel & Doherty, 1974). Another early observation was what was once called the 'immune response' (Ir) phenomenon, in which the ability of an animal to respond to certain antigens is controlled by the MHC molecules (Bevan, 1975). Finally, MHC antigens are noted to be associated with the rejection of tissue and graft-versus-host (GVH) reactions, either or both of which can occur when there is a mismatch between transplant donor and recipient MHC types (Benacerraf & McDevitt, 1972). Thus, these diverse phenomena are all associated with MHC molecules that are coded for by genes closely linked together on chromosomes 6 and designated HLA in humans, and chromosome 17 in mouse, where they are designated H-2.

A molecular understanding of the structure of MHC molecules has made clear their true function with respect to antigen recognition by T cells: MHC molecules are receptors for peptide antigens (Rammensee, Falk & Rotzsche, 1993b). MHC molecules are physically associated with peptide antigens and X-ray crystallographic data have indicated precisely how such an interaction occurs. The solution of the crystal structure of MHC class I and class III molecules has clarified the molecular structure of MHC molecules, specifically the way MHC molecules bind antigen (Bjorkman et al., 1987a, 1987b; Brown, Driscoll & Monaco, 1993). MHC molecules have peptide binding domains consisting of a deep groove which runs between two long α-helices found on the outward facing surface of the MHC molecule. In the case of class I molecules, X-ray crystallographic findings have since been refined and extended to include X-ray images of particular peptides lying in the cleft of MHC molecules (Fremont et al., 1992; Matsumura et al., 1992; Stura et al., 1992; Wilson & Fremont, 1993). These findings reveal that the peptides are bound in an extended conformation. More recently, the crystal structure of human class II MHC molecule HLA-DR1 complexed with a peptide from influenza virus hemagglutinin has been obtained (Stern et al., 1994). While the general architecture of the peptide-binding grooves are almost identical, there are critical differences that fundamentally change the way peptides are bound. Class I molecules bind shorter peptides of defined lengths (generally 8–10 residues) while class II molecules bind peptides that appear to be arbitrary in length (often 12–20 amino acids but occasionally longer). In fact, class II molecules often bind a core motif of an antigen that can extend in either direction by different lengths (also referred to as 'nested sets' of peptides). The binding cleft of class I molecules is closed at both ends, enabling the molecule to make hydrogen bonds with the bound peptides at both the N- and C-termini. Class II molecules, on the other hand, have a peptide-binding cleft that is open on both ends. In both the class I and class II molecules, peptides are bound by pockets in the binding site. Class II molecules generally have five major pockets compared with class I molecules, which usually have three major pockets (Stern et al., 1994; Young et al., 1994). While the peptides bound by class II molecules are generally thought to have an extended and straight orientation in the binding cleft, the peptides bound by class I molecules are usually arched and sometimes sharply kinked near the fourth residue from the amino terminus.

The nature of the contact between the TCR and the complex of peptide–MHC is important, because this influences whether the TCR is triggered, and also the consequences of triggering, such as T cell proliferation or cytokine production. Model systems have been studied that allow amino acid substitutions in each of the three elements involved with the binding: the MHC molecule, the peptide and the TCR (Jorgensen et al., 1992). Findings indicate that the affinity of the TCR for the peptide–MHC complex is much weaker than that of most antibody–antigen interactions, a property consistent with an important role for other antigen-independent T cell surface receptors acting as cofactors in the triggering process.

Sequence studies indicate that MHC class I and class II molecules are among the most highly polymorphic molecules in the genome. The extreme amount of polymorphism of MHC molecules is associated with their function as antigen receptors, and is concentrated in the peptide-binding domains of the class I and class II molecules (Barber & Parham, 1993; Parham, 1993). Specifically, the polymorphism of MHC molecules is concentrated in the pockets that bind the peptides in the grooves of MHC molecules. The polymorphisms form the molecular basis for the preference of different MHC alleles for different peptide-sequence motifs and they enable each MHC molecule to bind a different set of peptides. It has been demonstrated that MHC polymorphism causes differences in levels of human resistance to specific infections (Hill et al., 1991). MHC polymorphism ensures that, within a species, a broad ability to bind peptide derived from a pathogenic challenge will exist (Roy et al., 1989). MHC diversity is what makes the job of the transplant surgeon, and the role of the cancer or infectious disease immunotherapist more difficult.

## Differences Between MHC Class I and Class II Molecules

United by their function as receptors for antigenic peptides, the differences in structure and intracellular trafficking between class I and class

II molecules are critical. Class I and class II molecules differ structurally, have different genetic organization and tissue distribution, present bound peptides to different T cell subsets, and elicit different type of immune responses. Class I and class II molecules also differ in their requirements for binding of peptide antigens, and these peptides originate from different sources. Finally, the two types of MHC follow different intracellular routes on their way to the cell surface and noncovalently associate with peptides in different subcellular compartments.

The major subregions for class I genes are named A, B, and C in the human and K, D, and L in the mouse. Class II molecules originate from three major subregions in the human designated DP, DQ, and DR, and two in the mouse designated I-A and I-E. MHC molecules from these major subregions are codominantly expressed. The extent of MHC polymorphism present in the gene pool usually results in heterozygosity for most individuals at every major class I and class II locus. Since there are three different major class I loci and three different major class II loci in the human, most individuals express six different class I alleles and six different class II alleles. Thus, codominant expression in a single individual of MHC molecules originating from multiple loci enhances that individual's ability to present a variety of antigens.

Both class I and class II molecules are integral membrane glycoproteins. Class I molecules are composed of a 45-kDa $\alpha$-chain with a single transmembrane segment and a short carboxy-terminal cytoplasmic domain, which is noncovalently associated with $\beta_2$-microglobulin ($\beta_2$m). The $\beta_2$m molecule is not encoded within the MHC, has minimal polymorphism, and is highly conserved among species.

The $\alpha$-chains of class I molecules (also called heavy chains) are encoded in the genome in an eight-exon form. The first exon encodes a signal peptide or leader sequence that directs insertion of the rest of the nascent class I molecule into the endoplasmic reticulum (ER) during translation. The extracellular domain of the class I molecule is dominated by three $\alpha$-chain segments and $\beta_2$-microglobulin. The peptide-binding region is comprised of approximately 180 amino acids from the amino terminus of the $\alpha$-chain. These amino acids interact to form a three-dimensional structure that has an eight-stranded $\beta$-pleated sheet floor and an $\alpha$-helix (alpha segment one and two, exons 2 and 3) on either side. The cleft that is formed can fit peptides of between eight and ten amino acids, but more importantly it cannot accommodate globular proteins. This leads to the conclusion that these peptides are most likely the product of a single or series of proteolytic events occurring on the inside of the cell. The three large extracellular domains are encoded by exons 2–4 of the heavy-chain gene. The third $\alpha$-segment (exon 4) of the $\alpha$-chain shares close homology with the constant region of immunoglobulins and is highly conserved between MHC molecules. This Ig-like region is about 90 amino acids long and starts at the carboxy terminus of the $\alpha_2$-segment and extends to the surface of the cell. It contains the nonpolymorphic region recognized by CD8. $\beta_2$m also shares structural homology with Ig constant regions. Exon five encodes a 25-amino-acid transmembrane region that forms a hydrophobic $\alpha$-helix that anchors class I into the cell membrane but does not affect the conformation of the class I molecule. In fact, papain digestion of the class I molecule from the surface of the cell yields a soluble and stable molecule. Similarly, genetically engineered class I molecules truncated after exon 4 are not only stable but are functional (Mage et al., 1992). As the transmembrane region emerges on the inside of the cell, it is rich with basic amino acids that interact with the phospholipid heads of the inner ER membrane leaflet. The intracytoplasmic segment of the class I $\alpha$-chain spans 30 amino acids (exons 6, 7, and 8) and is most likely involved in the intracellular trafficking of class I molecules. It contains regions that interact with the cytoskeleton as well as residues that can be phosphorylated.

The $\alpha$-chain and $\beta_2$m are synthesized, and form a heterodimer in the ER membrane so that the potential peptide-binding cleft sticks into the lumen. Apparently before binding peptide it is transiently bound to calnexin, possibly serving to stabilize the $\alpha$-chain-$\beta_2$m heterodimer.

The heterodimer may not necessarily bind a 8–10-amino-acid long peptide initially. A longer peptide with the appropriate basic or hydrophobic carboxy terminus binds to the anchor residues in the cleft and that, after this peptide conforms to the binding requirements of the class I molecule, a exopeptidase in the ER or along the pathway to the surface of the cell trims the amino terminus so that there is no overhanging peptide. Unlike class II molecules, class I peptides at both the amino and carboxy termini are buried into the cleft allowing no overhanging peptide. This model also takes into account that the class I molecule itself may account for the binding of specific peptides. Human cells cotransfected with the mouse $K_b$ molecule and ovalbumin presented the same peptide, SIINFELK, as the C57/b16 thymoma EL4 transfected with the ovalbumin gene. Therefore, the repertoire of class I molecules, another advantage of vast polymorphism, may direct the ability to present certain antigens and not necessarily the ability to process them. The ability for human and mouse to process the same peptide suggests that the proteolytic machinery, MHC-dependent and MHC-independent, of the cell must be widely conserved. After peptide is bound, the class I-molecule passes through the Golgi complex, where it is further modified until it finally reaches the cell surface.

The class II molecule is very similar to the class I molecule in its general shape, but is composed of an $\alpha$-chain of 34 kDa and a $\beta$-chain of 28 kDa, both of which are integral membrane glycoproteins. These molecules also have transmembrane regions as well as short intracytoplasmic regions. The $\alpha_1$ and $\beta_1$ domains of the class II molecule correspond with the $\alpha_1$ and $\alpha_2$ domains of the class I molecule, and thus are directly involved in the binding of the presented peptide. The $\alpha_2$ domain of class II corresponds with the $\beta_2$m light chain of class I. Finally, the $\beta_2$ domain of class II corresponds with the $\alpha_2$ domain of class I.

### Recognition of MHC/Antigen Complexes by T Cell Subsets

There are many interactions involved in T cell activation but the specificity of T cell recognition of a cognate partner cell occurs via the interaction of the TCR with an MHC molecule to which is bound a peptide. Some peptide/MHC complexes, designated 'antigenic,' trigger a T cell response, which can consist of proliferation, up-regulation of surface molecules, activation of lytic machinery and/or secretion of cyclokines. The number of MHC molecules, which must be occupied by a particular peptide in order to activate a T cell, is thought to be extremely low: on the order of 0.03% of the total MHC or as few as 60 peptide/MHC complexes (Harding & Unanue, 1990; Demotz, Grey & Sette, 1990).

Thus far, no clear structural or sequence differences between TCR detecting class I from those detecting class II molecules have been found. However, a clear difference between the two sets of T cells is found in the ligands for the cell surface markers, CD4 and CD8, from which they derive their names. CD8 molecules bind to the $\alpha_3$ domain of the class I molecules on the target cell (Potter et al., 1989; Connolly et al., 1990; Salter et al., 1990) and CD4 molecules bind with the $\beta_2$ domain of the class II heterodimer on the target cell (Cammarota et al., 1992; Konig, Huang & Germain, 1992).

### Sources of Antigens Bound by MHC Class I and Class II Molecules

There is evidence that the antigens complexed with MHC class I and II molecules originate from two different sources (Figure 3.1). Class I molecules generally present antigens derived from intracellular sources. Class II molecules, though somewhat more versatile in their sources of antigens, generally present antigens derived from extracellular sources. The immunologically critical distinction between the two types of MHC molecules relates to differences in intracellular trafficking of these two molecules: class II molecules intersect endocytosed antigen whereas class I molecules do not. Class I molecules, on the other hand, are exposed to

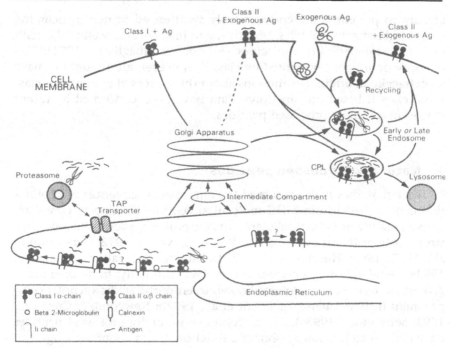

**Figure 3.1** Intracellular pathways for antigen processing and presentation by MHC class I and class II molecules.

intracellular antigens in the ER, whereas class II molecules are protected at this site (Yewdell & Bennink, 1992; Germain, 1994). As a test of the above stated distinction, antigen was supplied to a cell via different routes. When antigen was supplied from the outside of a cell, by an inactivated virus, it was presented to T lymphocytes by class II molecules. When antigen was generated inside the cell, for example, by an active viral infection, class I-restricted presentation occurred (Morrison et al., 1986).

Clear examples exist that contradict the distinction that class I molecules present only peptides derived from the cytosol (Weiss & Bogen, 1991), and some of the exceptions to the rule may have very specific functions, for example, the presentation of Ig V regions by class I molecules. The elicitation of tumor-specific CTL by antigen-presenting cells (APC) processing exogenous antigen has recently been reported. It is difficult to assess the significance of this interaction in vivo and its importance toward immunotherapy still remains unclear. However, the exceptions to the rule are sufficiently specialized that they do not require a revision of the stated paradigm. Class II molecules do appear systematically to present some endogenously synthesized proteins, including some viral antigens (measles, hepatitis, and influenza) as well as the cell's own histocompatibility molecules (Brodsky & Guagliardi, 1991). The majority of antigens presented by class II, however, are thought to have an extracellular origin. Distinctions about the sources of antigens for class I and class II based on functional data have been confirmed by recent studies of naturally processed peptides.

### Naturally processed peptides

Recent studies have examined the amino-acid sequences of peptides that can be eluted from MHC molecules. Peptides binding to class I are derived mainly from intracellular/cytosolic proteins, such as histones and stress proteins (Hunt et al., 1992a; Wei & Cresswell, 1992; Henderson et al., 1992, 1993; Huczko et al., 1993; Rammensee, Falk & Rotzschke, 1993a), while class II peptides are derived primarily from membrane glycoproteins or serum proteins known to enter the acidic vacuolar compartment in large quantities (Hunt et al., 1992b; Newcomb & Cresswell, 1993; Sette et al., 1993a). Thus, studies of naturally processed peptides have confirmed previously obtained functional data about the origins of peptides bound to MHC molecules.

The identification of naturally processed peptides has also provided clues to the structural requirements of peptide binding to MHC, as well as to how peptides might be cut from the protein molecules from which they are originally derived. Naturally processed peptides bind to MHC molecules with high affinity generally better than the micromolar range, and can even extend into the picomolar range. Naturally processed peptides bound to class I molecules are of a very specific size (8–10 amino acids) (Hunt et al., 1992a) and are smaller than those bound to class II molecules (12–20 amino acids) (Rudensky et al., 1991; Hunt et al., 1992b), which are much more variable and often nested.

Despite a restricted length of peptides presented by MHC class II molecules and the even more restricted length of those presented by class I, a tremendous amount of specificity can still occur. Note that it is possible to make at least $5 \times 10^{11}$ different peptides of nine amino acids, although the stringency required by class I binding may reduce this by several orders of magnitude. There appears to be less stringency for peptides bound to class II molecules than for class I (Stern et al., 1994; Young et al., 1994), that is, within a given protein there are more peptides that bind to class II than to class I. The molecular basis for this is probably due to the fact that class II molecules differ from class I molecules in the way that they bind peptides as described above.

It is now possible to forecast what epitopes within a protein will bind to particular class I molecules. Since class I molecules are so polymorphic, this epitope forecast will obviously be allele specific. Allele-specific epitope forecasting has now been done with a large number of human and murine MHC molecules (Rammensee et al., 1993a, 1993b) and is characterized by strong preferences for particular amino-acid side chains at some positions in the bound peptides, and a wide tolerance for amino acid side chains at other positions. Although the so-called anchor positions are of clinical importance in the prediction of what peptides will bind to particular class I molecules, the amino-acid side chains at other positions can play a role and should not be disregarded in an allele-specific epitope forecast (Rupper et al., 1993). Class II epitopes also have allele-specific motifs (Hammer et al., 1993; Sette et al., 1993b; Falk et al., 1994; Sidney et al., 1994) but it has been more difficult to characterize them because of the difficulty in aligning peptides of different lengths.

# ■ THE MHC CLASS I PATHWAY FOR ANTIGEN PROCESSING

Antigen processing is generally necessary for the expression of class I molecules at the cell surface. This is because first, class I $\alpha$-chains do not leave the ER in large quantities unless they are fully assembled with peptide and $\beta_2$m, and second, they need to bind a peptide in order to be thermodynamically stable. 'Empty' class I molecules appear to be unstable at 37°C but somewhat more stable at lower temperatures (Ljunggren et al., 1990). Such 'empty' class I molecules are short lived and subject to proteolysis, but nevertheless are expressed at relatively low levels by certain cells, especially those deficient in antigen processing. Since most nucleated cells express stable class I molecules on their cell surfaces, antigen processing is probably a universal characteristic of normal cells. Thus, the molecules involved in the processing of antigen are likely to be expressed ubiquitously as well.

$\beta_2$m plays an important role in the proper folding of the 45 kDa class I $\alpha$-chain. The mutant human cell line named Daudi expresses virtually no class I on its cell surface. It lacks $\beta_2$m and has class I $\alpha$-chain molecules, which do not fold properly, never leave the endoplasmic reticulum, and are rapidly degraded. $\beta_2$m-deficient mice have been found to express little, if any, functional class I antigen and have no mature CD8$^+$ T cells (Zijlstra et al., 1990). As shown in Figure 3.1 it is unclear as to whether $\beta_2$m binds to class 1 $\alpha$-chain before, or after, the peptide-antigen is complexed. In experiments using detergent lysates, Townsend and colleagues have found that the addition of peptide to 'empty' class I $\alpha$-chains (presumably derived largely from the ER) increases their affinity for $\beta_2$m

(Townsend et al., 1990). Although there is some conflicting evidence that suggests that α-chain molecules bind to $\beta_2$m before they bind peptide (Kozlowski et al., 1991), it is clear that peptide can induce the stable assembly of class I and $\beta_2$m. Whatever the sequence of events is in the assembly of class I molecules, the fully formed trimolecular complex of class I α-chain, peptide, and $\beta_2$m has greatly enhanced thermodynamic stability as well as resistance to proteolysis. It also appears that these fully formed trimolecular complexes are optimal for transport out of the endoplasmic reticulum, through the Golgi apparatus, and to the cell surface.

Key elements of the molecular apparatus involved in the cleavage and transport of peptides that are bound by class I have now been characterized. The task of generating these peptide fragments from intracellular proteins is probably achieved, in part, by a molecular complex known as the proteosome (Brown, Driscoll & Monaco, 1991, 1993; Goldberg & Rock, 1992; Driscoll et al., 1993; Michalek et al., 1993). The proteosome is a cylindrical and hollow structure believed to be composed of at least 16 individual subunits stacked in four hexagonal rings. Besides being conserved from archaebacterium, *Thermoplasma acidophilum*, to mammals, they are abundant, constituting 1% of the total soluble protein in cell extracts. Traditionally it is thought of as a cellular housekeeper; an endopeptidase (cleaving after basic, acidic and hydrophobic bonds) considered to mediate nonlysosomal protein turnover in eukaryotic cells.

Two proteosome component genes are coded for in the class II region of the MHC and are thought to function in the endogenous antigen presentation pathway to generate peptides presented by class I. These two genes, *LMP-1* and *LMP-2* (for low-molecular-weight proteins), were initially described a decade ago without knowledge of their functions. They have since been found to be the two polymorphic components of a complex consisting of 16 polypeptides. LMP-2 and LMP-7 are believed to have one or both of the following functions. Since they are incorporated into the proteosome, some investigators believe that they may serve as potential docking sites for TAP-1 and TAP-2. Alternatively, others argue that the proteosome is probably not a peptide chaperone or docking facility; rather, the LMP proteins must alter the proteolytic or endopeptidase activity of the proteosome in such a way as to facilitate the cleavage of proteins into the kind of peptide fragments that are most suited for binding into the cleft of class I molecules in the ER. Specifically, they should enhance the cleavage of peptides that leave a basic or hydrophobic amino acid as the carboxy-terminus anchor residue. To decipher these two functions, proteosomes were extracted and purified from LMP+ (721.45) and LMP− (721.174) cell lines and compared for their endopeptidase activity against substrates who had either basic, acidic, or hydrophobic amino acids immediately preceding (P1) the cleavage site. In these experiments LMP− proteosomes show decreased activity against basic and hydrophobic residues at P1, although the binding affinity of these substrates in unchanged. The LMP− activity against acidic, proline, and glycine residues at P1 is equivalent to the LMP+ proteosomes. Further studies show that the $V_{max}$ of the LMP+ protesomes is increased for basic and hydrophobic residues at P1; therefore, the authors suggest that the incorporation of LMP-2 and LMP-7 can accelerate the production of specific peptides. Further experiments go on to show that IFN-$\gamma$ can induce the expression of these LMP genes in a hepatoma cell line (H6), and that these proteosomes from cells treated with IFN-$\gamma$ for three days not only display a larger LMP+:LMP− ratio, but they also accelerate the cleavage of peptides with basic or hydrophobic amino acids at P1. They conclude that LMP-2 and LMP-7 subunit incorporation into the proteosome not only creates a larger pool of peptides that can bind class I, but that they produce peptides that bear an appropriate carboxy terminus for class I binding. Yet in T2 cells, which have lost both the transporter and proteosome subunit genes, stable class I molecules that are recognized by cytotoxic T lymphocytes can be generated solely by the transfection of TAP-1 and TAP-2 genes. This serves as a warning that not all INF-$\gamma$-induced proteosomes incorporate LMP-2 and LMP-7, and that there must be other non-MHC-linked proteosome subunits that can also generate these kinds of peptides.

IFN-$\gamma$ and LMPs have been shown to function not as accelerators of proteolysis, but as molecules that increase the efficiency of endopeptidase activity (Boes et al., 1994; Dick et al., 1994; Fruh et al., 1993; Patel et al., 1994). These findings help to explain MHC-independent activities of the proteosome that still produce peptides that can bind class I. Furthermore, these studies suggest that treatment with IFN-$\gamma$ and the subsequent incorporation of LMP subunits into the proteosome does not make the peptide 'pie' any larger, it redistributes the portion of the 'pie' devoted to peptides that have basic and hydrophobic amino acids at P1. The incorporation of MHC encoded gene products LMP-2 and LMP-7 into the proteosome, and their subsequent ability to accelerate proteolysis and enhance the cleavage of peptides preferentially leaving hydrophobic and basic carboxy termini, provide additional evidence that the proteosome may be involved in processing antigens for class I molecules.

It has been argued that ubiquitin-dependent targeting of proteins for proteolytic degradation by the proteosome plays a role in generating peptides for binding to MHC class I (Michalek et al., 1993). Ubiquitin is a 76-residue protein that is highly conserved (Tobias et al., 1991; Johnson et al., 1992; Varschavsky, 1992). Yeast and man differ at only three amino acids, even oat and man differ at only three amino acids. Of its numerous functions, it is believed to mark proteins for selective degradation, that is, elimination of defective protein variants that arise through mutation, transcriptional and translational errors, chemical damage, and heat denaturation. In general, it is implicated in cellular processes as various as DNA repair, cell cycle control, stress response, ribosome and peroxisome biogenesis, transcription, viral infection, neural/muscular degeneration, and cellular differentiation. Of particular interest is the role of the proteins that are degraded in an ATP-dependent manner by the 26S proteosome following ubiquitination. Presumably this form of proteolysis follows the N-end rule pathway where proteins are targeted for degradation by the identity of the N-terminus (arginine being least stable, and valine and methionine being most stable) and subsequent polyubiquitination. Natural substrates already identified include phytochrome, cyclin, and p53/E6. An increase in the presentation of influenza nucleoprotein has been observed after it had been targeted for the ubiquitin pathway (Townsend et al., 1988).

Peptide fragments may be transported across the membrane of the endoplasmic reticulum (ER) or some post-ER compartment by a specialized protein heterodimer composed of TAP-1 and TAP-2 (for transporter associated with antigen processing), which are related to the products of the multi-drug resistance gene (Deverson et al., 1990). These putative peptide transport protein genes are members of the ABC (ATP-binding cassette) superfamily of transmembrane transporters. The genes for TAP-1 and TAP-2, and LMP-2 and LMP-7 are found alternatively intermingled in the MHC class II region. Their close genomic linkage initially led people to believe that their functions may also be linked. In early publications, TAP were designated HAM (for histocompatibility antigen modifier) in the mouse, PSF (peptide supply factor) in the human, and *mtp* (for MHC-linked transporter protein) in the rat (Monaco et al., 1990; Parham, 1990; Spies et al., 1990; Glynne et al., 1991). The YAP transporters are ATP-dependent peptide pumps, which function as peptide transporters in the presentation of endogenous antigens by class I molecules. The mutant cell line RMA-S was shown to have a defect in the TAP-2 gene, since antigen processing and presentation capabilities was restored by the CDNA of the homologous rat transporter gene *mtp2*.

TAP molecules have recently been shown to be directly involved in the assembly of the class I $\alpha$-chain/$\beta_2$m/antigenic peptide trimolecular complex (Ortmann et al., 1994). TAP probably transfers peptides from the cytoplasm directly to newly synthesized class I molecules to which it is physically associated. This peptide transfer may also occur through another intermediate molecule. One candidate for such an intermediate molecule in the lumen of the ER is a member of the heat shock protein (HSPs) family of proteins called gp96, which can bind peptides in the ER that could be subsequently presented by class I molecules (Srivastava,

1993; Srivasta et al., 1994) (see Chapter 13). The genes for HSPs are located in the MHC and a putative peptide binding region of hsp70 shows sequence homology to the peptide-binding domains of MHC class I. On the outside of the ER hsp70 and hsp90 may serve as peptide chaperones that bring peptides to TAP, which in turn transfers the peptide to gp96. gp96 may help to stabilize unfolded class I heavy-chain molecules, then transfer antigenic peptides to these molecules, leading to the formation of the stable trimolecular complex of class I α-chain, $\beta_2$m, and peptide antigen. Each peptide binding and release step is ATP dependent and catalyzed through the ATPase activities of hsp70 and gp96. There is evidence that HSPs may be useful in the priming of CD8[+] and particularly useful in the generation of antitumor immune responses (Udono & Srivastava, 1993; Udono, Levey & Srivastava 1994). Calnexin, which has also been called P88 and IP90, is likely to function as a chaperone for MHC molecules in the ER. Calnexin is sometimes designated a 'quality control' molecule, since it prevents unfolded or misfolded molecules from exiting the ER (David et al., 1993; Ou et al., 1993; Hammond et al., 1994; Rajagopalan, Xu & Brenner, 1994). Calnexin has been shown to associate in the ER with nascent class I molecules. It prevents class I α-chains that have not yet fully assembled with $\beta_2$m and antigenic peptides from leaving the ER (Degen, Cohen-Doyle & Williams, 1992). Calnexin is probably involved in the folding of class I molecules, which is an essential step in quality control (Jackson et al., 1994; Sone et al., 1994). Calnexin also plays a similar role for other proteins, among them such immunologically important proteins as MHC class II (Schreiber et al., 1994) and the α/β chains of the TCR, which do not leave the ER until they are fully assembled with the CD3 complex (Rajagopalan et al., 1994).

Of the groups of molecules known to be required for the processing of endogenous antigens, many can be upregulated by IFN-γ. These include two proteosome component molecules, the peptide transporters, class I heavy chain, and $\beta_2$m. Note also that some HSPs are also inducible with IFN-γ. Thus, these groups of molecules appear to share regulatory elements, which allow them to be regulated in concert. Evidence of the related functions of these molecules is genetic as well. The putative peptide transporter proteins and the proteosome component molecules appear to be within the MHC region on chromosome 17 in the mouse and chromosome 6 in the human.

# ■ THE MHC CLASS II PATHWAY FOR ANTIGEN PROCESSING

The ability of a cell to process antigens via the class II pathway (Figure 3.1) is more specialized than the almost ubiquitous ability of nucleated cells to process antigen via the class I pathway. Specialized, class II-bearing cells include macrophages, dendritic cells, Langerhans cells, and B lymphocytes. These cells bear not only class II heterodimers, but also possess the invariant chain monomer, the requisite enzymatic machinery, and an important subcellular architecture used in the processing and presentation of antigens via the class II pathway.

The peptides ultimately presented by class II are derived from protein molecules, which are generally acquired from outside the cell (that is, exogenous) by endocytic vesicles. These vesicles change in composition as they move away from the periphery of the cell towards the nucleus, and become acidified and acquire high concentrations of proteolytic enzymes. Pharmacologic agents, such as chloroquine, which disrupt intracellular pH gradients, have been shown to inhibit antigen processing. Furthermore, mutant cell lines, defective in endosomal acidification, have been shown to have diminished antigen-processing abilities. In B cells, surface-bound Ig molecules may be involved in the acquisition of molecules for presentation. Protein molecules to be presented by the class II pathway are processed by denaturation and proteolysis to short linear segments, some of which fit into the antigen-binding groove of class II molecules. These peptides play a role in determining the structure of class II heterodimers.

Class II heterodimers, consisting of one $\alpha$- and $\beta$-chain, associate with the invariant chain polypeptide (Ii) in the ER soon after synthesis, but dissociate with the invariant chain prior to expression on the cell surface (Figure 3.1). Ii ranges in size from 31 to 43 kDa as a result of alternate splicing as well as alternate sites for translation initiation, and has a single transmembrane domain and an amino-terminal cytoplasmic tail. It is coded for on human chromosome 5 and mouse chromosome 18, and it therefore is not genetically linked with the MHC. The invariant chain is known to have three important functions. First, it protects the peptide-binding site from binding by peptides prior to the designated physiologic site. Second, it protects the class II molecule itself, since in the acidic, proteolytic environment where class II is likely to bind a peptide, it must rapidly acquire peptide or risk getting destroyed by proteolysis. Finally, Ii influences the cellular routing of the class II heterodimer. It has been postulated that Ii is disposed of by the same proteolytic, acidic environment that is responsible for the digestion of exogenous antigens, which results in the creation of peptides able to bind to class II. Class II $\alpha$ and $\beta$-

chains transfected into cells without Ii are assembled and expressed on the cell surface albeit with much lower efficiency than if Ii is present. However, class II molecules fold differently in the absence of Ii, as is revealed by differential reactivity with monoclonal antibodies. These studies suggest that, in addition to other functions, Ii may behave as a molecular chaperone, helping the class II molecule to fold properly. Thus, the Ii blocks binding of endogenous antigens to the class II molecules and stabilizes the unoccupied $\alpha/\beta$ heterodimers while escorting them through the biosynthetic pathway to the endosomal compartment. Once the Ii is removed in the acidic and proteolytic environment of the endosomal compartment, the class II molecules are available for the binding of peptides.

The cell biology of antigen processing for presentation via class II molecules is now known in significant detail. Recently, a unique endosome-related subcellular compartment has been identified in specialized APCs that naturally express class II. The question of where, exactly, the class II biosynthetic pathway meets the antigen-generating endosomal pathway involves a comprehensive understanding of the subcellular trafficking of the relevant molecules. Several independent groups have used a variety of different techniques (both biochemical and functional) to identify a unique and previously undescribed subcellular compartment in which class II peptide loading occurs (Schmid & Jackson, 1994; Amigorena et al., 1994; Tupl et al., 1994; West, Lucocq & Watts, 1994). It has been proposed that this compartment be designated the compartment(s) for peptide loading or CPL. Morphologically, the CPL are somewhat heterogeneous in structure. They are spherical and tubular, and contain internal membrane vesicles or infoldings, covered with class II $\alpha/\beta$. These infoldings presumably act to increase the surface area for class II and help optimize exposure to potentially antigenic peptides. The Ii probably targets the class II $\alpha/\beta/$Ii complex to the CPL, probably by a di-leucine motif in the cytoplasmic tail of the Ii. Since the FcRII-$\beta2$ receptor also contains a di-leucine motif, such a motif could be implicated in the specific delivery of Ag to the CPL as well. The molecular mechanisms involved in the release from the CPL of class II molecules that are loaded with peptides are as yet unelucidated.

# ■ ANTIGEN PROCESSING AND PRESENTATION IN MALIGNANCY

Most cells in the body express class I/peptide complexes, which are the ligands for CD8$^+$ T cells. Some tumors cells clearly present antigenic peptides in the context of class I, since specific recognition of tumor cells by CD8$^+$ T cells has been shown to result in their destruction in vitro and in vivo. The mechanisms involved in tumor destruction include direct cytotoxicity as well as the release of cytokines by the T cells. If tumor cells that present antigenic peptides in the context of class I on their surfaces can be eliminated by the immune system, tumor cells that fail to present antigen recognizable by T cells may enjoy a selective advantage, since they would not be eliminated by the immune system. As a possible example of this phenomenon, many naturally occurring tumors, especially those of epithelial derivation, either do not express, or display greatly reduced levels of class I molecules on their surfaces. These histologies include embryonal carcinomas, choriocarcinomas, cervical carcinomas, mammary carcinomas, small-cell carcinomas of the lung, neuroblastomas, some colorectal carcinomas, and some melanomas (Kourilsky et al., 1991; Ruiter et al., 1991; Ruiz-Cabello et al., 1991; Bodmer et al., 1993; Garrido et al., 1993). The failure of class I antigen expression is so uniform amongst some of these histologies, for example, small-cell carcinomas of the lung (Restifo et al., 1993a; Doyle et al., 1985), that it may be an essential requirement for tumor survival. However, it is clear that malignant cells can express class I antigens and still have defective presentation of endogenous antigens.

The impetus for studying antigen processing and presentation in malignancy comes from the observation that many tumors do not elicit clear T cell responses. Lack of a T cell response is associated with the inability of the tumor to protect against subsequent tumor challenge, and these tumors have been identified as nonimmunogenic. While there are many possible explanations for the phenomenon of nonimmunogenicity, it has been demonstrated that some of these tumors fail to present antigen in the context of restricting MHC molecules. This can result from a wide variety of molecular deficiencies (Ruiter et al., 1991; Bodmer et al., 1993). There is evidence that tumor cells evade recognition by T cells by failing to present tumor antigens, which were not absent but instead 'hidden' intracellularly (Restifo et al., 1991, 1992, 1993a; see also Restifo et al., 1993b).

Several molecular mechanisms by which tumor cells fail to process and present endogenous antigens to $T_{CD8+}$ have been hypothesized (Restifo et al., 1993b). Using isolates of tumor cells from patients at the National Institutes of Health to establish cell lines from in vitro studies and fresh tumor sections for immunohistochemical studies, and in vivo correlates, we have identified that at least three different mechanisms are operative. The first mechanism, found in five different melanoma cell lines (N.P. Restifo, in preparation) involves the loss of functional $\beta_2m$ expression. This antigen presentation defect is entirely correctable in these cell line studies by gene insertion of $\beta_2m$. Bodmer and colleagues have shown that human cancer cells, especially adenocarcinomas of the colon, can fail to express $\beta_2$m (Bodmer et al., 1993; Bicknell, Rowan & Bodmer, 1994). Ferrone has shown that two human melanoma cell lines, do not express class I as a result of mutations in $\beta_2$m (D'Urso et al., 1991; Maio et al., 1991; Wang et al., 1993). The loss or mutation of $\beta_2$m is a highly efficient mechanism for tumor escape, since stable presentation of peptide antigen by class I molecules does not occur in the absence of $\beta_2$m.

A second mechanism of tumor escape, also observed in melanoma, involves the loss of expression of particular MHC class I alleles or loci (Marincola et al., 1994a, 1994b), and is again correctable by gene insertion of the missing α-chain genes or, in the case of the down-regulation of the transcription of an α-chain gene, by treatment with IFN-γ. The third type of defect observed, originally in the small-cell lung cancer histology, involved the down-regulation of certain components (Restifo et al., 1993a). This mechanism is correctable with treatment with exogenous IFN-γ or with gene modification with the IFN-γ gene (Restifo et al., 1992).

There is evidence that some tumors express antigens that are recognized in the context of class II molecules by CD4$^+$ lymphocytes. However, tumor cells generally do not express detectable levels of class II molecules on their cell surfaces. In these cases, the recognition of tumor cell antigens by CD4$^+$ cells is thought to be indirect, with tumor antigens presented by macrophages, dendritic cells, B lymphocytes, or another class II-bearing cell. CD4$^+$ cells have been implicated as suppressors ($T_s$) of host responses and this is covered in detail in later sections. Melanoma is one tumor that is known to express class II molecules frequently in vivo.

## Presentation of Tumor-associated Antigens to CD4$^+$ T Cells

To process tumor antigens that are subsequently recognized by CD4$^+$ T cells, shed substances or cellular debris from tumor cells presumably are taken into the APC by pinocytosis or receptor-associated endocytosis. The material is then degraded within lysosomes, following which the peptide fragments selectively associate with MHC class II molecules (Bevan, 1987; Moller, 1988; Kourilsky & Claverie, 1989). Processing of antigens by APC is not restricted by the normal location of the antigenic protein in the parent cell, such as a tumor cell. Characteristic aspects of the model are that antigenic peptides destined for association with MHC class II molecules are usually derived from extracellular material and are processed in a cystolic pathway different from that associated with MHC class I molecules. An exception has been reported for processing of measles virus antigens, where endogenously produced and processed antigens appear capable of associating with MHC class II molecules (Long & Jacobson, 1989). Thus, there are at least two potential selection criteria for antigen binding to MHC class II molecules: whether the antigen is in the appropriate cytosolic pathway and whether the peptide has binding affinity for the MHC class II molecules produced by the APC.

There are several possible paths for activation of CD4$^+$ T cells by tumor antigens. Host APC could process exogenous sources of tumor antigen and generate MHC class II antigen complexes. The antigen-armed APC that also expressed the needed costimulatory ligands (for example, B7) and adhesion molecules could directly activate the CD4$^+$ T cells, as described above. The CD4$^+$ T cells activated against tumor anigens could be directly cytotoxic for tumor cells, for example, by releasing lymphotoxin in the immediate vicinity of tumor cells. Alternatively, they could act indirectly by releasing cytokines that induce inflammation, induce hemorrhagic necrosis, or help activate effector cells such as CD8$^+$ T cells, macrophages, NK cells, or neutrophils.

CD4$^+$ T cells could also be activated directly by tumor cells. Human melanoma cells, for example, frequently express MHC class II molecules. Melanoma cells could serve as APCs, if they also express co-stimulatory molecules, such as B7, and the required levels of adhesion molecules. Indeed, MHC-class II expressing melanoma cell lines established from melanomas early in the course of the disease effectively present antigen to autologous T cells (Alexander, Bennicelli & Guerry, 1989). The antigen-presenting function of the melanoma cells is inhibited by agents that disrupt lysosomes, such as ammonium chloride, suggesting that the tumor cells carry out processing of exogenous antigens much like classical host APCs. Of note is the fact that activated T cell infiltrates have been observed in early lesions of primary melanoma (Carbone et al., 1988).

## Presentation of Tumor-associated Antigens to CD8$^+$ T Cells

CD8$^+$ T cells that are precursors to cytoxic cells could also be activated by tumor antigens, albeit probably different tumor peptides from those that stimulate CD4$^+$ T cells. CD8$^+$ T cells commonly receive their first signal for activation upon binding to antigen presented in association with cell-surface MHC class I molecules. There are several possible pathways whereby this might occur against tumor cells (Jelachich & Biddison, 1989; Kourilsky & Claverie, 1989; Townsend & Bodmer, 1989). First, many of the antigens associated with MHC class I arise endogenously, in constrast with the antigens of exogenous origin that associate with MHC class II. Foreign proteins made in tumor cells might be destined for a cellular location other than the cell surface. However, irrespective of the normal location of the foreign protein, endogenously synthesized and degraded products are able to enter a cytosolic pathway that links with MHC class I molecules destined for the cell surface.

Thus, by the first path, CD8[+] T cells would receive the initial signal for activation not on antigen-presenting host cells but rather on tumor cells. Additional signals needed for stimulation of cytotoxic T cell precursors, such as IL-2 and the B7 ligand, could be provided by activated CD4[+] helper T cells and APC, respectively. Alternatively, the stimulation of CD28 receptors on CD8[+] cells by B7 ligands on APC might stimulate sufficient IL-2 production by the CD8[+] T cells to avoid the need for CD4[+] T helper cell support.

A second possible pathway for activation of CD8[+] T cells is suggested by reports that not all antigens presented with class I arise endogenously (Bevan, 1987; Carbone et al., 1989; Jelachich & Biddison, 1989). One explanation for this observation is that extracellular antigenic peptides or proteins not requiring fragmentation for binding to class I molecules may bind directly to cell-surface class I molecules. In this case, CD8[+] T cells could bind to host APC and directly receive each of the required additional signals. Of note, primary stimulation of the TCR by tumor antigens and cost-stimulation of the same T cell by B7 can be from different cells; however, signaling is far more efficient if both are delivered by the same ancillary cell.

### Collaboration of CD4[+] and CD8[+] T Cells in an Antitumor Response

An efficient mechanism for providing CD8[+] CTL precursors with both primary activation signals and secondary support from CD4[+] T cells is for individual APC to express both MHC class I- and II-associated antigens. This mechanism for generating CTL, which has been referred to as 'epitope linking,' makes efficient use of the short range of action of helper cytokines (Mitchison & O'Malley, 1987). The situation could occur with tumor cells expressing both MHC class I and II molecules, and serving as APC. It could also occur if some of the tumor antigens destined for MHC class I presentation on the tumor cells were released from the tumor cells in a form capable of binding to the MHC class I molecules on host APC. Recent evidence from analysis of a mouse tumor model shows that CD8[+] CLT precursor cells indeed can be sensitized in situ against MHC class I-restricted tumor antigens presented by host APCs rather than by the tumor cells (Huang et al., 1994). Tumor antigens destined for MHC class II presentation would also need to be effectively processed and presented by the APC, if the CD8[+] T cells were not capable of providing 'help,' such as IL-2.

The site of T cell activation by tumor antigens within the tumor-bearing host is an important issue. One possiblity is that the antigen processing and presentation to T cells may both occur at the tumor site. Macrophages and T cells, CD4$^+$ and CD8$^+$, have been observed among host cell infiltrates in melanomas, for example (Brocker et al., 1988). Alternatively, tumor antigens could be processed by APC in regional lymph nodes or other sites distant from the tumor, and presented to CD4$^+$ and/or CD8$^+$ T cells there or at the tumor site. In either case, homing of the APC expressing tumor antigens or homing of activated CD4$^+$ and/or CD8$^+$ T cells to the tumor site would be necessary for antitumor effects, because of the short range of cytotoxic activity of CD4$^+$ and CD8$^+$ CTL.

## ■ RECOMBINANT AND SYNTHETIC ANTICANCER VACCINES

Designing tumor vaccines is particularly well positioned to benefit from the burgeoning knowledge of cellular immune responses in general, and antigen processing and presentation in particular. The possible applications of this technology include the development of vaccines based on known tumor antigens, on synthetic peptides modeled after naturally processed antigenic tumor peptides, and on the ability to enhance antigen processing and presentation genetically or pharmacologically. Where the antigenic tumor peptides are not known, peptide structures can be identified as likely to be immunogenic on the basis of amino acid or nucleotide sequence data (Berzofsky, 1988). Tumor antigens can be genetically engineered into constructs capable of producing large quantities of the desired recombinant antigen (Restifo et al., 1994). Such recombinant vaccines may be based on a variety of constructs including vaccinia virus (Moss, 1991, 1993, 1992a, 1992b), adenovirus (Berkner, 1992), and fowlpox virus (Baxby & Paoletti, 1992). This approach generally depends upon tumor antigens in the vaccine being processed in vivo to antigenic fragments, which then may be presented by the individual's own MHC-restriction elements. Using techniques in virology, molecular biology, and synthetic protein chemistry, the immunotherapist can now potentially control the quantity and kinetics of tumor-antigen expression, the intracellular compartment in which these antigens are expressed, and what tissues or cell types are used to express the antigens in vivo.

The identification of immunodominant T cell epitopes from tumor antigens has greatly expedited the development of peptide-based vaccines. In addition, antitumor T cell cultures can be efficiently stimulated with artificially synthesized peptide fragments and are now helping immunotherapists in the laboratory to grow antitumor T cells much more efficiently. Finally, immunodominant T cell epitopes from tumor antigens can be expressed by recombinant vectors in forms that exploit our understanding of antigen processing and presentation. For example, synthetic oligonucleotides can be constructed that express fragments of tumor antigens directly into the endoplasmic reticulum where they can bind very efficiently with nascent class I molecules, as has been demonstrated in the case of an antiviral response. Synthetic and recombinant strategies aimed at eliciting antitumor cells are becoming so powerful that the immunotherapist may in time be able to treat tumor histologies not previously thought to be susceptible to T cell-based immunotherapies.

## SUMMARY

Important concepts have emerged from studies of antigen processing and presentation concerning how the human cellular immune system can recognize and respond to autologous tumors. T cells can recognize peptide fragments presented by specialized molecules of the MHC, called H-2 in the mouse and HLA in the human, on the surfaces of tumor cells. These peptides are generally protolytic fragments of antigenic proteins. Detailed structural knowledge of MHC–antigen complexes has gained from X-ray crystallography studies. With an understanding of how the peptides are processed and expressed by normal cells, recent studies have identified a variety of shortcomings and defects in general antigen processing by a wide assortment of tumor cells. The study and use of specific tumor antigens is now possible, as several tumor-associated antigens recognized by autologous T cells from melanoma patients have been cloned, and have generally been found to be normal, nonmutated 'self' antigens. One of the key challenges facing immunotherapists is how to activate the T cell responses against tumors. Gene therapy, and recombinant and synthetic anticancer vaccines, in particular, offer new approaches to immunotherapists for treating cancer. Understanding how antigens are processed and presented, and how cellular immune responses normally occur, has provided a rational basis for designing new therapeutic strategies.

## ACKNOWLEDGMENT

The authors would like to thank Maria J. Ionata for helpful discussions.

## REFERENCES

Alexander M.A., Bennicelli J. & Guerry D. (1989) Defective antigen presentation by human melanoma cell lines cultured from advanced, but not biologically early, disease. *Journal of Immunology*, **142**, 4070–8.

Amigorena S., Drake J.R., Webster P. & Mellman I. (1994) Transient accumulation of new class II MHC molecules in a novel endocytic compartment of B lymphocytes. *Nature (London)*, **369**, 113–120.

Bach F.H., Widmer M.B., Bach M.L. & Klein, J. (1972) Serologically defined and lymphocyte-defined components of the major histocompatibility complex in the mouse. *Journal of Experimental Medicine*, **136**, 1430–44.

Barber L.D. & Parham P. (1993) Peptide binding to major histocompatibility complex molecules. *Annual Review of Cell Biology*, **9**, 163–206.

Barth R.J., Mule J.J., Spiess P.J. & Rosenberg S.A. (1991) Interferon gamma and tumor necrosis factor have a role in tumor regressions mediated by murine CD8+ tumor-infiltrating lymphocytes. *Journal of Experimental Medicine*, **173** 647–58.

Baxby D. & Paoletti E. (1992) Potential use of non-replicating vectors as recombinant vaccines. *Vaccine*, **10**, 8–9.

Benacerraf B. & McDevitt H.O. (1972) Histocompatibility-linked immune response genes. *Science*, **175**, 273–9.

Berkner K.L. (1992) Expression of heterologous sequences in adenoviral vectors. *Current Topics in Microbiology and Immunology*, **158**, 39–66.

Berzofsky J.A. (1988) Structural basis of antigen recognition by T lymphocytes: implications for vaccines. *Journal of Clinical Investigation*, **82**, 1811–7.

Bevan M.J. (1975) The major histocompatibility complex determines susceptibility to cytotoxic T cells directed against minor histocompatibility antigens. *Journal of Experimental Medicine*, **142**, 1349–64.

Bevan M.J. (1987) Antigen recognition. Class discrimination in the world of immunology. *Nature*, **325**, 192–4.

Bicknell D.C., Rowan A. & Bodmer W.F. (1944) Beta 2-microglobulin gene mutations: a study of established colorectal cell lines and fresh tumors. *Proceedings of the National Academy of Sciences USA*, **91**, 4751–6.

Bjorkman P.J., Saper M.A., Samraoui B., Bennett W.S., Strominger J.L. & Wiley D.C. (1987) Structure of the human class I histocompatibility antigen, HLA-A2. *Nature (London)*, **329**, 506–12.

Bodmer W.F., Browning M.J., Krausa P., Rowan A., Bicknell D.C. & Bodmer, J.G. (1993) Tumor escape from immune response by variation in HLA expression and other mechanisms. *Annals of the New York Academy of Sciences*, **690**, 42–9.

Boes B., Hengel H., Ruppert T., Multhaup G., Koszinowski U.H. & Kloetzel P.M. (1994) Interferon gamma stimulation modulates the proteolytic activity and cleavage site preference of 20S mouse proteasomes. *Journal of Experimental Medicine*, **179**, 901–9.

Brocker E.B., Zwadlo G., Holzmann B., Macher E. & Sorg C. (1988) Inflammatory cell infiltrates in human melanoma at different stages of tumor progression. *International Journal of Cancer*, **41**, 562–7.

Brodsky F.M. & Guagliardi L.E. (1991) The cell biology of antigen processing and presentation. *Annual Review of Immunology*, **9**, 707–44.

Brown J.H., Jardetzky T.S., Gorga J.C., Stern L.J., Urban R.G., Strominger J.L. & Wiley D.C. (1993) Three-dimensional structure of the human class II histocompatibility antigen HLA-DR1. *Nature (London)*, **364**, 33–9.

Brown M.C., Driscoll J. & Monaco J.J. (1991) Structutal and serological similarity of MHC-linked LMP and proteasone (multicatalytic proteinase) complexes. *Nature (London)*, **353**, 355.

Brown M.G., Driscoll J. & Monaco J.J. (1993) MHC-linked low-molecular mass polypeptide subunits define distinct subsets of proteasomes. Implications for divergent function among distinct proteasome subsets. *Journal of Immunology*, 151, 1193–204.

Cammarota G., Scheirle A., Takacs B., Doran D.M., Knorr R., Bannwarth W., Guardiola J. & Sinigaglia F. (1992) Identification of a CD4 binding site on the beta 2 domain of HLA-DR molecules. *Nature (London)*, 356, 799–801.

Carbone F.R., Moore M.W., Sheil J.M. & Bevan M.J. (1988) Induction of cytotoxic T lymphocytes by primary in vitro stimulation with peptides. *Journal of Experimental Medicine*, 167, 1767–79.

Connolly J.M., Hansen T.H., Ingold A.L. & Potter T.A. (1990) Recognition by CD8 on cytotoxic T lymphocytes is ablated by several substitutions in the class I alpha 3 domain: CD8 and the T-cell receptor recognize the same class I molecule. *Proceedings of the National Academy of Sciences USA*, 87, 2137–41.

David V., Hochstenbach F., Rajagopalan S. & Brenner M.B. (1993) Interaction with newly synthesized and retained proteins in the endoplasmic reticulum suggests a chaperone function for human integral membrane protein IP90 (calnexin). *Journal of Biological Chemistry*, 268, 9585–92.

Degen E., Cohen-Doyle M.F. & Williams D.B. (1992) Efficient dissociation of the p88 chaperone from major histocompatibility complex class I molecules requires both beta 2-microglobulin and peptide. *Journal of Experimental Medicine*, 175, 1653–61.

Demotz S., Grey H.M. & Sette A. (1990) The minimal number of class II MHC-antigen complexes needed for T cell association. *Science*, 249, 1028–30.

Deverson E., Gow I.R., Coadwell W.J., Monaco J.J., Butcher G.W. & Howard J.C. (1990) MHC class II region encoding proteins related to the multidrug resistance family of transmembrane transporters. *Nature (London)*, 348, 738–41.

Dick L.R., Aldrich C., Jameson S.C. et al. (1994) Proteolytic processing of ovalbumin and beta-galactosidase by the proteasome to a yield antigenic peptides. *Jounral of Immunology*, 152, 3884–94.

Doyle A., Martin W.J., Funa K. et al. (1985) Markedly decreased expression of class I histocompatibility antigens, protein, and mRNA in human small-cell lung cancer. *Journal of Experimental Medicine*, 161, 1135–44.

Driscoll J., Brown M.G., Finley D. & Monaco J.J. (1993) MHC-linked LMP gene products specifically alter peptidase activities of the proteasome. *Nature (London)*, 365, 262–4.

D'Urso C.M., Wang Z.G., Cao Y., Tatake R., Zeff R.A. & Ferrone S. (1991) Lack of HLA class I antigen expression by cultured melanoma cells FO-1 due to a defect in B2m gene expression. *Journal of Clinical Investigation*, 87, 284–92.

Falk, K., Rotzschke O., Stevanovic S., Jung G. & Rammensee H.G. (1994) Pool sequencing of natural HLA-DR, DQ, and DP ligands reveals detailed peptide motifs, constraints of processing, and general rules. *Immunogenetics*, 39, 230–42.

Fremont D.H., Matsumura M., Stura E.A., Peterson P.A. & Wilson I.A. (1992) Crystal structures of two viral peptides in complex with murine MHC class I H-2K$^b$. *Science*, 257, 919–27.

Fruh K., Gossen M., Wang K., Bujard H., Peterson P.A. & Yang Y. (1994) Displacement of housekeeping proteasome subunits by MHC-encoded LMPs: a newly discovered mechanism for modulating the multicatalytic proteinase complex. *EMBO Journal*, 13, 3236–44.

Garrido F., Cabrera T., Concha A., Glew, S., Ruiz-Cabelloe F. & Stern P.L. (1993) Natural history of HLA expression during tumor development. *Immunology Today*, 14, 491–9.

Germain R.N. (1994) MHC-dependent antigen processing and peptide presentation: providing ligands for T lymphocyte activation. *Cell*, **76**, 287–99.

Glynne R., Powis S.H., Beck S., Kelly A., Kerr L.-A. & Trowsdale J. (1991) A proteosome-related gene between the two ABC transporter loci in the class II region of the human MHC. *Nature (London)*, **353**, 357–60.

Goldberg A.L. & Rock K.L. (1992) Proteolysis, proteasomes and antigen presentation. *Nature (London)*, **357**, 375–9.

Greenberg P.D. (1991) Adoptive T cell therapy of tumots: mechanisms operative in the recognition and elimination of tumor cells. *Advances in Immunology*, **49**, 281–355

Greenberg P.D., Cheever M.A. & Fefer A. (1981) H-2 restriction of adoptive immunotherapy of advanced tumors. *Journal of Immunology*, **126**, 2100–3.

Hammer J., Valsasnini P., Tolba K., Bolin D., Higelin J., Takacs B. & Sinigaglia F. (1993) Promiscuous and allele-specific anchors in HLA-DR-binding peptides. *Cell*, **74**, 197–203.

Hammond C., Braakman I. & Helenius A. (1994) Role of N-linked oligosaccharide recognition, glucose trimming, and calnexin in glycoprotein folding and quality control. *Proceedings of the National Academy of Sciences USA*, **91**, 913–17.

Hansen T.H., Carreno B.M. & Sachs D.H. (1993) The major histocompatibility complex. In W. Paul (ed) *Fundamental immunology*, pp. 577–628. New York, Raven Press.

Harding C.V. & Unanue E.R. (1990) Quantitation of antigen-presenting cell MHC class II/peptide complexes necessary for T-cell stimulation. *Nature (London)*, **346**, 574.

Henderson, R.A., Cox A.L., Sakaguchi K., Appella E., Shananowitz J., Hunt D.F. & Engelhard V.H. (1993) Direct identification of an endogeneous peptide recognized by multiple HLA-A2.1-specific cytotoxic T cells. *Proceedings of the National Academy of Sciences USA*, **90**, 10275–9.

Henderson, R.A., Michel H., Sakaguchi K., Shabanowitz J., Appella E., Hunt D.F. & Engelhard V.H. (1992) HLA-A2.1-associated peptides from a mutant cell line: a second pathway of antigen presentation. *Science*, **255**, 1264–6.

Hill, A.V., Allsopp C.E., Kwiatkowski D. et al. (1991) Common west African HLA antigens are associated with protection from severe malaria. *Nature (London)*, **352**, 595–600.

Huang A.Y.C., Golumbek P., Ahmadzadeh M., Jaffee E., Pardoll D. & Levitsky H. (1994) Role of bone marrow-derived cells in presenting MHC class I-restricted tumor antigens. *Science*, **264**, 961–5.

Huczko E.L., Bodnar W.M., Benjamin D. et al. (1993) Characteristics of endogenous peptides eluted from the class I MHC molecule HLA-B7 determined by mass spectrometry and computer modeling. *Journal of Immunology*, **151**, 2572–87.

Hunt D.F., Henderson R.A., Shabanowitz J. et al., (1992a) Characterization of peptides bound to the class I MHC molecule HLA-A2.1 by mass spectrometry. *Scienc*, **255**, 1261–3.

Hunt D.F., Michel H., Dickenson T.A. et al. (1992b) Peptides presented to the immune system by the murine class II major histocompatibility complex molecule I-A$^d$. *Science*, **256**, 1817–20.

Itoh K., Platsoucas D.C. & Balch C.M. (1988) Autologous tumor-specific cytotoxic T lymphocytes in the infiltrate of human metastatic melanomas: activation by interleukin 2 and autologous tumor cells and involvement of the T cell receptor. *Journal of Experimental Medicine*, **168**, 1419–41.

Jackson M.R., Cohen-Doyle M.F., Peterson P.A. & Williams D.B. (1994) Regulation of MHC class I transport by the molecular chaperone, calnexin (p.88, IP90). *Science*, **263**, 384–7.

Jelachich M.L. & Biddison W.E. (1989) Class I antigen presentation. *Yearbook of Immunology*, **4**, 41–58.

Johnson E.S., Bartel B., Seufert W. & Varsjavsky A. (1992) Ubiquitin as a degradation signal. *EMBO Journal*, **11**, 497–505.

Jorgensen J.L., Reay P.A., Ehrich E.W. & Davis M.M. (1992) Molecular components of T-cell recognition. *Annual Review of Immunology*, **10**, 835–73.

Klein G., Sjogren H.O., Klein, E. & Hellstrom K.E. (1960) Demonstration of resistance against methylcholanthrene-induced sarcomas in the primary autochthonous host. *Cancer Research*, **20**, 1561–9.

Konig R., Huang L.Y., & Germain R.N. (1992) MHC class II interaction with CD4 mediated by a region analogous to the MHC class I binding site for CD8. *Nature (London)*, **356**, 796–8.

Kourilsky P. & Claverie J.M. (1989) MHC-antigen interaction: what does the T cell receptor see. *Advances in Immunology*, **45**, 107–93.

Kozlowski S., Takeshita T., Boehncke W.-H. et al. Excess $\beta_2$ microglobulin promoting functional peptide association with purified soluble class I MHC molecules. *Nature (London)*, **359**, 74–7.

Ljunggren H.-G., Stam N.J., Ohlen C. et al. (1990) Empty MHC class I molecules come out in the cold. *Nature (London)*, **346**, 476–80.

Long E.O. & Jacobson S. (1989) Pathways of viral antigen processing and presentation to CTL: defined by the mode of virus entry. *Immunology Today*, **10**, 45–8.

Mage M.G., Lee L., Ribaudo R.K., Corr M., Kozlowski S., McHugh L. & Marguiles D.H. (1992) A recombinant, soluble, single-chain class I major histocompatibility complex molecule with biological activity. *Proceedings of the National Academy of Sciences USA*, **89**, 10658–62.

Maio M., Altomonte M., Tatake R., Zeff R.A. & Ferrone S. (1991) Reduction in susceptibility to natural killer cell-mediated lysis of human FO-1 melanoma cells after induction of HLA class I antigen expression by transfection with $\beta_2$m gene. *Journal of Clinical Investigation*, **88**, 282–9.

Marincola F.M., Shamamian P., Alexander R.B. et al. Loss of HLA haplotype and B locus down-regulation in melanoma cell lines. *Journal of Immunology*, **153**, 1225–37.

Marincola F.M., Shamamian, P., Simonis T.B. et al. Locus-specific analysis of human leukocyte antigen class I expression in melanoma cell lines. *Journal of Immunotherapy with Emphasis on Tumor Immunology*, **16**, 12–23.

Matsumura M., Fremont D.H., Peterson P.A. & Wilson I.A. (1992) Emerging principles for the recognition of peptide antigens by MHC class I molecules. *Science*, **257**, 927–34.

Michalek M.T., Grant E.P., Gramm C., Goldberg A.L. & Rock K.L. (1993) A role for the ubiquitin-dependent proteolytic pathway in MHC class I-restricted antigen presentation. *Nature (London)*, **363**, 552–4.

Mitchison N.A. & O'Malley C. (1987) Three-cell-type clusters of T cells with antigen-presenting cells best explain the epitope linkage and noncognate requirements of the in vivo cytolytic response. *European Journal of Immunology*, **17**, 1579–83.

Moller G. (1988) *Antigen processing*. Immunological Reviews, Vol. 106. Copenhagen, Munksgaard.

Monaco J.J., Cho S. & Attaya M. (1990) Transport protein genes in the murine MHC: possible implications for antigen processing. *Science*, **250**, 1723–6.

Morrison L.A., Lugo J.P., Braciale V.L., Fan D.P. & Braciale T.J. (1986) Differences in antigen presentation ot MHC class I- and class II-restricted influenza virus-specific cytolytic T lymphocyte clones. *Journal of Experimental Medicine*, **163**, 903–21.

Moss B. (1991) Vaccinia virus: a tool for research and vaccine development. *Science*, 252, 1662–7.

Moss B. (1992a) Vaccinia virus vectors. *Biotechnology*, 20, 345–62.

Moss B. (1992b) Poxvirus expression vectors. *Current Topics in Microbiology and Immunology*, 158, 25–38.

Moss B. (1993) Poxvirus vectors: cytoplasmic expression of transferred genes. *Current Opinions in Genetics Development*, 3, 86–90.

Ortmann B., Androlewicz M.J., & Cresswell P. (1994) MHC class I/beta 2-microglobulin complexes associate with TAP transporters before peptide binding. *Nature (London)*, 368, 854–7.

Ou W.J., Cameron, P.H., Thomas D.Y. & Bergerson J.J. (1993) Association of folding intermediates of glycoproteins with calnexin during protein maturation. *Nature (London)*, 364, 771–6.

Parham P. (1990) Transporters of delight. *Nature (London)*, 348, 674–5.

Parham P. (1993) HLA, anthropology, and transplantation. *Transplantation Proceedings*, 25, 159–61.

Patel S.D., Monaco J.J. & McDevitt H.O. (1994) Delineation of the subunit composition of human proteasomes using antisera against the major histocompatibility complex-encodes LMP2 and LMP7 subunits. *Proceedings of the National Academy of Sciences USA*, 9, 296–300.

Potter T.A., Rajan T.V., Dick R.F., II & Bluestone J.A. (1989) Substitution at residue 227 of H-2 class I molecules abrogates recognition by CD8-dependent, but not CD8-independent, cytotoxic T lymphocytes. *Nature (London)*, 337, 73–5.

Prehn R. T. & Main J.M. 1957) Immunity to methylcholanthrene-induced sarcomas. *Journal of the National Cancer Institute*, 18, 769–81.

Rajagopalan S., Xu Y. and Brenner M.B. (1994) Retention of unassembled components of integral membrane proteins by calnexin. *Science*, 263, 387–90.

Rammensee H.G., Falk K. & Rotzsckke O. (1993a) Peptides naturally presented by MHC class I molecules. *Annual Review of Immunology*, 11, 213–44.

Rammensee H.G., Falk, K. & Rotzschke O. (1993b) MHC molecules as peptide receptors. *Current Opinion in Immunology*, 5, 35–44.

Restifo N.P., Esquivel F., Asher A.L. et al. (1991) Defective presentation of endogenous antigens by a murine sarcoma: implications for the failure of an anti-tumor immune response. *Journal of Immunology*, 147, 1453–9.

Restifo N.P., Esquivel F., Kawakami, Y. et al. (1993a) Identification of human cancers deficient in antigen processing. *Journal of Experimental Medicine*, 177, 265–72.

Restifo N.P., Kawakami Y., Maricola F. et al. (1993b) Molecular mechanisms of escape of tumor from immune recognition: immunogenetherapy and the cell biology of MHC class I. *Journal of Immunotherapy*, 142, 182–90.

Restifo N.P., Minev B.R., Taggarse A.S., McFarland B.J., Wang M., & Irvine K.R. (1994) Enhancing the recognition of tumor associated antigens. *Folio Biologica (Praha)*, 40,1–15.

Restifo N.P., Spiess P.J., Karp S.E., Mule J.J. & Rosenberg S.A. (1992) A nonimmunogenic sarcoma transduced with the cDNA for interferon gamma elicits CD8+ T cells against the wild-type tumor: correlation with antigen presentation capability. *Journal of Experimental Medicine*, 175, 1423–31.

Rosenberg, S.A., Packard B.S., Aebersold P.M. et al. (1988) Use of tumor infiltrating lymphocytes and interleukin-2 in the immunotherpy of patients with metastatic melanoma. Preliminary report. *New England Journal of Medicine*, 319, 1676–80.

Rosenberg S.A., Spiess P. & Lafreniere R. (1986) A new approach to the adoptive immunotherapy of cancer with tumor-infiltrating lymphocytes. *Science*, **233**, 1318–21.

Roy S., Scherer M.T., Briner T.J., Smith J.A. & Gefter M.L. (1989) Murine MHC polymorphism and T cell sepcificities. *Science*, **244**, 572–5.

Rudensky A.Y., Preston-Hurlburt P., Hong S.C., Barlow A. & Janeway C.A., Jr. (1991) Sequence analysis of peptides bound to MHC class II molecules. *Nature (London)*, **353**, 622–7.

Ruiter D.J., Mattijssen V., Broecker E.B. & Ferrone S. (1991) MHC antigen in human melanomas. *Seminars in Cancer and Biology*, **2**, 34–45.

Ruiz-Cabello F., Perez-Ayala M., Gomez O. et al. (1991) Molecular analysis of MHC-class-I alterations in human tumor cell lines. *International Journal of Cancer*, **6** (Suppl.), 123–30.

Ruppert J., Sidney J., Celis E., Kubo R.T., Grey H.M. & Sette A. (1993) Prominent role of secondary anchor residues in peptide binding to HLA-A2.1 molecules. *Cell*, **74**, 929–37.

Salter R.D., Benjamin R.J., Wesley P.K. et al. (1990) A binding site for the T-cell co-receptor CD8 on the $\alpha_3$ domain of HLA-A2. *Nature (London)*, **345**, 41–6.

Schmid S.L. & Jackson M.R. (1994) Making class II presentable. *Nature (London)*, **369**, 103–4.

Schreiber H., Ward P.L., Rowley D.A. & Stauss H.J. (1988) Unique tumor-specific antigens. *Annual Review of Immunology*, **6**, 465–83.

Schreiber K.L., Bell M.P., Huntoon C.J., Rajagopalan S., Brenner M.B. & McKean D.J. (1994) Class II histocompatibility molecules associate with calnexin during assembly in the endoplasmic reticulum. *International Immunology*, **6**, 101–11.

Sette A., DeMars R., Grey H.M. et al. (1993a) Isolation and characterization of naturally processed peptides bound by class II molecules and peptides presented by normal and mutant antigen-presenting cells. *Chemical Immunology*, **57**, 152–65.

Sette A., Sidney J., Oseroff et al. (1993b) HLA DR4w4-binding motifs illustrate the biochemical basis of degeneracy and specificity in peptide-DR interactions. *Journal of Immunology*, **151**, 3163–70.

Shimizu K. & Shen F.-W. (1979) Role of different T cell set in the rejection of syngeneic chemically induced tumors. *Journal of Immunology*, **122**, 1162–5.

Sidney J., Oseroff C., del Guercio M.F. et al. (1994) Definition of a DQ3.1-specific binding motif. *Journal of Immunology*, **152**, 4516–25.

Spies T., Bresnhan M., Bahram S., Arnold D., Blanck G., Mellins E., Pious D. & DeMars R. (1990) A gene in the human major histocompatibility complex class II region controlling the class I antigen presentation pathway. *Nature (London)*, **348**, 744–7.

Srivastava P.K. (1993) Peptide-binding heat shock proteins in the endoplasmic reticulum: role in immune response to cancer and in antigen presentation. *Advances in Cancer Research*, **62**, 153–77.

Srivastava P.K., Udono H., Blachere N.E. & Li Z. (1994) Heat shock proteins transfer peptides during antigen processing and CTL priming. *Immunogenetics*, **39**, 93–8.

Stern L.J., Brown J.H., Jardetzky T.S., Gorga J.C., Urban R.G., Strominger J.L., & Wiley D.C. (1994) Crystal structure of the human class II MHC protein HLA-DR1 complexed with an influenza virus peptide. *Nature (London)*, **368**, 215–21.

Stura E.A., Matsumura M., Fremont D.H., Saito Y., Peterson P.A. & Wilson I.A. (1992) Crystallization of murine major histocompatibility complex class I H-2Kb with single peptides. *Journal of Molecular Biology*, **288**, 975–82.

Tobias J.W., Shrader T.E., Rocap G. & Varshavsky A. (1991) The N-end rule in bacteria. *Science*, **254**, 1374–7.

Topalian S.L., Solomon D. & Rosenberg S.A. (1989) Tumor-specific cytolysis by lymphocytes infiltrating human melanomas. *Journal of Immunology*, **142**, 3714–25.

Townsend A. & Bodmer H. (1989) Antigen recognition by class I-restricted T lymphocytes. *Annual Review of Immunology*, **7**, 601–24.

Townsend A., Bastin J., Gould K. et al. (1988) Defective presentation to class I-restricted cytotoxic T lymphocytes in vaccinia-infected cells is overcome by enhanced degradation of antigen. *Journal of Experimental Medicine*, **168**, 1211–24.

Townsend A., Elliot T., Cerundolo V., Foster L., Barber B. & Tse A. (1990) Assembly of MHC class I molecules analyzed in vitro. *Cell*, **62**, 285–95.

Tulp A., Verwoerd D., Dobberstein B., Ploegh H.L. & Pieters J. (1994) Isolation and characterization of the intracellular MHC class II compartment. *Nature (London)*, **369**, 120–6.

Udono H., Levy D.L. & Srivastava P.K. (1994) Cellular requirements for tumor-specific immunity elicited by heat shock proteins: tumor rejection antigen gp96 primes CD8[+] T cells in vivo. *Proceedings of the National Academy of Sciences USA*, **91**, 3077–81.

Udono H. & Srivastava P.K. (1993) Heat shock protein 70-associated peptides elicit specific cancer immunity. *Journal of Experimental Medicine*, **178**, 1391–6.

Varshavsky A. (1992) The N-end rule. *Cell*, **69**, 725–35.

Wang Z., Cao Y., Albino A.P., Zeff R.A., Houghton A. & Ferrone S. (1993) Lack of HLA class I antigen expression by melanoma cells SK-MEL-33 caused by a reading frameshift in beta 2-microglobulin messenger RNA. *Journal of Clinical Investigation*, **91**, 684–92.

Wei M.L. & Cresswell P. (1992) HLA-A2 molecules in an antigen-processing mutant cell contain signal sequence-derived peptides. *Nature (London)*, **356**, 443–6.

Weiss A. & Bogen B. (1991) MHC class II-restricted presentation of intracellular antigen. *Cell*, **64**, 767–76.

West M.A., Lucocq J.M. & Watts C. (1994) Antigen processing and class II MHC peptide-loading compartments in human B-lymphoblastoid cells. *Nature (London)*, **369**, 147–51.

Wilson I.A. & Fremont D.H. (1993) Structural analysis of MHC class I molecules with bound peptide antigens. *Seminars in Immunology*, **5**, 75–80.

Yewdell J.W. & Bennink J.R. (1992) Cell biology of antigen processing and presentation to major histocompatibility complex class I molecule-restricted T lymphocytes. *Advances in Immunology*, **52**, 1–123.

Young A.C., Zhang W., Sacchettini J.C. & Nathenson S.G. (1994) The three-dimensional structure of H-2D[b] at 2.4 A resolution: implications for antigen-determinant selection. *Cell*, **76**, 39–50.

Zijlstra M., Bix M., Simister N.E., Loring J.M., Raulet D.H. & Jaenisch R. (1990) B2-Microglobulin deficient mice lack CD4[−] CD8[+] cytolytic T cells. *Nature (London)*, **344**, 742–6.

Zinkernagel R.M. & Doherty P.C. (1974) Restriction of in vitro T cell-mediated cytotoxicity in lymphocytic choriomeningitis within a syngeneic or semiallogeneic system. *Nature (London)*, **248**, 701–2.

# ──4────────────────────────────────

# The Role of MHC Class I in Tumour Immunity

MICHAEL BROWNING

## ■ INTRODUCTION

Defining the role that the immune system plays in the surveillance and elimination of cancer has been a long and often problematic process. The ability of the host to reject malignant cells was demonstrated four decades ago by the experiments of Foley (1953), and Prehn & Main (1957) using transplantable tumours in syngeneic mice. It was not until the last fifteen years or so, however, that the mechanisms by which tumour cells may be killed or rejected have been elucidated, and a role for MHC class I antigens in mediating tumour rejection has been established.

The classical experiments of Zinkernagel & Doherty in the 1970s (1975, 1979) demonstrated that the reactivity of cytotoxic T lymphocytes (CTL) was restricted by surface molecules encoded by genes of the class I region of the major histocompatibility complex (MHC), and led to the idea that these molecules might also be of relevance in the host's defence against tumours. In the 1980s Townsend and colleagues showed that CTL recognize short peptides derived from intracellular proteins presented in association with MHC class I molecules (Townsend, Gotch & Davey, 1985; Townsend et al., 1986). These observations greatly widened the range of potential tumour antigens that the immune system might recognize. In addition to these advances in cellular immunology, it became apparent that the development of a cancer represents a multi-step process, which is characterized by the accumulation of genetic events, including mutations in proto-oncogenes and tumour suppressor genes (Fearon & Vogelstein, 1990), as well as in other cellular genes. The products of these mutated genes represent potential targets for tumour-specific immune responses. Thus a model of a tumour cell was established that was consistent with the concept that T lymphocytes could recognize tumour cells as 'foreign' and, under appropriate circumstances, could mediate their rejection. Direct evidence for a role of MHC class I molecules in the rejection of syngeneic tumour cells came from a variety of animal models. In humans, however, evidence for a role of HLA class I in

**69**

tumour rejection has been harder to come by. The identification of HLA class I-restricted, tumour-specific CTL in a proportion of patients with melanoma (Knuth et al., 1984; Herin et al., 1987; Topalian et al., 1989) and more recently with other tumours (Ioannides et al., 1991; Schendel et al., 1993; Yasumura et al., 1993) suggests that, in humans also, MHC class I molecules may be involved in the immune response to at least some cancers, but the extent to which they might mediate tumour rejection remains unresolved. For the majority of spontaneous human tumours, direct evidence of HLA class I restricted T cell responses is still lacking. The loss or down-regulation of HLA class I expression observed on a wide variety of tumour types (reviewed by Moller & Hammerling, 1992; Garrido et al., 1993) has been interpreted as indirect evidence for HLA class I-restricted responses to these malignancies. In this respect, the loss of HLA class I expression may represent a means by which tumour cells escape from immune attack by tumour-specific CTL.

Several chapters in this volume deal in detail with specific areas of the interaction between T lymphocytes and tumour cells. The aim of this chapter is to provide an overview of the evidence that supports a role of MHC class I molecules in tumour rejection, and of the mechanisms and significance of loss or down-regulation of HLA expression on tumour cells, in tumour immunity and immunotherapy. Whilst reference is made to lessons learned from animal models, the emphasis of the chapter is on the role of HLA class I in the immune response to tumours in humans.

## ■ MHC CLASS I MOLECULES

### Antigen Presentation by MHC Class I Molecules

Human and murine MHC class I molecules are polymorphic cell surface proteins, which act as antigen-presenting molecules for $CD8^+$ T lymphocytes, principally antigen-specific CTL. The class I molecule consists of a heterodimer of heavy and light glycoprotein chains, noncovalently associated with a short, cell-derived peptide. The polymorphic heavy chain spans the cell membrane, and is encoded, in humans, by the three 'classical' HLA class I genes, HLA-A, HLA-B, and HLA-C, of the major histocompatibility complex on the short arm of chromosome 6. The extensive polymorphism of the class I heavy-chain genes means that, in outbred populations, the majority of individuals will express six different class I molecules, each of which is capable of associating with and presenting a different array of peptides (reviewed by Rammensee, Friede & Stevanovic, 1995). The class I light chain is the monomorphic $\beta_2$ microglobulin ($\beta_2$m). Peptides derived from both self and foreign cytosolic proteins bind MHC class I molecules, and are presented at the cell surface to antigen-specific receptors on T lymphocytes. MHC complexes involving self-derived peptides are normally tolerated, whilst those involving peptides derived from foreign (for example, viral) proteins may be stimulatory to the immune system. Through the presentation of cell-derived peptides at the cell surface by MHC class I molecules, the array of intracellular proteins expressed in somatic cells, both self and foreign, is continuously surveyed by the immune system. Thus the HLA class I molecules expressed by an individual play a critical role in determining the range of antigens and/or peptide epitopes that are presented to the individual's immune system. The structure, biosynthesis, and assembly of MHC class I molecules are discussed in detail in Chapter 3 of this volume, and are not described further here.

### Regulation of MHC Class I Expression

MHC class I molecules are expressed constitutively on the great majority of somatic cells, although levels of expression vary between different cell types; in general, levels of class I expression are highest on cells of lymphoid origin. In several cell lineages, such as hepatocytes, skeletal muscle, and lymph vessel endothelium, expression of HLA class I is absent or very low under physiological conditions, but can be up-regulated at sites of inflammation (David-Watine, Israel & Kourilsky, 1991). Several exogenous stimuli have been shown to up-regulate expression of MHC class I. These include the interferons, especially interferon-$\gamma$ (IFN-$\gamma$), and tumour necrosis factor-$\alpha$. In addition, a number of virus infections, including oncogenic viruses, have been shown to modulate HLA expression on cells (Schrier et al., 1983; del Val, Hengel & Hacker, 1992). At the molecular level, regulation of MHC class I genes is mediated by a variety of *trans*-acting factors, which bind to regulatory elements on the *cis*-MHC genes. The molecular basis of MHC class I expression and regulation has been reviewed by Singer & Maguire (1990) and by David-Watine, Israel & Kourilsky (1991).

### ■ MHC CLASS I AND IMMUNITY TO TUMOURS

The ability of the immune system to reject tumour cells was first demonstrated in the 1950s using chemically induced tumours transplanted into syngeneic mice (Foley 1953; Prehn & Main, 1957). Subsequent experiments confirmed the role of MHC antigens in the rejection of tumour cells, and identified a number of mechanisms by which T cells mediate tumour rejection (Greenberg, 1991). In particular, the ability of MHC class I-restricted tumour-specific T lymphocytes to lyse tumour cells in vitro, and to mediate tumour rejection in vivo, under certain conditions at least, supported a role for MHC class I molecules in tumour immunity.

## MHC Class I and Tumour Rejection in Animal Models

The antitumour activity of CD8$^+$ CTL has been demonstrated in a variety of animal models, including lymphomas and leukaemias, sarcomas, glioma, mastocytoma, melanoma, and others (Boon et al., 1980; Dailey, Pillemer & Weissman, 1982; Mills & North, 1983; Rosenstein, Eberlein & Rosenberg, 1984; Yamasaki et al., 1984; Greenberg, 1986; Lynch & Miller, 1991). In the majority of these models, however, whilst the tumour was capable of inducing specific effector cells, these cells did not reject the primary tumour. The disparity between induction of a specific immune response and tumour rejection was clearly demonstrated by the experiments of Klein and colleagues (1960), in which tumours were induced in mice with the chemical mutagen methylcholanthrene. The primary tumours were rarely rejected and grew progressively. If the primary tumour was removed surgically, however, and the host was then challenged with cells derived from the same tumour, the tumour cell challenge was rejected. This rejection was specific for the immunizing tumour, and displayed two key features of the cognitive immune response, namely specificity and memory. It was subsequently shown that the principal effector cell population that mediated tumour rejection was CD8$^+$, MHC class I-restricted CTL.

The failure of the CTL to reject a heterologous tumour cell challenge in these models suggested that each individual tumour expressed unique tumour antigens, even when induced in the same cell type and by the same mutagen. This led Boon and colleagues to study the specificity of tumour rejection, using the murine mastocytoma cell line P815. Exposure of the tumour cell line to chemical mutagens was used to generate tumour cell variants, which were no longer able to form progressive tumours (termed 'tum$^-$' variants) (Boon, 1983) and which induced populations of MHC-restricted, tumour-specific CTL. In an analysis of 15 independent tum$^-$ variants of the P815 tumour line, none of the antigens that were recognized by the CTL was expressed by more than one tum$^-$ variant (Boon et al., 1980). The potential significance of this observation for human disease was that, if every tumour expressed unique antigens, then the possibility of vaccination against cancer would be remote. From this point of view it was important to study human tumours, not only to identify whether they induced HLA class I-restricted CTL, but also to investigate the extent to which different tumours expressed shared tumour antigens.

## HLA Class I Restricted Responses to Human Tumours

Whilst a role for MHC class I in tumour immunity has been well documented in animal models, the definition of a role for HLA-restricted CTL in the immune response to the majority of human tumours is less clear. A wide variety of human malignant diseases have been studied for their ability to stimulate tumour-specific CTL in vivo, by testing peripheral blood, tumour infiltrating or draining node lymphocytes from tumour-bearing patients for their ability to lyse autologous and heterologous tumor cells in vitro (Anichini, Fossati & Parmiani, 1987). Whilst effector cells with lytic activity against autologous tumour cell lines have been derived and in some cases cloned from patients with a variety of tumours, many of these cells have not been restricted by HLA class I molecules, and have shown MHC-unrestricted reactivity against tumour cells lines of diverse type.

One significant exception to this is melanoma, for which evidence has accumulated over a number of years that patients can respond immunologically to their own tumours by the induction of tumour-specific, HLA class I-restricted CTL (Hellstrom & Hellstrom, 1974; Herin et al., 1987; Anichini et al., 1989; Knuth et al., 1989; Topalian et al., 1989). By repeated stimulation of peripheral blood or tumour infiltrating lymphocytes from melanoma patients with autologous tumour cells in the presence of interleukin-2 in vitro, it was possible to derive individual CTL clones and to maintain these in long-term culture (Herin et al., 1987). As with the animal models described above, in spite of the presence of tumour specific effectors, the tumours were rarely rejected by the hosts from whom the tumour-specific CTL were derived. The establishment of tumour-specific CTL lines and clones in vitro, however, has allowed detailed study of the antigens that they recognize and the definition of the HLA class I molecules that present these antigens. Several studies showed that melanoma-specific CTL lines or clones were capable of lysing not only autologous tumour cells but also (some) heterologous tumour cell lines that shared HLA class I specificities with the autologous tumour (Darrow, Slingluff & Seigler, 1989; Topalian et al., 1989; Wolfel et al., 1989; Kawakami et al., 1992). In addition, using melanoma-specific CTL lines, which were restricted by HLA-A2, Kawakami and colleagues showed that transfection of a melanoma cell line from an HLA-A2-negative individual with the HLA-A2 gene resulted in recognition of the tumour cells by the CTL (Kawakami et al., 1992). These results clearly demonstrated the existence of shared tumour antigens in diverse melanoma cell lines (and in some cases in non-melanoma tumour cell lines), which were presented to antigen-specific CTL by self MHC class I molecules.

The demonstration that different tumour cell lines expressed shared tumour-associated antigens led to a concerted effort to identify the target antigens that were recognized by the CTL. Two principal approaches were used in these studies. Using a genetic approach, Boon and colleagues (van der Bruggen et al., 1991; Brichard et al., 1993; Coulie et al., 1994) identified and cloned the genes encoding a number of melanoma antigens, and confirmed the ability of a single tumour cell to present several tumour antigens independently through different class I molecules on the cell surface (described in detail by Coulie in Chapter 5). More recently, Cox and colleagues (1994) described a biochemical approach to the identification of a melanoma-associated antigen. These authors acid-eluted the peptides that were bound to HLA-A2 on a melanoma cell line, which was recognized and lysed in vitro by tumour-specific, HLA-A2-restricted CTL lines. By a process of repeated high-performance liquid chromatography (HPLC) separation of the eluted peptides and the ability of individual, exogenously added peptide fractions to confer susceptibility of HLA-A2$^+$ target cells to lysis by the CTL clone, a single fraction containing three candidate peptides was identified. The sequences of the peptides were elucidated by tandem mass spectrometry and a single peptide was identified, which constituted the CTL epitope (Cox et al., 1994).

The ability to identify individual antigens that encode shared tumour-specific CTL epitopes has considerable implications for the development of candidate tumour vaccines. It is interesting to note, however, that of the human tumour antigens which have been identified so far, almost all have been the products of non-mutated cellular genes, rather than the result of mutations in genes (see Table 5.2). Furthermore, these naturally occurring tumour-associated CTL epitope peptides have generally shown a relatively low binding affinity for the HLA class I molecules by which they are presented, as compared with the binding affinities of naturally occurring peptide epitopes from 'foreign' antigens such as viral proteins. The likely explanation is that CTL clones that recognize high-affinity HLA-binding peptides derived from self proteins are deleted in the thymus as part of the process of self-tolerance (Lo, 1992), and only low-affinity interactions between self-derived peptides and MHC escape this negative selection.

Recently, HLA-restricted tumour-specific CTL have been described in several tumour types other than melanoma. Ioannides and colleagues described tumour-specific CTL derived from malignant ascites of patients with ovarian cancer (Ioannides et al., 1991, 1993). These CTL were specific for tumour cells which expressed HLA-A2 and the proto-oncogene

HER-2/neu, and also recognized HLA-A2$^+$ target cells pulsed with synthetic peptides corresponding to amino acids 971–980 of the HER-2/neu protein (Ioannides et al., 1993; Yoshino et al., 1994). In addition, tumour-specific HLA-restricted CTL have been described in renal cell cancer (Schendel et al., 1993; Bernhard et al., 1994), and in squamous cell cancers of the head and neck (Yasumura et al., 1993) and lung (Slingluff et al., 1994). From these examples, it seems reasonable to assume that, as our ability to circumvent the technical difficulties associated with studying tumour-specific immune responses improves, further examples of HLA class I-restricted, tumour-specific CTL will be demonstrated and more tumour antigens will be identified. The proportion of individual patients who respond to their tumour by mounting specific CTL responses remains to be seen. The identification of shared tumour antigens that encode HLA-restricted CTL epitopes gives rise, however, to the possibility of developing tumour vaccines for prevention or therapy of specific cancers. The search for such vaccines is currently an area of considerable scientific research (see Chapters 5–7).

## MHC Class I and Virally Induced Tumours

The ability of HLA class I-restricted CTL to mediate tumour rejection in animal models and in humans has been further demonstrated by studies of virally induced tumours. Kast and colleagues (1989) demonstrated that cloned MHC class I-restricted CTL specific for the adenovirus type 5 E1A antigen, upon passive transfer to syngeneic nude mice bearing Ad5 E1-induced tumours, were capable of rejecting large tumour masses. Similar experiments in mice have indicated that the viral oncogenes E6 and E7 of human papilloma virus type 16 also can act as tumour rejection antigens in mice (Chen et al., 1991). Following from these studies, Feltkamp and colleagues (1993) recently showed that vaccination of C57BL/6 mice with an MHC binding peptide encoding a CTL epitope of E7 induced a CTL response capable of lysing E7 transformed cells in vitro, and rendered the mice resistant to a subsequent challenge with HPV 16 transformed tumour cells in vivo. These studies raised the possibility of using MHC class I binding peptides derived from tumour-associated antigens as vaccines against cancer (Chapter 6).

Viral gene products have been shown to act as target antigens in humans also, limiting the spread of oncogenic viruses and the growth of virally induced tumours. Perhaps the best characterized oncogenic virus in humans is the Epstein–Barr virus (EBV), which has been associated with a variety of tumours, including Burkitt and other B cell lymphomas and nasopharyngeal carcinoma. In most individuals infected with EBV, a vigorous CTL response can be detected (reviewed by Rickinson et al., 1992), which controls the infection and restricts the potential outgrowth of EBV-associated tumours. In immunosuppressed individuals, however, the incidence of EBV-associated tumours is greatly increased, indicating a role for immunosurveillance against EBV-induced tumours. Furthermore a recent report (Papadopoulos et al., 1994) suggests that EBV-specific CTL may be capable of mediating rejection of established EBV-associated tumours in vivo. The authors treated five patients, in whom EBV-associated lymphoma complicated allogeneic bone-marrow transplantation, with infusions of non-irradiated leucocytes from the original marrow transplant donors. Following infusion of donor lymphocytes, there was objective clinical and histological evidence of tumour regression in all patients, and long-term remission from tumour was induced in three patients. Whilst the mechanism responsible for tumour regression in this study was not established, it was proposed that donor-derived, EBV-reactive T cells played a critical role in tumour rejection (Papadopoulous et al., 1994). Further studies will be required to validate this hypothesis. Regardless of the mechanism, however, this study represents a remarkable example of the immune system's potential to reject established tumours.

Given the ability of MHC class I-restricted CTL to lyse tumour cells expressing viral antigens, it is relevant to ask why the immune system fails to reject virally induced tumours completely. One explanation is that the causative viruses have evolved a variety of ways of evading the immune response. In the case of oncogenic adenoviruses, this may be achieved through the down-regulation of MHC class I on the surface of the cell. The viral oncogene E1A of adenovirus type 12 has been shown to exert a strong down-regulatory effect on HLA expression (Bernards et al., 1983; Schrier et al., 1983). Down-regulation of HLA is seen also in cytomegalovirus infection, although in this case the effect is mediated through inhibition of the transport of HLA molecules through the medial Golgi to the cell surface (del Val, Hengel & Hacker, 1992). Other viruses, such as EBV and human papilloma virus (HPV), are able to maintain latent infection of cells whilst expressing a minimum number of viral genes. For instance in EBV-associated Burkitt lymphoma, the only viral gene expressed in the cell is the EBNA-1 antigen (Rickinson et al., 1992). Recent evidence (Levitskaya et al., 1995) has shown an internal glycine-alanine repeat region of this antigen which effectively inhibits its processing for presentation by HLA class I. Thus, in this latent form, EBV can maintain infection in the absence of EBV-encoded antigens being presented at the cell surface.

## MHC Expression and Tumour Immunogenicity

The expression of mutated gene products or the disregulated expression of normally silent genes in tumour cells gives rise potentially to the association of novel peptide/MHC complexes, which the immune system can recognize as foreign. The expression of such complexes on a tumour cell does not equate, however, with its ability to induce a T cell response. There is a distinction between a tumour cell's antigenicity (that is, its ability to present an antigen to effector T lymphocytes) and its immunogenicity (that is, its ability to induce a primary T lymphocyte response). Several factors play a role in this distinction. A number of animal studies have suggested that the level and nature of MHC expression may play a role in determining the ability of a tumour to induce an immune response. Several groups have shown that the introduction and expression of allogeneic MHC class I genes in poorly immunogenic tumour cells results in enhanced tumour immunogenicity, and the induction of specific CTL directed not only against the allogeneic class I molecule, but also against tumour-associated antigens presented through autologous MHC class I molecules on the parent cell line (Gelber et al., 1989; Isobe et al., 1989; Ostrand-Rosenberg et al., 1991). The mechanism by which expression of allo-MHC class I enhances immunogenicity in these models is not clear, but it may be pertinent to the mixed allogeneic human melanoma tumour cell vaccine studies described elsewhere in this volume (see Chapter 11). In addition, in one of these models (Ostrand-Rosenberg et al., 1991), transfection of the tumour with syngeneic MHC class II was associated with enhanced immunogenicity of the tumour. The explanation in this case was that the constitutive expression of MHC class II on the tumour cell allowed it to present antigen not only to CTL (through MHC class I), but also directly to tumour-specific CD4$^+$ helper T cells, thus bypassing the need for 'professional' (constitutive MHC class II positive) antigen-presenting cells in the induction of the tumour specific immune response. This may be something of an oversimplification, as it is now recognized that, in addition to the T cell receptor interaction with antigen/MHC complexes on the antigen-presenting cell, co-stimulatory signals mediated through the interaction of other cell surface receptors on the T cell and their ligand molecules on the antigen-presenting cell are required for the induction of the primary T cell response (discussed below).

In addition to the nature of the MHC molecules expressed, the level of MHC class I expression on the tumour cell may also influence the immunogenicity of a tumour. Koeppen and colleagues (1993), using an ultraviolet irradiation-induced tumour transfected with an allogeneic MHC class I molecule, showed that tumour cells that expressed high levels of allo-MHC class I were immunogenic, whilst tumour cells expressing low levels of the allo-Class I molecule failed to induce CTL, but were still sensitive to lysis by tumour-specific CTL. Two recent models (Seung, Urban & Schreiber, 1993; Huang et al., 1994), however, suggest that, in certain instances, host antigen-presenting cells (dendritic cells, macrophages) may take up and present tumour antigens to induce antigen-specific, MHC Class I restricted CTL, thus bypassing antigen presentation by the tumour cell itself in the induction of a tumour-specific immune response. The relative roles of the tumour cell and professional antigen presenting cells in priming the tumour-specific immune response remain to be clearly defined.

In general, stimulation of a naive CTL precursor by antigen/MHC requires signals in addition to T cell receptor (TCR): antigen/MHC interaction, usually involving cytokine(s), for example, interleukin-2 (IL-2), secreted by antigen-specific helper T cells, and a co-stimulatory signal delivered by the interaction of the CD28/CTLA4 receptors on the T cell and their ligand molecule, B7, on the antigen-presenting cell (June et al., 1994). The majority of tumour cells do not express co-stimulatory ligand molecules. The lack of appropriate co-stimulatory signals at the time of first interaction of a T cell with an appropriate antigen/MHC complex may result in the induction of clonal anergy rather than clonal stimulation. Recent studies in mice, using poorly immunogenic tumour cells transfected with cytokine genes or with the co-stimulatory receptor ligand B7 (Fearon et al., 1990; Chen et al., 1992, 1994; Linsley & Hellstrom, 1993; Hock et al., 1993; Townsend & Allison, 1993; Columbo & Forni, 1994), have emphasized the role of these second signals in priming the tumour-specific immune response. These studies are described in greater detail elsewhere in this volume (see Chapters 8 and 9).

Taken together, the studies described above show that, whilst MHC class I molecules play a central role in both the induction and elicitation of tumour-specific CTL responses through the presentation of tumour-associated antigens to the immune system, the relationship between MHC class I and tumour immunity is complex, and there remain a number of unanswered questions.

# ■ MHC CLASS I EXPRESSION ON TUMOUR CELLS

## Abnormalities of HLA Expression on Tumours

Loss or down-regulation of expression of MHC class I molecules has been described on a wide variety of tumours, and has stimulated the hypothesis that this might represent a mechanism of tumour escape from the immune response (Bodmer et al., 1993).

Immunohistochemical studies indicate that abnormalities of HLA expression are a relatively common finding on a wide variety of tumour types, including breast, ovarian, lung, colon, melanoma, and cervical malignancies (Fleming et al., 1981; Kabawat et al., 1983; Doyle et al., 1985; Momburg et al., 1986; Moller et al., 1987; Natali et al., 1989; Smith et al., 1989; Kageshita et al., 1993; Cromme et al., 1994). These abnormalities range from lack of expresson of all class I antigens (complete loss) to selective loss of expression of individual alleles. A number of mechanisms have been implicated in loss of HLA class I expression on tumour cells. These are discussed below, and are illustrated in Figure 4.1. Broadly the mechanisms can be separated into two major groups: those involving abnormal regulation of otherwise normal HLA and associated genes, and those which involve structural mutations in HLA genes and gene products.

## Mechanisms Underlying Abnormalities of MHC Class I Expression on Tumour Cells

The production of functional HLA class I molecules involves a number of different gene products and a complex biosynthetic pathway (see Chapter 3). The mechanisms that underlie alterations in the expression of HLA class I molecules on tumour cells target almost every stage in the production of HLA molecules, from mutations in the genes themselves to the transport of the mature class I complex to the cell surface.

**Genetic Mutations and Deletions**  It has been known for many years that cancer cells display abnormal genomes, including chromosomal rearrangements and aneuploidy (Nowell, 1976), as well as mutations in individual genes. A number of genetic mutations have been described in HLA and associated genes, which lead to abnormal expression of HLA class I in tumour cells. Complete loss of HLA class I expression has been associated in a number of tumour types with mutations or deletions in $\beta_2$m genes (Klein et al., 1967; Rosa et al., 1983; d'Urso et al., 1991; Gatton-Celli et al., 1992; Bicknell et al., 1994). By this process, loss

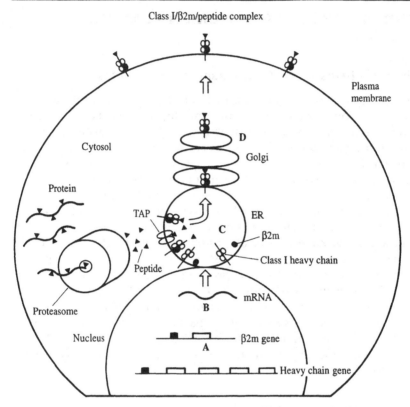

**Figure 4.1** Mechanisms of loss or down-regulation of HLA class I expression on tumour cells. (A) Mutations in HLA and related genes including mutations in $\beta_2$m and class I heavy-chain genes and promoter regions. (B) Decreased transcription and translation due to abnormal methylation status of DNA, and lack of stimulatory or presence of inhibitory *trans*-acting DNA binding factors including cellular and viral oncogenes. (C) Deficient assembly and peptide binding due to lack of $\beta_2$m or heavy-chain gene product, or to deficient peptide transport into the ER due to TAP gene down-regulation or mutation. (D) Defective glycosylation and transport of the class I molecule, due to binding of viral gene products to class I molecules, or aberrant glycosylation in tumour cells.

of expression of all HLA class I molecules can be achieved in two cumulative genetic events, if each of these mutations results in the loss of expression of a functional $\beta_2$m gene product. The phenomenon was first observed in the Burkitt lymphoma cell line Daudi (Klein et al., 1967), in which one copy of the $\beta_2$m gene was lost, and a point mutation in the initiating codon of the other $\beta_2$m gene resulted in failure to translate the mRNA (Rosa et al., 1983). In colorectal and melanoma tumour cell lines, a variety of mutations have been described in $\beta_2$m genes, leading to failure to express a functional gene product (d'Urso et al., 1991; Gattoni-Celli et al., 1992; Bicknell et al., 1994). Studies of $\beta_2$m genes in colorectal tumour cells and cell lines identified a short sequence of four CT nucleotide repeats in exon 1 of the gene which appeared to act as a 'hot spot' for mutations in the gene, accounting for four of seven $\beta_2$m gene mutations identified. Interestingly, the colorectal tumour cells with mutations in $\beta_2$m genes or other abnormalities of HLA expression also exhibited the mutator phenotype (Branch et al., 1995), which was described recently in association with defects in DNA mismatch repair in colorectal cancer (Ionov et al., 1993; Bronner et al., 1994). Whilst further studies are required to confirm this association, it is possible that HLA loss may be associated, in some tumours at least, with deficient DNA mismatch repair mechanisms.

The recent description of DNA based techniques for defining HLA class I genes (Browning et al., 1993a; Krausa, Bodmer & Browning, 1993) has allowed for a more detailed analysis of the underlying basis of loss of expression of some or all HLA class I molecules on a tumour or tumour cell line, by comparision of tumour cell HLA genotype with 'normal' DNA from the same patient. Loss of a complete HLA haplotype has recently been demonstrated in a melanoma cell line (Marincola et al., 1994), and in the colorectal tumour cell line PC/JW (Browning et al., unpublished observations). In addition, in a study of over 30 colorectal tumour cell lines genotyped for HLA-A, HLA-B, and HLA-DR by PCR, a further five cell lines were identified (where normal tissue was not available for comparison) which were homozygous at each locus (Browning et al., unpublished observations), strongly suggesting the loss of a complete HLA haplotype in these cell lines. In one other colorectal tumour cell line (LS411), HLA genotyping showed the absence of one HLA-A gene as compared with normal tissue (Browning et al., 1993b), whilst 2 HLA-B and 2 HLA-DR genes were identified in both tumour cell and normal DNA, suggesting a break point or deletion within the HLA region itself.

Several other studies have reported the selective loss of expression of individual HLA specificities on a variety of tumour cell types, by comparison of surface HLA expression on tumour cells with expression on normal tissue from the same individuals (Versteeg et al., 1989; Wang et al., 1991; Browning et al., 1993b; Vegh et al., 1993; Imreh et al., 1995). The basis for the selective loss of expression of individual class I alleles has not been identified in most cases. To date, there is no direct evidence for mutations in the heavy chain genes themselves, however, several observations suggest that this may occur in at least certain cases. One of the most striking examples of selective HLA class I loss is the high frequency of loss of expression of HLA-A11 on Burkitt lymphoma cell lines derived from HLA-A11 individuals (Mascucci et al., 1987). The frequency of down-regulation of HLA-A11 in Burkitt lymphoma is suggestive of a selective pressure acting against the expression of this allele, possibly through a dominant HLA-A11-restricted CTL response to EBV-encoded antigens (Rickinson et al., 1992). A study of five such Burkitt cell lines suggested several different mechanisms that affected expression of HLA-A11, including lack of transcription factors and mutations in the promoter regions of the genes (Imreh et al., 1995). In two colorectal tumour cell lines, HCA 7 and LS 174T, there was selective loss of expression of a single HLA class I molecule (HLA-A1 and HLA-A2, respectively), in spite of the presence of the genes encoding these HLA molecules in cell-derived genomic DNA (Browning et al., 1993b). In both these cell lines mRNA was detected by allele-specific reverse transcriptase polymerase chain reaction, indicating that the class I heavy-chain genes were being transcribed. In addition, in HCA 7, expression of HLA-A1 was restored by transfection of the cell line with a genomic HLA-A1 clone. These results suggest a structural genetic defect rather than a defect of HLA gene regulation. Cloning and sequencing of the class I heavy chain genes should clarify whether this is the case.

**Gene Regulation**   Whilst genetic mutations account for a proportion of cases of abnormal HLA expression on tumour cells, they do not account for all. A variety of mechanisms affecting transcriptional regulation of HLA and related genes may be involved in down-regulation of HLA expression on tumour cells. Both the constitutive and inducible levels of MHC class I expression are regulated by *trans*-acting factors binding to *cis*-acting regulatory sequences in the 5'-untranslated portion of the MHC gene (David-Watine, Israel & Kourilsky, 1991). Mechanisms that affect chromatin structure or methylation status of these *cis*-acting elements may affect transcription of MHC genes (Bonal et al., 1986; Maschek, Pulm & Hammerling, 1989), and down-regulation of MHC class I expression has been associated with a decrease in binding of *trans*-acting factors to enhancer regions in MHC genes (Blanchet et al., 1991). In this respect, HLA locus-specific transcriptional factors and regulatory elements have been described (Soong & Hui, 1991; Cereb & Yang, 1994). Levels of HLA expression in tumour cells have been shown in a number of studies to correlate with intracellular levels of mRNA (Esteban et al., 1989; Blanchet et al., 1991; Ruiz-Cabello et al., 1991).

Modulation of MHC class I expression on tumour cells may be associated with the expression of certain viral and cellular oncogenes. The transforming oncogene E1A of adenovirus type 12 is a potent down-regulator of MHC class I expression in adenovirus-associated tumours (Schrier et al., 1983; Bernards, Dessain & Weinberg, 1983), and

Rous sarcoma virus infection has been associated with reduced HLA class I expression in transformed human fibroblasts (Gogusev et al., 1988). The role of activated cellular oncogenes on HLA expression in tumour cells is less clear. The oncogene v-ras in transformed murine fibroblasts, and N- and c-myc genes in neuroblastoma and melanoma cells have been associated with down-regulation of HLA expression in some studies (Bernards et al., 1986; Versteeg et al., 1988; Lu et al., 1991). However, other studies of c-myc activation in non-small cell lung carcinoma and neuroblastoma have failed to support these observations (Feltner et al., 1989; Redondo et al., 1991). Recent studies have indicated that c-myc may selectively down-regulate HLA gene expression in a locus-specific manner (Versteeg et al., 1989), whilst N-myc down-regulates all HLA class I genes equally.

## Defective antigen processing in tumour cells

The expression of HLA class I molecules at the cell surface requires the expression not only of heavy-chain and $\beta_2$m gene products, but also of other gene products involved in the intracellular processing of antigen, such as the peptide transporters (TAP) (Suh et al., 1994). Absent or deficient TAP gene expression results in the failure to transport peptides from the cytosol into the endoplasmic reticulum (ER). As a result, MHC class I molecules fail to bind peptide and are retained within the ER. This phenotype was first described in the murine tumour cell line RMA-s (Karre et al., 1986) and in the human cell line 721.134 (de Mars et al., 1985), which were subsequently shown to have deletions within the MHC class II region where the TAP genes are encoded. Recently, lack of HLA expression on tumour cells has been shown to be associated with lack of expression of TAP gene products in a variety of tumours, including non-small cell lung cancer, cervical carcinoma and colorectal cancer (Restifo et al., 1993; Cromme et al., 1994; Kaklamanis et al., 1994). In the case of nonsmall cell lung cancer cells, the expression of HLA class I was restored by treatment of the cells with interferon-$\gamma$ (IFN-$\gamma$) indicating a regulatory rather than a structural defect in TAP gene expression.

## Significance of HLA Loss on Tumour Cells

In spite of the wealth of data that have accumulated in recent years on the frequency of abnormal HLA class I expression on tumour cells and the mechanisms that underlie it, the biological significance of HLA loss on tumour cells remains uncertain. The relatively high frequency of HLA loss on tumour cells suggests that loss of HLA expression is associated with some selective advantage for growth. Given our understanding of the function of MHC, the most obvious explanation is that the loss of MHC class I expression allows the cell to evade or escape from attack by MHC class I-restricted CTL (Bodmer et al., 1993). It is certainly clear that immunoselection of HLA loss mutants can be mediated by CTL. MHC loss mutants have been generated under selection by CTL both in vitro (van der Bruggen et al., 1991) and in vivo (Urban & Schreiber, 1992; Ward et al., 1990). The extent to which immunoselection mediates HLA loss on most human tumours, however, is assumed rather than established. In general, the frequency of HLA loss is not significantly higher in tumours for which there is direct evidence of tumour-specific CTL responses (such as melanoma) than in tumours for which there is not direct evidence of immune response (such as colorectal cancer). In addition, at the level of the individual tumour, HLA class I loss has been demonstrated in tumours in which there is little or no lymphocytic infiltrate (Kaklamanis & Hill, 1992), suggesting that the immune response may not be directly involved in HLA loss in these tumours. The possibility that HLA loss may be associated with some other mechanism that confers a selective advantage on the cell should not be dismissed. For example, the loss of a complete HLA haplotype may reflect a selective pressure for loss of heterozygosity of a gene or genes with which the HLA region is in linkage disequilibrium. The recent identification of a tumour suppressor gene, WAF-1, at 6p21.2 on chromosome 6 (El-Deiry et al., 1993), close to the HLA region on 6p21.3, raises the possibility that deletion of the WAF-1 gene might represent a cause of chromosomal instability in this region of chromosome 6 in tumour cells. The crucial question that remains unanswered is whether HLA and associated genes show a higher rate of mutation than other cellular genes, which are not essential for tumour growth. For the time being, immunoselection remains the only explanation of HLA loss for which there is direct evidence.

Just as it is uncertain whether immunoselection is the only explanation for HLA loss on tumours, the biological significance of this loss also remains unclear. In a recent study of over 700 tumours of several types, and corresponding normal tissues, little or no HLA loss was observed on premalignant tumours or carcinoma *in situ* (Garrido et al., 1993), although it is recognised that a number of (potentially antigenic) mutations in cellular genes are likely to have already occurred by this stage (Fearon & Vogelstein, 1990). An association between HLA loss and poor differentiation state has been described for a number of tumour types (Esteban et al., 1990; Tomita et al., 1990), and a higher incidence of HLA loss on metastatic deposits than on the primary tumour has been reported (Cordon-Cardo et al., 1991; Pantel et al., 1991). Overall, however, there is no clear correlation between lack of HLA expression on tumour cells and patient survival. For example, Concha et al. (1991), in study of 94 patients with breast cancer, found a significant association between tumour HLA expression and survival, whilst Wintzer, Benzing & von Kleist (1990) found no correlation between HLA expression and either disease-free or overall survival in patients with breast cancer. Similarly, there was no correlation between disease-free survival and tumour HLA expression in a series of 152 patients with curatively resected colorectal tumours followed for a mean period of 48 months (Stein et al., 1988; Moller et al., 1991). A variety of other studies have yielded similarly inconclusive results on the prognostic significance of HLA loss on tumour cells. These studies have been based largely on the presence or absence of HLA class I expression (that is, only complete loss of HLA expression was assessed). A recent study of HLA expression in cervical carcinoma has reported a correlation between the loss of expression of HLA-B7 and poor patient survival (Keating et al., 1995; Ellis et al., 1995). Although this study remains to be substantiated by further reports, it may be that more discriminating methods of assessing HLA expression will be required in order to assess the biological significance of HLA loss accurately.

The most obvious consequence of HLA loss on tumour cells is that any cell that fails to express appropriate HLA molecules on its surface will be unable to present antigenic peptides to antigen-specific CTL. Regardless of the mechanism of loss of HLA expression on a tumour cell, the frequency of HLA loss that has been observed on tumours in vivo may represent a signficant barrier to the effective use of immunotherapeutic protocols aimed at stimulating tumour-specific CTL responses in patients. In this respect, the distinction between regulatory and structural genetic mechanisms of HLA loss may be important, in that regulatory mechanisms may potentially be overcome by appropriate up-regulatory stimuli, whilst reversal of genetic mutations can be achieved only by replacement of the affected gene.

The expression of HLA class I on a tumour cell, however, is not necessarily required for tumour rejection. Paradoxically, it has been shown that cells that lack HLA expression are more susceptible to lysis by NK cells than HLA class I-positive tumour cells (Karre et al., 1986; Ljunggren & Karre, 1990), and transfection and expression of HLA class I genes into tumour cell lines that had lost class I expression was associated with reduced susceptibility to NK-mediated lysis (Storkus et al., 1989; Maiao et al., 1991). Recent studies have identified peptide sequences in the HLA class I heavy chains, which are associated with inhibition of lysis by NK cells from individuals who express these motifs (Colonna et al., 1993). These findings support the idea that 'lack of self MHC' is part of the means by which NK cells recognize their targets. Thus the loss of HLA expression on a tumour may allow escape from a tumour-specific CTL response, but may result in increased susceptibility to NK-mediated lysis. The ability of the immune response to recognize and reject an MHC class I $^-$ tumour was recently emphasized by Levitsky et al. (1994), who demonstrated that immunisation of mice with a MHC class I $^-$ tumour cell line transfected with granulocyte–macrophage colony-stimulating factor (GM-CSF) resulted in the induction of an immune response, which was capable of rejecting a subsequent challenge with the (class I $^-$) tumour cell line. This response was dependent on CD4$^+$ T cells and NK cells, but only minimally on CD8$^+$ T cells. The relationship between the tumour cell, MHC class I, and the immune response is more complex, therefore, than might appear at first.

# ■ SUMMARY AND CONCLUSIONS

In the last few years, a number of major advances have been made in our understanding of the relationship between tumour cells and the immune system. In humans, a role for HLA class I in the presentation of tumour-associated antigens has been established for melanoma and other cancers, and recent studies suggest that immune T lymphocytes may be capable of rejecting tumours in patients with EBV-associated lymphomas. Methods have been established for identifying antigenic epitopes recognized by tumour-specific CTL, raising hopes of tumour vaccines capable of stimulating tumour-specific CTL. Animal models involving transfection of poorly immunogenic tumours with cytokine or T cell co-stimulatory ligand genes have suggested new immunotherapeutic strategies by which more effective tumour-specific immune responses, including MHC class I-restricted CTL, may be induced. With recent advances in our understanding of the mechanisms that are associated with the oncogenic process and the induction of MHC class I-restricted CTL, the prospects for vaccination or immunotherapy (including gene therapy) of cancer are better than ever before. The question 'to what extent does HLA class I expression regulate tumour growth or rejection in the natural course of disease?', however, remains open.

### REFERENCES

Anichini A., Fossati G. & Parmiani G. (1987) Clonal analysis of the cytolytic T cell response to human tumors. *Immunology Today*, **8**, 385–9.

Anichini A., Mazzochi A., Fosatti G. & Parmiani G. (1989) Cytotoxic T lymphocyte clones from peripheral blood and from tumor site detect intratumor heterogeneity of melanoma cells: analysis of specificity and mechanisms of interaction. *Journal of Immunology*, **142**, 3692–701.

Bernards R., Dessain S.K. & Weinberg R.A. (1986) N-myc amplification causes down modulation of MHC Class I antigen expression in neuroblastoma. *Cell*, **47**, 667–74.

Bernards R., Schrier P.I., Houweling A. et al. (1983) Tumourogenicity of cells transformed by adenovirus type 12 by evasion of T cell immunity. *Nature (London)*, 305, 776–9.

Bernhard H., Karback J., Wolfel T. et al. (1994) Cellular immune response to human renal-cell carcinomas: definition of a common antigen recognized by HLA-A2-restricted cytotoxic T-lymphocyte (CTL) clones. *International Journal of Cancer*, 59, 837–42.

Bicknell D.C., Rowan A. & Bodmer W.F. (1994) β2-Microglobulin mutations: a study of established colorectal cell lines and fresh tumours. *Proceedings of the National Academy of Sciences*, 91, 4751–5.

Blanchet O., Bourge J.F., Zinszner H., Tatari Z., Degos L. & Paul P. (1991) DNA binding of regulatory factors interacting with MHC Class I gene enhancer correlates with MHC Class I transcriptional level in Class I defective cell lines. *International Journal of Cancer*, 6 (Suppl.), 138–45.

Bodmer W.F., Browning M.J., Krausa P., Rowan A., Bicknell D.C. & Bodmer J.G. (1993) Tumor escape from immune response by variation in HLA expression and other mechanisms. *Annals of the New York Academy of Science*, 690, 42–9.

Bonal F.J., Pareja E., Martin J., Romero C. & Garrido F. (1986) Repression of Class I H-2K, H-2D antigens on GR9 methylcholanthrene induced tumour cell clones is related to the level of DNA methylation. *Journal of Immunogenetics*, 13, 179–86.

Boon T. (1983) Antigenic tumour cell variants obtained with mutagens. *Advances in Cancer Research*, 39, 121–51.

Boon T., van Snick J., van Pel A., Uytenhove C. & Marchand M. (1980) Immunogenic variants obtained by mutagenesis of mouse mastocytoma P815. II. T lymphocyte mediated cytolysis. *Journal of Experimental Medicine*, 152, 1184–93.

Branch P., Rowan A., Bicknell D.C., Bodmer W.F. & Karran P. (1995) Immune surveillance in colorectal carcinoma. *Nature Genetics*, 9, 231–2.

Brichard V., Van Pel A., Wolfel T. et al. (1993) The tyrosinase gene codes for an antigen recognized by autologous cytolytic T lymphocytes on HLA-A2 melanomas. *Journal of Experimental Medicine*, 178, 489–95.

Bronner C.E., Baker S.M., Morrison P.T. et al. (1994) Mutation in the DNA mismatch repair gene homologue hMLH1 is associated with hereditary non-polyposis colon cancer. *Nature (London)*, 368, 258–61.

Browning M.J., Krausa P., Rowan A., Bicknell D.C., Bodmer J.G. & Bodmer W.F. (1993a) Tissue typing the HLA-A locus from genomic DNA by sequence specific PCR: comparison of HLA genotype and surface expression on colorectal tumour cell lines. *Proceedings of the National Academy of Sciences USA*, 90, 2842–5.

Browning M.J., Krausa P., Rowan A. et al. (1993b) Loss of human leukocyte antigen expression on colorectal tumor cell lines: implications for anti-tumor immunity and immunotherapy. *Journal of Immunotherapy*, 14, 163–8.

Cereb N. & Yang S.Y. (1994) The regulatory complex of HLA Class I promoters exhibits locus specific conservation with limited allelic variation. *Journal of Immunology*, 152, 3873–83.

Chen L., Ashe S., Brady W.A. et al. (1992) Costimulation of antitumor immunity by the B7 counterreceptor for the T lymphocyte molecules CD28 and CTLA-4. *Cell*, 71, 1093–102.

Chen L., Linsley P.S. & Hellstrom K.E. (1993) Costimulation of T cells for tumor immunity. *Immunology Today*, 14, 483–6.

Chen L., McGowan P., Ashe S., Johnston J., Li Y., Hellstrom I. & Hellstrom K.E. (1994) Tumor immunogenicity determines the effect of B7 costimulation on T cell mediated tumor immunity. *Journal of Experimental Medicine*, 179, 523–32.

Chen L., Thomas E.K., Hu S.-L., Hellstrom I. & Hellstrom K.E. (1991) Human papilloma virus type 16 nucleoprotein E7 is a tumor rejection antigen. *Proceedings of the National Academy of Sciences USA*, **88**, 110–4.

Colombo M.P. & Forni G. (1994) Cytokine gene transfer in tumour inhibition and tentative tumour therapy: where are we now? *Immunology Today*, **15**, 48–51.

Colonna M., Brooks E.G., Falco M., Ferrara G.B. & Strominger J.L. (1993) Generation of allospecific natural killer cells by stimulation across a polymorphism of HLA-C. *Science*, **260**, 1121–4.

Concha A., Cabrera T., Ruiz-Cabello F. & Garrido F. (1991) Can the HLA phenotype be sued as a prognostic factor in breast carcinoma? *International Journal of Cancer*, **6** (Suppl.), 146–54.

Cordon-Cardo C., Fuks Z., Drobnjak M., Moreno C., Eisenbach L. & Feldman M. (1991) Expression of HLA-A,B,C antigens on primary and metastatic tumor cell populations of human carcinomas. *Cancer Research*, **51**, 6372–80.

Coulie P.G., Brichard V., Van Pel A. et al. (1994) A new gene coding for a differentiation antigen recognized by autologous cytolytic T lymphocytes on HLA-A2 melanomas. *Journal of Experimental Medicine*, **180**, 35–42.

Cox A.L., Skipper J., Chen Y. et al. (1994) Identification of a peptide recognised by five melanoma specific human cytotoxic T cell lines. *Science*, **264**, 716–9.

Cromme F.V., Airey J., Heemals M.T. et al. (1994) Loss of transporter protein, encoded by the TAP-1 gene is highly correlated with loss of HLA expression in cervical carcinomas. *Journal of Experimental Medicine*, **179**, 335–40.

Dailey M.O., Pillemer E. & Weissman I.L. (1982) Protection against syngeneic lymphoma by a long lived cytotoxic T cell clone. *Proceedings of the National Academy of Sciences USA*, **79**, 5384–7.

Darrow T.L., Slingluff C.L. & Seigler H.F. (1989) The role of HLA Class I antigens in recognition of melanoma cells by tumor specific cytotoxic T lymphocytes. Evidence for shared tumor antigens. *Journal of Immunology*, **142**, 3329–35.

David-Watine B., Israel A. & Kourilsky P. (1991) The regulation and expression of MHC Class I genes. *Immunology Today*, **11**, 286–92.

del Val M., Hengel H. & Hacker H. (1992) Cytomegalovirus prevents antigen presentation by blocking the transport of peptide loaded major histocompatibility complex Class I molecules into the medial-Golgi compartment. *Journal of Experimental Medicine*, **176**, 729–38.

de Mars R., Rudersdorf R., Xhang C. et al. (1985) Mutations that impair a post-transcriptional step in expression of HLA-A and -B antigens. *Proceedings of the National Academy of Sciences USA*, **82**, 8183–7.

d'Urso C.M., Wang Z., Cao Y., Tatake R., Zeff R.A. & Ferrone S. (1991) Lack of HLA Class I antigen expression by cultured melanoma cells FO-1 due to a defect in β2m gene expression. *Journal of Clinical Investigation*, **87**, 284–92.

Doyle A., Martin J., Funa K. et al. (1985) Markedly decreased expression of Class I histocompatibility antigens, protein and mRNA in human small cell lung cancer. *Journal of Experimental Medicine*, **161**, 1135–51.

El-Deiry W.S., Tokino T., Velculescu V.E. et al. (1993) WAF-1, a potential mediator of p53 tumor suppression. *Cell*, **75**, 817–25.

Ellis J.R.M., Keating P.J., Baird J. et al. (1995) The association of an HPV16 oncogene variant with HLA-B7 has implications for vaccine design in cervical cancer. *Nature Medicine*, **1**, 464–70.

Esteban F., Concha A., Huelin C. et al (1989) Histocompatibility antigens in primary and metastatic squamous cell carcinoma of the larynx. *International Journal of Cancer*, **43**, 436–42.

Esteban F., Concha A., Delgado M., Perez-Ayala M., Ruiz-Cabello F. & Garrido F. (1990) Lack of MHC Class I antigens and tumour aggressiveness of squamous cell carcinoma of the larynx. *British Journal of Cancer*, **62**, 1047–51.

Fearon E.R., Pardoll D.M., Itaya T. et al. (1990) Interleukin-2 production by tumor cells bypasses T helper function in the generation of an antitumor response. *Cell*, **60**, 397–403.

Fearon E.R. & Vogelstein B. (1990) A genetic model for colorectal tumorigenesis. *Cell*, **61**, 759–67.

Feltkamp M.C.W., Smits H.L., Vierboom M.P.M. et al. (1993) Vaccination with cytotoxic T lymphocyte epitope containing peptide protects against a tumor induced by human papillomavirus type 16 transformed cells. *European Journal of Immunology*, **23**, 2242–9.

Feltner D.E., Cooper M., Weber J., Israel M.A. & Thiele C.J. (1989) Expression of Class I histocompatibility antigens in neuroectodermal tumours is independent of the expression of a transfected neuroblastoma myc gene. *Journal of Immunology*, **143**, 4292–9.

Fleming K., McMichael A., Morton J., Woods J. & McGee J. (1981) Distribution of HLA Class I antigens in normal human tissue and in mammary cancer. *Journal of Clinical Pathology*, **34**, 779–84.

Foley E.J. (1953) Antigenic properties of methylcholanthrene-induced tumours in mice of the strain of origin. *Cancer Research*, **13**, 835–7.

Garrido F., Cabera T., Concha A., Glew S., Ruiz-Cabello F. & Stern P. (1993) Natural history of HLA expression during tumour development. *Immunology Today*, **14**, 491–9.

Gattoni-Celli S., Kirsch K., Timpane R. & Isselbacher K.J. (1992) β2-microglobulin gene is mutated in a human colon cancer cell line (HCT) deficient in the expression of H1A Class I antigens on the cell surface. *Cancer Research*, **52**, 1201–4.

Gelber C., Plaksin D., Vadai E., Feldman M. & Eisenbach L. (1989) Abolishment of metastasis formation by murine tumour cells transfected with foreign H-2 K genes. *Cancer Research*, **49**, 2366–73.

Gogusev J., Teutsch B., Morin M.T. et al. (1988) Inhibition of HLA Class I antigen mRNA expression induced by Rous sarcoma virus in transformed human fibroblasts. *Proceedings of the National Academy of Sciences USA*, **85**, 203–9.

Greenberg P.D. (1986) Therapy of murine leukaemia with cyclophosphamide and immune Lyt2⁺ cells: cytolytic T cells can mediate eradication of disseminated leukaemia. *Journal of Immunology*, **136**, 1917–22.

Greenberg P.D. (1991) Adoptive T cell therapy of tumours: mechanisms operative in the recognition and elimination of tumour cells. *Advances in Immunology*, **49**, 281–355.

Hellstrom K.E. & Hellstrom I. (1974) Lymphocyte mediated cytotoxicity and blocking serum activity to tumor antigens. *Advances in Immunology*, **18**, 209–77.

Herin H., Lemoine C., Weynants P. et al. (1987) Production of stable cytolytic T cell clones directed against autologous human melanoma. *International Journal of Cancer*, **39**, 390–6.

Hock H., Dorsch M., Kunzendorf U., Qin Z., Diamantstein T. & Blankenstein T. (1993) Mechanisms of rejection induced by tumour cell targeted gene transfer of interleukin-2, interleukin-4, interleukin 7, tumor necrosis factor or interferon gamma. *Proceedings of the National Academy of Sciences USA*, **90**, 2774–8.

Huang A.Y.C., Golumbek P., Ahmadzadeh M., Jaffee E., Pardoll D. & Levitsky H. (1994) Role of bone marrow derived cells in presenting MHC Class I restricted tumor antigens. *Science*, **264**, 961–5.

Imreh M.P., Zhang Q.J., de Campos Lima P.O. et al. (1995) Mechanisms of allele selective down-regulation of HLA class I in Burleiff's lymphoma. *International Journal of Cancer*, **62**, 90–6.

Ioannides C.G., Fisk B., Fan D, Biddison W.E., Wharton J.T. & O'Brian C.A. (1993) Cytotoxic T cells isolated from ovarian malignant ascites recognise a peptide derived from the HER-2/neu proto-oncogene. *Cellular Immunology*, **151**, 225–34.

Ioannides C.G., Freedman R.S., Platsoucas C.D., Rashed S. & Kim Y.-P. (1991) Cytotoxic T cell clones isolated from ovarian tumor infiltrating lymphocytes recognize multiple antigenic epitopes on autologous tumor cells. *Journal of Immunology*, **146**, 1700–7.

Ionov Y., Peinado M.A., Malkhosyan S., Shibia D. & Perucho M. (1993) Ubiquitous somatic mutations in simple repeated sequences reveal a new mechanism for colon carcinogenesis. *Nature (London)*, **363**, 558–61.

Isobe K.-I., Hasegawa Y., Iwamoto T. et al. (1989) Induction of antitumor immunity in mice by allo-major histocompatibility complex Class I gene transfectant with strong antigen expression. *Journal of the National Cancer Institute*, **81**, 1823–8.

June C.H., Bluestone J.A., Nadler L.M. & Thompson C.B. (1994) The B7 and CD28 receptor families. *Immunology Today*, **15**, 321–31.

Kabawat S., Bast R.J., Welch W., Knapp R. & Bhan A. (1983) Expression of major histocompatibility antigens and nature of inflammatory cellular infiltrate in ovarian neoplasms. *International Journal of Cancer*, **32**, 547–54.

Kageshita T., Wang Z., Calorini L. et al. (1993) Selective loss of human leukocyte Class I allospecificities and staining of melanoma cells by monoclonal antibodies recognizing monomorphic determinants of Class I human leukocyte antigens. *Cancer Research*, **53**, 3349–54.

Kaklamanis L. & Hill A.B. (1992) MHC loss in colorectal tumours: evidence for immunoselection. *Cancer Surveys*, **13**, 155–71.

Kaklamanis L., Townsend A., Doussis-Anagnostopoulou I.A., Mortensen N., Harris A.L. & Gatter K.C. (1994) Loss of major histocompatibility complex-encoded transporter associated with antigen presentation (TAP) in colorectal cancer. *American Journal of Pathology*, **145**, 505–9.

Karre K., Ljunggren H.G., Piontek G. & Kiessling R. (1986) Selective rejection of H-2 deficient lymphoma variants suggests alternative immune defence strategy. *Nature (London)*, **324**, 575–7.

Kast W.M., Offringa R., Peters P.J. et al. (1989) Eradication of adenovirus E1-induced tumors by E1A specific cytotoxic T lymphocytes. *Cell*, **59**, 603–14.

Kawakami Y., Zakut R., Topalian S.L., Stotter H. & Rosenberg S.A. (1992) Shared human melanoma antigens. Recognition by tumor infiltrating lymphocytes in HLA-2.1 transfected melanomas. *Journal of Immunology*, **148**, 638–43.

Klein E., Klein G., Nadkarni J.S. et al. (1967) Surface IgM specificity on cells derived from a Burkitt's lymphoma. *Lancet*, ii: 1068–70.

Klein G., Sjogren H.O., Klein E. & Hellstrom K.E. (1960) Demonstration of resistance against methylcholanthrene-induced sarcomas in the primary autochthonous host. *Cancer Research*, **20**, 1561–72.

Knuth A., Danowski B., Oettgen H.F. & Old L.J. (1984) T cell mediated cytotoxicity against autologous malignant melanoma: analysis with interleukin-2 dependent T cell cultures. *Proceedings of the National Academy of Sciences USA*, **86**, 3511–15.

Knuth A., Wolfel T., Klehmann E., Boon T. & Meyer zum Buschenfelde K.-H. (1989) Cytolytic T cell clones against an autologous human melanoma: specificity study and definition of three antigens by immunoselection. *Proceedings of the National Academy of Sciences USA*, **86**, 2804–8.

Koeppen H., Acena M., Drolet A., Rowley D.A. & Schreiber H. (1993) Tumours with reduced expression of a cytotoxic T lymphocyte recognized antigen lack immunogenicity but retain sensitivity to lysis by cytotoxic T lymphocytes. *European Journal of Immunology*, 23, 2770–7.

Krausa P., Bodmer J.G. & Browning M.J. (1993) Defining the common subtypes of HLA-A9, A10, A28 and A19 by use of ARMS PCR. *Tissue Antigens*, 43, 91–9.

Levitskaya J., Coram M., Levitsky V. et al. (1995) Inhibition of antigen processing by the internal repeat region of the Epstein-Barr virus nuclear antigen-1. *Nature (London)*, 375, 685–8.

Levitsky H.I., Lazenby A., Hayashi R.J. & Pardoll D.M. (1994) In vivo priming of two distinct antitumor effector populations: the role of MHC Class I expression. *Journal of Experimental Medicine*, 179, 1215–24.

Ljunggren H.G. & Karre K. (1990) In search of the 'missing self': MHC molecules and NK recognition. *Immunology Today*, 11, 237–44.

Lo D. (1992) T cell tolerance. *Current Opinion in Immunology*, 4, 711–5.

Lu Y.Y., Blair D.G., Segal S., Shih T.Y. & Clanton D.J. (1991) Tumorogenicity, metastasis and suppression of MHC Class I expression in murine fibroblasts transformed by mutant v-ras deficient in GTP binding. *International Journal of Cancer*, 13, 45–53.

Lynch D.H. & Miller R.E. (1991) Immunotherapeutic elimination of syngeneic tumours in vivo by cytotoxic T lymphocytes generated in vitro from lymphocytes from the draining lymph nodes of tumor-bearing mice. *European Journal of Immunology*, 21, 1403–10.

Maio M., Altomonte M., Tatake R., Zeff R.A. & Ferrone S. (1991) Reduction in susceptibility to natural killer cell mediated lysis of human FO-1 melanoma cells after induction of HLA Class I antigen expression by transfection with β2m gene. *Journal of Clinical Investigation*, 88, 282–9.

Marincola F.M., Shamanian P., Alexander R.B. et al. (1994) Loss of HLA haplotype and B locus downregulation in melanoma cell lines. *Journal of Immunology*, 153, 1225–37.

Maschek U., Pulm W. & Hammerling G.J. (1989) Altered regulation of MHC Class I genes in different tumour cell lines is reflected by distinct sets of DN'ase I hypersensitive sites. *EMBO Journal*, 8, 2297–304.

Masucci M.G., Torsteinsdottir S., Colombani J., Brautbar C., Klein E. & Klein G. (1987) Down regulation of Class I HLA antigens and of the Epstein–Barr-virus-encoded latent membrane protein in Burkitt lymphoma cell lines. *Proceedings of the National Academy of Sciences USA*, 84, 4567–71.

Mills C.D. & North R.J. (1983) Expression of passively transferred immunity against an established tumor depends on generation of cytolytic T cells in recipient. Inhibition by supressor T cells. *Journal of Experimental Medicine*, 157, 1448–60.

Moller P. & Hammerling G.J. (1992) The role of surface HLA-A,B,C molecules in tumour immunity. *Cancer Surveys*, 13, 101–84.

Moller P., Herrmann B., Moldenhauer G. & Momburg F. (1987) Defective expression of MHC Class I antigens is frequent in B cell lymphomas of high grade malignancy. *International Journal of Cancer*, 40, 32–9.

Moller P., Momberg F., Koretz K. et al. (1991) Influence of major histocompatibility complex Class I and Class II antigens on survival in colorectal carcinoma. *Cancer Research*, 51, 729–36.

Momburg F., Degener T., Bacchus L., Moldenhauer G., Hammerling G. & Moller P. (1986) Loss of HLA-A,B,C and de novo expression of HLA-D in colorectal cancer. *International Journal of Cancer*, 37, 179–84.

Natali P., Nicotra M., Bigotti A. et al. (1989) Selective changes in expression of HLA Class I polymorphic determinants in human solid tumours. *Proceedings of the National Academy of Sciences USA*, **86**, 6719–23.

Nowell P.C. (1976) The clonal evolution of tumour cell populations. *Science*, **194**, 23–8.

Ostrand-Rosenberg S., Roby C., Clements V.K. & Cole G.A. (1991) Tumour-specific immunity can be enhanced by transfection of tumour cells with syngeneic MHC Class II genes or allogeneic MHC Class I genes. *International Journal of Cancer*, **6** (Suppl.), 61–8.

Pantel K., Schlimok G., Kutter D. et al. (1991) Frequent down regulation of major histocompatibility Class I antigen expression on individual micrometastatic carcinoma cells. *Cancer Research*, **51**, 4712–5.

Papadopoulos E.B., Ladanyi M., Emanuel D. et al. (1994) Infusion of donor leukocytes to treat Epstein–Barr virus associated lymphoproliferative disorders after allogeneic bone marrow transplantation. *New England Journal of Medicine*, **330**, 1185–91.

Prehn R.T. & Main J.M. (1957) Immunity to methylcholanthrene-induced sarcomas. *Journal of the National Cancer Institute*, **18**, 769–78.

Rammensee H.-G., Friede T. & Stevanovic, P. (1995) MHC ligands and peptide motifs: first listing. *Immunogenetics*, **41**, 178–228.

Redondo M., Ruiz-Cabello F., Concha A. et al. (1991) Altered HLA Class I expression in non small cell lung cancer is independent of c-myc activation. *Cancer Research*, **51**, 2463–8.

Restifo N.P., Esquivel F., Kawakami Y. et al. (1993) Identification of human cancers deficient in antigen processing. *Journal of Experimental Medicine*, **177**, 265–72.

Rickinson A.B., Murray R.J., Brooks J., Griffin H., Moss D.J. & Masucci M.G. (1992) T cell recognition of Epstein–Barr virus associated lymphomas. *Cancer Surveys*, **13**, 53–80.

Rosa F., Berissi H., Weissenbach J., Maroteaux L., Fellous M. & Revel M. (1983) The $\beta$2 microglobulin in RNA in human Daudi cells has a mutated initiation codon but is still inducible by interferon. *EMBO Journal*, **2**, 239–43.

Rosenstein M., Eberlein T. & Rosenberg S.A. (1984) Adoptive immunotherapy of established syngeneic solic tumors: role of T lymphoid subpopulation. *Journal of Immunology*, **132**, 2117–22.

Ruiz-Cabello F., Perez-Ayala M., Redondo M., Concha A., Cabrera T. & Garrido F. (1991) Molecular analaysis of MHC Class I alterations in human tumour cell lines. *International Journal of Cancer*, **6** (Suppl.), 123–30.

Schendel D.J., Gansbacher B., Obernader R. et al. (1993) Tumor specific lysis of human renal cell carcinomas by tumor infiltrating lymphocytes. I. HLA-A2 restricted recognition of autologous and allogeneic tumor cell lines. *Journal of Immunology*, **151**, 4209–20.

Schrier P.I., Bernards R., Vaessen R.T.M.J., Houweling A. & van der Eb A.J. (1983) Expression of Class I MHC switched off by highly oncogenic adenovirus 12 in transformed rat cells. *Nature (London)*, **305**, 771–5.

Seung S., Urban J.L. & Schreiber H. (1993) A tumour escape variant that has lost one major histocompatibility complex Class I restriction element induces specific CD8[+] T cells to an antigen that no longer serves as a target. *Journal of Experimental Medicine*, **178**, 933–40.

Singer D.S. & Maguire J.E. (1990) Regulation of the expression of Class I MHC genes. *Critical Reviews in Immunology*, 10, 235–57.

Slingluff C.L., Cox A.L., Stover J.M. Jr., Moore M.M., Hunt D.F. & Engelhard V.H. (1994) Cytotoxic T lymphocyte response to autologous squamous cell cancer of the lung: epitope reconstitution with peptides extracted from HLA-Aw68. *Cancer Research*, **54**, 2731–7.

Smith M.E.F., Marsh S.G.E., Bodmer J.G., Gelsthorpe K. & Bodmer W.F. (1989) Loss of HLA-A,B,C allele products and lymphocyte function associated antigen 3 in colorectal neoplasia. *Proceedings of the National Academy of Science USA*, **86**, 5557–61.

Soong T.W. & Hui K.M. (1991) Identification of locus specific DNA binding factors for the regulation of HLA Class I genes in human colorectal cancer. *International Journal of Cancer*, **6** (Suppl.), 131–7.

Stein B., Momburg F., Schwarz V., Schlag P., Moldenhauer G. & Moller P. (1988) Reduction or loss of HLA-A,B,C antigens in colorectal carcinoma appears not to influence survival. *British Journal of Cancer*, **57**, 364–8.

Storkus W.J., Alexander J., Payne J.A., Dawson J.R. & Cresswell P. (1989) Reversal of natural killing susceptibility in target cells expressing transfected Class I HLA genes. *Proceedings of the National Academy of Science USA*, **86**, 2361–4.

Suh W.K., Cohen-Doyle M.F., Fruh K., Wang K., Peterson P.A. & Williams D.B. (1994) Interaction of MHC Class I molecules with the transporter associated with antigen processing. *Science*, **264**, 1322–6.

Tomita Y., Matsumoto Y., Nishiyama T. & Fujiwara M. (1990) Reduction of major histocompatibility complex Class I antigens on invasive and high grade transitional cell carcinoma. *Journal of Pathology*, **162**, 157–64.

Topalian S.L., Solomon D. & Rosenberg S.A. (1989) Tumor specific cytolysis by lymphocytes infiltrating human melanomas. *Journal of Immunology*, **142**, 3714–25.

Townsend A.R.M., Gotch F.M. & Davey J. (1985) Cytotoxic T cells recognise fragments of influenza nucleoprotein. *Cell*, **42**, 457–67.

Townsend A., Rothbard J., Gotch F., Bahadur G., Wraith D. & McMichael A. (1986) The epitopes of influenza nucleoprotein recognised by cytotoxic T lymphocytes can be defined with short synthetic peptides. *Cell*, **44**, 959–68.

Townsend S.E. & Allison J.P. (1993) Tumor rejection after direct costimulation of CD8$^+$ T cells by B7-transfected melanoma cells. *Science*, **259**, 368–70.

Urban J.L. & Schreiber H. (1992) Tumour antigens. *Annual Review of Immunology*, **10**, 617–44.

van der Bruggen P., Traversari C., Chomez P. et al. (1991) A gene encoding an antigen recognised by cytolytic T lymphocytes on a human melanoma. *Science*, **254**, 1643–7.

Vegh Z., Wang P., Vanky F. & Klein E. (1993) Selectively downregulated expression of MHC Class I alleles in human solid tumors. *Cancer Research*, **53**, 2416–20.

Versteeg R., Kruse-Volters K.M., Plomp A.C. et al. (1989) Suppression of Class I human histocompatibility leukocyte antigen by c-myc is locus specific. *Journal of Experimental Medicine*, **170**, 621–35.

Versteeg R., Noordermeer I.A., Kruse-Walters M., Ruiter D.J. and Schrier P.I. (1988) C-myc downregulates Class I HLA expression in human melanomas. *EMBO Journal*, **7**, 1023–9.

Ward P.L., Koeppen H.K., Hurteau T., Rowley D.A. & Schreiber H. (1990) Major histocompatibility complex Class I and unique antigen expression by tumors that escaped from CD8$^+$ T cell dependent surveillance. *Cancer Research*, **50**, 3851–8.

Wang P., Vanky F., Li S.L., Vegh Z., Persson U. & Klein E. (1991) Expression of MHC Class I antigens in human carcinomas and sarcomas analyzed by isoelectric focusing. *International Journal of Cancer*, **6** (Suppl.), 106–16.

Wintzer H.O., Benzing M. & von Kleist S. (1990) Lacking prognostic significance of $\beta$2-microglobulin, MHC Class I and Class II antigen expression in breast carcinomas. *British Journal of Cancer*, **62**, 289–95.

Wolfel T., Klehmann E., Muller C. et al. (1989) Lysis of human melanoma cells by autologous cytolytic T cell clones. Identification of human histocompatibility leukocyte antigen-A2 as a restriction element for three different antigens. *Journal of Experimental Medicine*, **170**, 797–810.

Yamasaki T., Handa H., Yamashita J., Wantanabe Y., Namba Y. & Hanaoke M. (1984) Specific adoptive immunotherapy with tumour specific cytotoxic T lymphocyte clone for murine malignant gliomas. *Cancer Research*, **44**, 1776–83.

Yasumura S., Hirabayashi H., Schwartz D.R. et al. (1993) Human cytotoxic T cell lines with restricted specificity for squamous cell carcinoma of the head and neck. *Cancer Research*, **53**, 1461–8.

Yoshino I., Peoples G.E., Goedegeburre P.S., Maziarz R. & Eberlein T.J. (1994) Association of HER-2/neu expression with sensitivity to tumor specific CTL in human ovarian cancer. *Journal of Immunology*, **152**, 2394–400.

Zinkernagel R.M. & Doherty P.C. (1975) H-2 compatibility requirement for T cell mediated lysis of target cells infected with lymphocytic choriomeningitis virus. *Journal of Experimental Medicine*, **141**, 1427–36.

Zinkernagel R.M. & Doherty P.C. (1979) MHC restricted cytotoxic T cells: studies on the biological role of polymorphic major transplantation antigens determining T cell restriction specificity, function and responsiveness. *Advances in Immunology*, **27**, 51–177.

# 5

# Human Tumor Antigens Recognized by Cytolytic T Lymphocytes

PIERRE G. COULIE

## ■ INTRODUCTION

Tumor immunology has been changing rapidly since tumor antigens recognized by cytolytic T lymphocytes (CTL) were first identified. The number of characterized antigens is steadily increasing and several are sufficiently tumor specific to qualify them as candidate anticancer vaccines in patients. The current list of tumor antigens comprises five categories: antigens encoded by genes expressed in tumors but not in most normal tissues; differentiation antigens; antigens derived from structurally abnormal proteins; viral antigens; and mucins. Several of those categories are very well covered in other sections of this book and will be described here only briefly. The author wishes to present here an updated account of what has been learned about human tumor antigens using a genetic approach to facilitate their identification. In order to provide a fairly comprehensive picture, results obtained with other approaches as well will be mentioned. Why the identification of these antigens gives rise to so much hope for patients but also why caution should still temper our dreams about anticancer vaccines will then be discussed.

## ■ TUMOR ANTIGENS RECOGNIZED BY AUTOLOGOUS T LYMPHOCYTES

It is now a common observation that T lymphocytes from cancer patients can be stimulated in vitro to produce CTL that show specificity for autologous tumor cells (Livingston et al., 1979; Vanky & Klein, 1982; Vose & Bonnard, 1982; Knuth et al., 1984). Establishment of autologous mixed lymphocyte–tumor cell cultures (MLTC) consists of incubating tumor cells, killed by irradiation or by treatment with mitomycin-C, with blood mononuclear cells or tumor-infiltrating lymphocytes obtained from the same patient (Figure 5.1). Cells are incubated in the

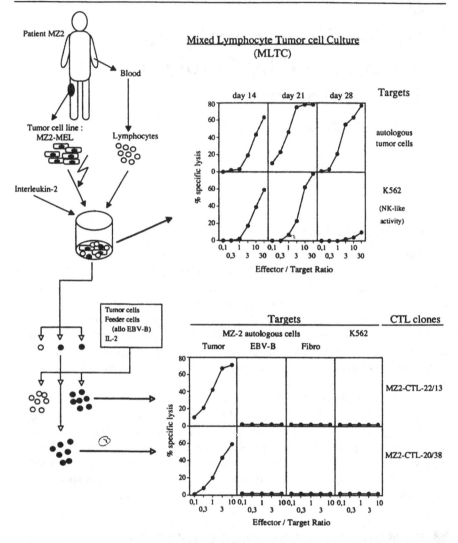

**Figure 5.1** Generation of autologous antitumour CTL clones from the blood of a melanoma patient.

presence of various T cell growth factors, the most important of which is interleukin-2 (IL-2). The cultures are restimulated every week by the addition of fresh tumor cells and IL-2. Lymphocytes proliferate and their lytic activity can be tested after two or three re-stimulations. Usually a significant lytic activity can be measured against the tumor cells but it is largely nonspecific. Owing to the presence of IL-2, mandatory for CTL growth in this system, natural killer (NK)-like cytolytic effector cells also proliferate in MLTC. They lyse not only the tumor cells but also a vast array of sensitive targets, the prototype of which is the myeloid leukemia cell line, K562. However, on further stimulation of the lymphocytes, the lytic activity becomes quite specific, mostly because the appropriately stimulated antitumor T cells proliferate better than the NK-like cells. A lytic activity can then be measured that is tumor specific inasmuch as available control targets are not recognized. These usually include K562, autologous Epstein–Barr virus (EBV)-transformed B cells, and sometimes autologous fibroblasts. The resulting CTL populations are mostly CD8$^+$ T lymphocytes that recognize antigens presented by HLA class I molecules. Most of the antitumor CTL obtained so far in autologous MLTC have been generated against melanomas, simply because metastatic melanoma cells are relatively easy to adapt to culture, providing cell lines that are convenient stimulator and target cells for the CTL. Some anti-tumor CTL populations have also been obtained against other types of tumors, such as sarcomas (Slovin et al., 1986), ovarian cancers (Ioannides et al., 1992), pancreatic carcinomas (Wölfel et al., 1983b), lung tumors (Slingluff et al., 1994), renal carcinoma (Schendel et al., 1993), or head and neck carcinomas (Yasumura et al., 1993).

It is possible to derive clones from the responder CTL populations obtained in MLTC (Mukherji & MacAlister 1983; Anichini, Fossati & Parmiani, 1985; Hérin et al., 1987; Wölfel et al., 1989). Limiting numbers of responder cells are re-stimulated in microwells by the addition of tumor cells and feeder cells. The limiting dilution conditions ensure that lymphocytes proliferate in only a minority of the wells and that most of these proliferating populations arise from a single lymphocyte. Because these CTL clones can be maintained for long periods of time, they are tools of crucial importance to describe and identify tumor antigens. CTL clones made it possible to select antigen-loss variants of the tumor cells (Figure 5.2). Typically, five to thirty million cells of a CTL clone are mixed with a similar number of melanoma cells until nearly all the targets have been killed. The CTL are washed off the adherent tumor cells and a few surviving melanoma cells proliferate. After two or three rounds of this immunoselection, the resulting tumor cells can be tested for their sensitivity to lysis by the CTL: they often prove to be resistant. If the antigen-loss variant remains sensitive to lysis by another CTL clone, it indicates that the latter CTL recognizes an antigen that is different from the one recognized by the selecting CTL. By extending this approach to several CTL clones with the same tumor cells, the number of different antigens recognized by CTL on a tumor cell line can be estimated. Such detailed analyses have been carried out with three melanoma cell lines. One of them is melanoma MZ2-MEL, derived from the tumor of patient

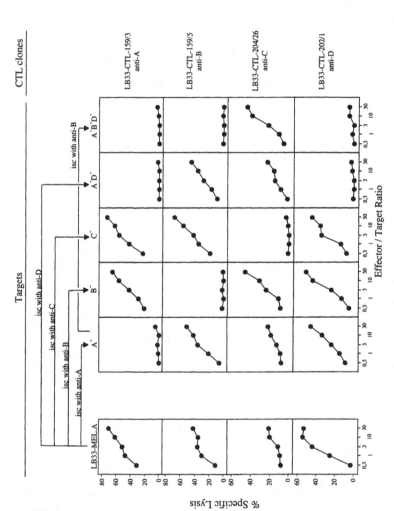

**Figure 5.2** Lytic activity of autologous antitumor CTL clones on several antigen-loss variants derived from a melanoma cell line. Four antitumor CTL clones were derived from MLTC performed with blood lymphocytes of melanoma patient LB33. They were used in vitro to select variants of melanoma cells LB33-MEL.A that resisted lysis by the CTL. The results indicate that tumor cells LB33-MEL.A express four distinct antigens, which were named A, B, C, and D.

MZ2. Immunoselection experiments with CTL led to the identification of six distinct CTL-defined antigens expressed by the tumor cells and designated MZ2-A to MZ2-F (Van den Eynde et al., 1989). A similar number of antigens was found to be expressed on melanoma SK29-MEL (Wölfel et al., 1993a), and recently on melanoma LB33-MEL (Lehmann et al., 1995). As discussed below, this multiplicity of antigens has important consequences for the development of antitumor immunotherapy.

# ■ EXPERIMENTAL APPROACHES TO THE IDENTIFICATION OF TUMOR ANTIGENS

Three different experimental approaches have led to the identification of antigens recognized by antitumor CTL obtained in vitro. The genetic approach consists of producing libraries of DNA or cDNA prepared from the antigenic tumor cells. The library is transfected into a cell that is not recognized by the CTL but expresses the presenting HLA molecule. The antitumor CTL clone is then used for the detection of the transfectant that expresses the gene encoding the antigen. Gene MAGE-1 was identified in this way after transfecting into an antigen-loss variant a genomic library prepared with DNA from the tumor cells. The stable transfectants were tested for the expression of the relevant antigen. A modified genetic approach was used subsequently to identify several other tumor antigens: this is based on the method developed by Seed (Seed & Aruffo, 1987), using transient transfection into COS-7 cells of cDNA libraries cloned into expression vectors carrying the SV40 origin of replication (Brichard et al., 1993; Coulie et al., 1994). In this system, transfectants transiently express large amounts of the transfected cDNA. Once the gene has been identified, the portion coding for the antigenic peptide can be narrowed down until synthetic peptides can be tested for recognition by the CTL.

The second approach is purely biochemical. The peptides bound to the major histocompatibility complex (MHC) class I molecules of the tumor cells are eluted with acid and fractionated with reversed-phase high-performance liquid chromatography and mass spectrometry. The fractions containing the antigenic peptide are incubated with mutant cells expressing empty class I molecules and these peptide-loaded cells are tested for lysis by the CTL. The peptides in the positive fractions are fractionated further by mass spectrometry until individual peptides can be tested and sequenced (Cox et al., 1994). The immunological approach differs from the two others in that the starting point is a postulated antigenic peptide that binds to a given HLA molecule. The peptide is used to stimulate in vitro lymphocytes from patients or from normal individuals in order to obtain CTL that specifically recognize the peptide–HLA combination. To demonstrate that the peptide is a genuine tumor antigen, tumor cells that express the relevant HLA class I molecule and the gene encoding the peptide have to be recognized by the CTL. This methodology is used to identify antigens encoded by proteins that are structurally altered during tumoral transformation or to define new epitopes encoded by normal proteins that are expressed specifically by tumor cells, such as the MAGE proteins.

# ■ IDENTIFICATION OF HUMAN TUMOR ANTIGENS

## The MAGE Gene Family

The first tumor antigen that was identified is antigen MZ2-E, expressed by melanoma cell line MZ2-MEL. The gene encoding antigen MZ2-E was discovered by following a gene transfection approach that had been successfully used for the identification of several antigens recognized by CTL on mouse mastocytoma P815 (De Plaen et al., 1988; Boon et al., 1992). A gene library prepared with the DNA of MZ2-MEL cells was constructed into cosmids. The library was cotransfected with a plasmid containing a gene conferring geneticin resistance into an E$^-$ antigen-loss variant of the melanoma, and the transfectants that integrated DNA were selected with geneticin. The procedure of identification of a transfectant that expressed antigen MZ2-E was based on the observation that a population of cells containing only one cell in thirty that expressed antigen MZ2-E stimulated the anti-E CTL clone to release a detectable amount of tumor necrosis factor (TNF). The secreted TNF was assayed by its cytotoxic effect on a subclone of WEHI-164 cells, a murine fibrosarcoma exquisitely senstive to TNF (Espevik & Nissen-Meyer, 1986; Traversari et al., 1992b). Therefore groups of thirty transfectants were distributed into microwells, the cultures were amplified and duplicated, anti-MZ2-E CTL clone was added to the wells, and the amount of TNF secreted in the medium was measured after 24 hours of stimulation. One pool of transfectants was found to stimulate the CTL. The duplicate pool was subcloned and from a positive transfectant it was possible to retrieve a cosmid that contained the gene encoding antigen MZ2-E. The gene was named MAGE-1, for melanoma antigen (van der Bruggen et al., 1991).

Gene MAGE-1 is 5 kb long and contains three exons (Figure 5.3). An open reading frame coding for a protein of 309 amino acids is located in the third exon. The sequence of the gene shows no significant homology with known human genes, with the exception of other members of the MAGE gene family. Gene MAGE-1 is not altered in melanoma MZ2-MEL:

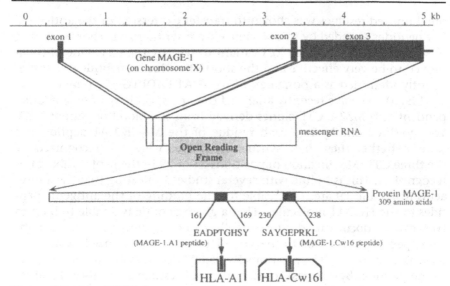

**Figure 5.3**   The MAGE-1 gene, protein, and antigenic peptides.

its sequence is the same in the DNA of the melanoma cells as in that of lymphocytes of patient MZ2.

MAGE-1 is a member of a family of at least twelve closely related genes (De Plaen et al., 1994). Their intron–exon organization is similar, and the third exon of MAGE-1 is 64–85% identical to that of the other MAGE genes. Despite these similarities, only gene MAGE-1 codes for antigen MZ2-E. All MAGE genes are located on the long arm of chromosome X and several of them appear to be closely linked. The MAGE proteins have no signal sequence. The distribution of hydrophilic and hydrophobic domains is conserved across the family and shared with mouse protein necdin, with which the MAGE-10 protein is 31% identical. Necdin is a nuclear protein expressed in neurally differentiated embryonal carcinoma cells and in the brain of adult mice (Maruyama et al., 1991). The function of the MAGE proteins is unknown.

The MZ2-E antigen was found to be presented by HLA-A1, because among MAGE-1-positive melanoma cell lines sharing one HLA class I allele with patient MZ2, only those expressing HLA-A1 were recognized by the CTL. This conclusion was verified by transfecting mouse P815 cells with HLA-A1 and MAGE-1: they were lysed by the anti-MZ2-E CTL clone derived from the patient. HLA-A1 is expressed by 20% of Caucasian individuals.

The antigenic peptide was identified by first transfecting small fragments of the third exon of MAGE-1. When a sequence encoding about one hundred residues was shown to transfer expression of the antigen, a few peptides encoded by this sequence were synthesized. They were used to sensitize the E⁻ antigen-loss variant to lysis by the CTL. One of them proved to be very effective and the shortest antigenic peptide was subsequently identified as a nonamer: MAGE-1.A1:EADPTGHSY (Traversari et al., 1992a). We have recently analyzed the fine specificity of several independent anti-MZ2-E CTL clones derived from the blood of patient MZ2. We modified one by one each residue of the MAGE-1.A1 peptide and tested whether these new synthetic peptides were still recognized by the three CTL. Modification of positions P3 or P9 in the peptide abrogates recognition. This is in line with several studies indicating that the amino acids in P3 and P9 are responsible for the binding of the antigenic peptides to the HLA-A1 molecules. That a given peptide is unable to bind to HLA can be documented by its inability to compete with another antigenic peptide that binds to the same HLA and is recognized by another CTL. The amino acids in positions P3 and P9 thus constitute the agretope of the peptide. By contrast, modification of residue at position P5 abrogated recognition by the CTL without affecting the binding of the peptide to HLA-A1. This amino acid is thus recognized by the receptor of the CTL: it is a part of the epitope of the peptide. We observed that our different CTL clones actually recognized slightly different epitopes: for example, one of them did not recognize a peptide with the proline at position P4 modified to alanine, whereas the others recognized it as well as the unmodified peptide. Altogether each CTL clone displayed a fine specificity that differed from those of the two other CTL. DNA sequencing of the α- and β-chains of the T cell receptors of these CTL showed that these were different in different clones. These results indicate that the same HLA-A1+MAGE-1.A1 peptide combination expressed several epitopes that can be recognized by distinct CTL (Romero et al., manuscript in preparation).

After the initial observation that MAGE-1 coded for antigen MZ2-E, it was found that other tumor antigens recognized by autologous CTL were also encoded by members of the MAGE gene family. Several antitumor CTL clones of patient MZ2 were found to recognize an antigen, which was named MZ2-Bb after immunoselection experiments with CTL in vitro. The MZ2-Bb antigen was subsequently found to be presented by HLA-Cw16. This HLA-C allele was previously designated HLA-C.clone-10 and recently renamed Cw*1601. It is expressed by approximately 7% of Caucasian individuals. When COS-7 cells were cotransfected with HLA-Cw16, and either MAGE-1, MAGE-2 or MAGE-3, only the transfectants expressing MAGE-1 stimulated the CTL to produce TNF. The antigenic peptide MAGE-1.Cw16 was identified and was shown to be a nonamer, different from the MAGE-1.A1 peptide. Thus two different peptides derived from the same MAGE-1 protein can bind to different HLA class I molecules within the same cells, and constitute two antigens recognized by different CTL (van der Bruggen et al., 1994b).

Yet another antitumor CTL clone (MZ2-D) of patient MZ2 was found to recognize tumors that expressed HLA-A1 and MAGE-3 when tested on a panel of melanoma cell lines. Moreover, COS-7 cells cotransfected with HLA-A1 and MAGE-3 stimulated the CTL. The MAGE-3.A1 antigenic peptide was identified as EVDPIGHLY. As expected, it shares with the MAGE-1–A1 peptide residues at positions P3 and P9, aspartic acid (D) and tyrosine (Y), respectively, which dock the peptide into the antigen-presenting groove of HLA-A1. Interestingly gene MAGE-6, which is 99% identical to MAGE-3, did not transfer the expression of the antigen after transfection into COS-7 cells. The MAGE-6 peptide, which is homologous to the MAGE-3.A1 peptide, differs from it at position P8 only. This MAGE-6 peptide also binds to HLA-A1 but is not recognized by the CTL. Thus the leucine residue in position P8 of peptide MAGE-3.A1 is recognized by the TCR of the anti-MZ2-D CTL clones (Gaugler et al., 1994).

The MAGE-3.A1 antigenic peptide was independently identified by other investigators who searched the sequence of the MAGE-3 protein for a peptide that fitted the consensus motif of binding to HLA-A1:D in position 3 and Y in position 9. The peptide was synthesized and it was first verified that it could indeed bind to HLA-A1 molecules in vitro. The next step required the generation of CTL against the peptide. This was achieved by a primary in vitro stimulation of blood lymphocytes from normal donors with autologous B cell blasts incubated with the peptide. The responder cells were cloned and an anti-MAGE-3.A1 CTL clone was obtained that recognized HLA-A1[+] tumor cells expressing gene MAGE-3 (Celis et al., 1994).

Because MAGE-3 is more often expressed by melanomas than MAGE-1 (65% and 36%, respectively), it has a wider applicability for specific antitumor immunization of melanoma patients. Moreover, all melanomas that express MAGE-1 also express MAGE-3, making it possible to attempt to immunize patients against both the MAGE-1 and MAGE-3 antigens simultaneously. As discussed below, this should reduce the likelihood of tumor escape, owing to the emergence of antigen-loss variants.

Another antigenic peptide derived from gene MAGE-3 was recently identified using the immunological approach. Because the consensus motif of binding to HLA-A2 is well characterized and because HLA-A2 is the most frequently expressed HLA class I allele (49% of Caucasians), we searched the MAGE-3 sequence for peptides that fitted with the A2-binding motif. Nine such peptides were localized and synthesized. They were tested in vitro for their capacity to bind to HLA-A2 and the three best binders were used for in vitro stimulation of blood lymphocytes of normal HLA-A2$^+$ individuals. The responder cells were cloned and CTL were identified that specifically lysed HLA-A2$^+$ cells incubated with the relevant peptide, but not in the absence of peptide. These CTL also recognized HLA-A2 melanoma cells expressing gene MAGE-3 (van der Bruggen et al., 1994a).

In view of their capacity to encode tumor antigens, the expression of MAGE genes was evaluated by reverse transcription and PCR amplification of RNA extracted from normal tissues and from tumors (Table 5.1) Several sets of primers were chosen that are specific for each MAGE gene. The primers of each set are located in different exons, so it is possible to distinguish by the size of the amplified product whether it derives from mRNA or from DNA that could contaminate the RNA preparation. A panel of normal adult tissues and a few tissues from > 20-week-old fetuses were tested for the expression of the MAGE genes. None of the MAGE genes were expressed by any of the normal tissues except for testis and placenta. Most of the MAGE genes are expressed in testis, probably by germinal cells because some expression is found also in sperm. The expression in testis is quantitatively significant. Placenta expresses MAGE-3 and MAGE-4.

Genes MAGE-1, 2, 3, 4, 6 and 12 are expressed by variable proportions of tumors of different histological types (Table 5.1) (van der Bruggen et al., 1991; De Smet et al., 1994; Gaugler et al., 1994). MAGE-1 is expressed by 40%, and MAGE-2 or MAGE-3 are expressed by 65% of melanoma

## Table 5.1    Expression of the MAGE Genes in Tumor Samples

| | Percentage of tumors positive for MAGE | | | | |
|---|---|---|---|---|---|
| | 1, 2, 3 or 4 | 1 | 2 | 3 | 4 |
| Melanomas ($n = 148$) | 75 | 36 | 63 | 65 | 23 |
| Head and neck squamous cell carninoma ($n = 44$) | 68 | 25 | 29 | 48 | 50 |
| Lung carcinomas ($n = 55$) | 53 | 34 | 33 | 31 | 36 |
| Sarcomas ($n = 18$) | 50 | 11 | 22 | 22 | 28 |
| Mammary carcinomas ($n = 146$) | 26 | 18 | 8 | 11 | 5 |
| Colorectal carcinomas ($n = 32$) | 25 | 0 | 9 | 16 | 16 |
| Prostatic carcinomas ($n = 20$) | 20 | 15 | 15 | 15 | 0 |
| Renal carcinomas ($n = 49$) | 0 | 0 | 0 | 0 | 0 |
| Bladder carcinomas ($n = 59$) | 42 | 19 | 29 | 34 | 31 |
| Leukemias–lymphomas ($n = 27$) | 0 | 0 | 0 | 0 | 0 |
| Brain ($n = 9$) | 0 | 0 | | 0 | 0 |

MAGE gene expression was assessed by PCR amplification of reverse transcribed RNA extracted from tumor samples frozen immediately after surgery.

samples, respectively. When MAGE-1 is expressed, MAGE-2 or MAGE-3 are almost invariably expressed as well. MAGE-1, 2, 3 and 4 are more often expressed by metastatic melanomas than by primary tumors. MAGE-1, 2 and 3 are expressed by 35% of nonsmall-cell lung carcinomas: adenocarcinomas or squamous carcinomas. Some small-cell lung cancers score positive as well. MAGE genes are expressed by 20–60% of bladder carcinomas, more often by invasive than by superficial tumors (Patard et al., 1995). Significant proportions of other types of tumors also express several MAGE genes: breast adenocarcinomas (Brasseur et al., 1992), sarcoma, as well as glioblastoma cell lines (Rimoldi, Romero & Carrel, 1993). On the contrary, leukemias have been consistently negative (Chambost et al., 1993), and colon or renal carcinomas are rarely positive.

The levels of expression are quite variable among the positive samples as well as among the different tumor cell lines. In a small survey of melanoma cell lines whose MAGE-1 gene expressions were quantitatively measured, it was estimated that a level of expression below 5–10% of that of the MZ2-MEL line could not produce sufficient antigen density to allow recognition by the anti-MZ2-E CTL clone (Lethé, unpublished observations). Therefore, since the expression of an antigen is ultimately the expected information, the conditions of PCR amplification do not need to be too sensitive for the analysis of expression of these genes by tumor samples. Owing to the absence of appropriate antibodies, there is no information yet about the distribution of the expression of these genes within the tumors. There is also a dearth of information on the localization of the physiological expression of the MAGE genes. One possibility is that they are expressed during fetal development, possibly by few cells or only for a short time. The expression of MAGE genes by tumor cells would then be reminiscent of the oncofoetal hypothesis, according to which tumors would re-express genes normally transcribed only during early embryonal development.

Two other new genes, unrelated to MAGE, were recently found to encode tumor antigens expressed by the melanoma cell line, MZ2-MEL. Like MAGE, these genes are expressed by several types of tumors but not by normal tissues except testis. Because this pattern of expression was similar to that of the MAGE genes, these two new genes were given names phonetically similar to MAGE. They were named BAGE and GAGE (Van Den Eynde et al., 1995; van der Bruggen et al., 1994a,b).

## Melanocyte Differentiation Antigens

Several groups have obtained from autologous MLTC CTL clones that lyse not only the stimulator tumor cells but also tumor cells of the same histological type derived from other individuals. The first indication of the existence of such common tumor antigens was obtained with sarcomas (Slovin et al., 1986), but most results were obtained with melanomas, and more precisely with HLA-A2$^+$ melanomas (Anichini et al., 1985; Crowley et al., 1990; Hom et al., 1991; Viret et al., 1993). Many antimelanoma CTL clones restricted by HLA-A2 recognized several allogeneic melanomas provided that they shared the expression of HLA-A2, or even non-A2 melanoma lines when they were transfected with an HLA-A2 gene (Kawakami et al., 1992). Some of these CTL recognized HLA-A2 melanocytes, suggesting that the target antigens were expressed not only by melanoma cells but also by normal cells of the melanocytic lineage (Anichini et al., 1993).

The first melanoma common antigen that was characterized proved to be encoded by the tyrosinase gene (Brichard et al., 1993). The gene was identified by cotransfecting COS-7 cells with a plasmid encoding HLA-A2 and with a cDNA library prepared with mRNA from the tumor cells. A cDNA clone was obtained that transferred the expression of the antigen and its sequence was almost identical to that of tyrosinase. Allelic variations probably accounted for the minor differences that were noted between the sequences. Tyrosinase converts tyrosine into dihydroxyphenylalanine (DOPA), the precursor of melanin. The gene is expressed in melanocytes and in no normal tissue; another enzyme, tyrosine hydroxylase, produces DOPA for the synthesis of catecholamines in adrenal cells and adrenergic neurons. Tyrosinase was expressed in virtually all melanoma samples that were tested but in only 70% of melanoma cell lines. This is in accordance with the common observation that many melanoma cell lines lose their pigmentation after a few weeks or months in culture. No tumors other than melanomas express tyrosinase.

Two antigenic peptides derived from the tyrosinase protein were subsequently identified (Wölfel et al., 1994). They were recognized by two CTL clones derived from two different HLA-A2$^+$ melanoma patients. One peptide is encoded by the first nine amino acids of the signal sequence of tyrosinase. The other corresponds to amino acids 368–376 of the protein. Both peptides are nonamers that bind to HLA-A2.

Since tyrosinase is a large protein of more than 500 amino acids, it is likely that other antigenic peptides, binding to HLA molecules other than A2, can also be the target of autologous antimelanoma CTL responses. A first such tyrosinase antigen is presented by HLA-A24 and is recognized by a CTL line derived from tumor-infiltrating lymphocytes (TIL) (Robbins et al., 1994). A second one is presented on HLA-B44 (Brichard et al., manuscript in preparation). Moreover, tyrosinase also contains an antigen presented on HLA class II molecules and recognized by CD4$^+$ CTL derived from TIL (Topalian et al., 1994). The presence in the tyrosinase protein of antigenic peptides that can be recognized by T lymphocytes on either

HLA class I or class II molecules suggests a fairly high immunologic potential in vivo due to the interplay between tyrosinase-specific CD4$^+$ helper T cells and CD8$^+$ cytolytic T cells.

Using similar approaches, another gene was identified that encodes a common melanoma antigen presented by HLA-A2. This new gene is 18 kb long and contains five exons (Figure 5.4). An open reading frame spanning exons 2–5 encodes a putative protein of 118 amino acids. The pattern of expression of the gene is similar to that of the tyrosinase gene: among normal tissues it is expressed only by melanocytes, and nearly all melanoma samples and 50% of melanoma cell lines score positive. We wished the name of the gene to be reminiscent of this melanocytic expression and designated it Melan-A (Coulie et al., 1994). The same cDNA was identified as coding for an antigen recognized by an A2-restricted CTL line derived from melanoma TIL and named MART-1 (Kawakami et al., 1994a). The antigenic peptide was subsequently localized (Kawakami et al., 1994c). It was recognized by nine out of ten CTL lines derived from the TIL of different HLA-A2$^+$ melanoma patients, and thus appeared to be a very common melanoma epitope.

Yet another CT1 epitope was identified in the glycoproteins Pmel17 and gp100, which are specifically expressed in melanocytes (Kwon et al., 1991; Adema et al., 1993). Both proteins originate from the same gene via

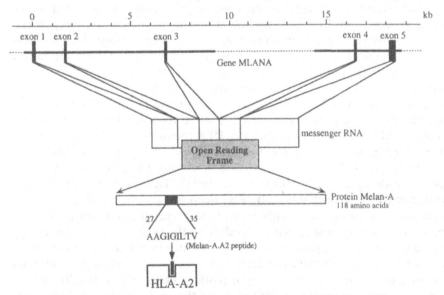

**Figure 5.4** The Melan-A gene, protein, and antigenic peptide. The Melan-A gene has been named MLANA following a proposal of the HUGO Nomenclature Committee of the Genome Data Base.

alternative splicing: mature gp100 contains 641 aminoacids, and Pmel17 has an additional stretch of seven amino acids inserted in position 567 (Adema et al., 1994). A CTL cell line, established with TIL obtained from a metastatic melanoma, recognized most HLA-A2$^+$ melanomas as well as HLA-A2$^+$ cultured melanocytes. A cDNA clone encoding the gp100 protein was transfected into an HLA-A2$^+$ melanoma line, which was previously unable to stimulate the CTL. The transfectants were specifically recognized by the T cells, implying that gp100 was the target antigen. A 10-amino-acid peptide in the protein was subsequently identified as the antigen (Bakker et al., 1994; Kawakami et al., 1994b).

Independently, another group used a biochemical approach to identify an antigenic peptide eluted from HLA-A2 molecules extracted from melanoma cells. The peptide, which is a nonamer, was recognized by CTL lines derived from five HLA-A2$^+$ melanoma patients. Its sequence was included into that of the Pmel17/gp100 protein and proved different from that of the previously identified gp100 antigenic peptide. The nonamer bound to HLA-A2 molecules in vitro with a low affinity, suggesting that the corresponding CTL have a high affinity for this peptide-HLA combination (Cox et al., 1994).

## Polymorphic Epithelial Mucins

Polymorphic epithelial mucins are large, heavily glycosylated molecules expressed and secreted by ductal epithelial cells of a variety of tissues, and by tumors of the same histological origin. They are made of a long polypeptide core surrounded by numerous carbohydrate moieties linked to the protein. Pioneering work by O. Finn and colleagues brought mucins into the limelight as tumor antigens. They derived antitumor CTL lines from breast and pancreatic cancer patients. These CD8$^+$ CTL showed specificity for the tumor cells, were inhibited by anti-CD3 antibodies, but recognized their targets without any HLA restriction (Brand et al., 1988, 1989; Jerome et al., 1991). The antigen recognized by these CTL proved to be the mucin molecule and the epitope was found to be expressed by the polypeptide core itself (Jerome et al., 1991). The latter, in mucin associated with breast and pancreatic adenocarcinomas, is encoded by a gene designated MUC-1 and mainly consists in a variable number of tandem repeats of twenty amino acids (Gendler et al., 1988). The epitope recognized by the CTL is a nine-amino-acid sequence in the repeat. It is masked on normal mucins by glycosylation and uncovered on malignant mucins because of incomplete glycosylation (Girling et al., 1989). It is likely that the antimucin CTL are activated through the cross linking of their T cell receptors by the highly repeated, regulatory spaced T cell epitopes. Cells transfected with a construct containing several tandem repeats could stimulate CTL in vitro (Jerome, Domenech & Finn, 1993). Such cells may be good immunogens to vaccinate patients. Mucins, expressed by numerous types of tumors, have recently been identified as the target antigen of CTL directed against an ovarian carcinoma (Ionnides et al., 1993). The role of mucins in tumor immunology is dealt with in greater detail in Chapter 12.

## Antigens Encoded by Abnormal Genes

The analysis of tumor antigens recognized by CTL on the murine mastocytoma P815 demonstrated that point mutations located in regions coding directly for antigenic peptides could generate new epitopes leading to very strong tumor rejection responses (Uyttenhove, Van Snick & Boon, 1980; Boon 1992). The modified amino acid either enabled the peptide to bind to a class I molecule (new agretope) or constituted a new epitope recognized by a CTL (Lurquin et al., 1989; Sibille et al., 1990). It is therefore possible that mutations affecting any transcribed gene may generate new antigens recognized by T cells. Point mutations that activate oncogenes in tumors can thus be studied in terms of their potential immunogenicity; this work is covered in greater detail in another section of this book (see Chapter 7). One should note here that the experimental approach differs totally from that which has thus far been described: in this case, the potential antigenic peptide is the starting point and the difficulty resides in producing in vitro T lymphocytes that specifically recognize the peptide as well as tumor cells expressing the mutated gene and the relevant HLA molecule.

Human CD4$^+$ lymphocytes have been produced that respond to stimulation with peptides encompassing the position 12, 13, or 61 mutations of p21 *ras*, but not with the normal *ras* peptide (Jung & Schluesener 1991; Gedde-Dahl et al., 1993; Fossum et al., 1995; Gedde-Dahl et al., 1994). Similar results have been obtained with p53: CD8$^+$ HLA-A2-restricted CTL could be derived from normal blood lymphocytes stimulated with cells loaded with peptide (Houbiers et al., 1993). Other potential sources of antigens comprise the HER2/neu oncogene, a peptide of which is presented by HLA-A2 and recognized by CTL from nonsmall-cell lung cancer patients (Yoshino et al., 1994), or the chimeric BCR-ABL protein of chronic myelogenous leukemia (Chen et al., 1992).

We have recently characterized antigen LB33-B expressed on melanoma cell line LB33-MEL and recognized by HLA-B44-restricted autologous CTL clones. The antigenic peptide is derived from a new gene that is ubiquitously expressed. By comparing the DNA sequence corresponding to the peptide in the melanoma cells with that present in lymphocytes of the patient, we observed that the gene of the tumor contained a point mutation that modified one amino acid in the antigenic peptide. The normal peptide is not recognized by the CTL, implying that the mutation is responsible for the expression of the antigen. This mutation appears to be present only in the melanoma cells of patient LB33: we did not find the mutated gene among twenty-odd tumors from other patients. Therefore the mutation, unlike those that activate oncogenes, has probably no role in the tumoral transformation. The mechanism leading to the expression of this melanoma antigen is akin to the tum$^-$ antigens of mouse mastocytoma P815; point mutations, in apparently any transcribed gene, modify the sequence of a peptide, which then becomes antigenic to T cells. These results illustrate the immune system's ability to monitor the integrity of any transcribed gene.

### Viral Antigens

Human tumors associated with viral transformation may express viral antigens. It is obvious, however, that very immunogenic antigens will most probably not be expressed on tumor cells. A remarkable example is EBV-positive tumors, in which the expression of all EBNA genes is repressed. These genes encode several strong antigens recognized by CTL on EBV-transformed B cells (Gavioli et al., 1992; Murray et al., 1992). Only EBNA-1 is expressed in those tumors but no CTL has ever been found that could recognize it. On the contrary, the EBV-induced lymphomas that occur in immunosuppressed patients express many EBV antigens and they regress when immunosuppression is relaxed (Rickinson et al., 1992). An interesting target for antitumor responses is human papillomavirus type 16, present in 90% of cervical carcinomas. The possibility of raising immunity against the E7 nucleoprotein of this virus (Kast, Brandt & Melief, 1993) is discussed in another section of this book (see Chapter 6). HTLV-infected cells have also been studied: CTL against them were obtained from T cell leukemia or tropical spastic paraplegia patients (Kannagi et al., 193; Mitsuya et al., 1983; Jacobson et al., 1991)

### ■ SPECIFIC IMMUNOTHERAPY OF CANCER

### New Strategies Made Possible by the Identification of Tumor Antigens

A few remarkable successes among so many setbacks – a terse expression that could as well summarize the outcome of numerous anticancer immunization attempts. The recent identification of a handful of poten-

Table 5.2.    The HLA–Peptide Combinations of Defined Tumor
Antigens Recognized by HLA Class I-restricted CTL

| Gene/ protein | Peptide | HLA | Reference for peptide identification | Tumors | Normal tissues |
|---|---|---|---|---|---|
| MAGE-1 | EADPTGHSY | A1 | Traversari et al. (1992a) | Several | Testis |
| | SAYGEPRKL | Cw16 | van der Bruggen et al. (1994b) | Several | Testis |
| MAGE-3 | EVDPIGHLY | A1 | Gaugler et al (1994) Celis et al. (1994) | Several | Testis |
| | FLWGPRALV | A2 | van der Bruggen et al. (1994a) | Several | Testis |
| BAGE | [a] | Cw16 | [a] | Several | Testis |
| GAGE | [a] | Cw6 | [a] | Several | Testis |
| Tyrosinase | MLLAVLYCL | A2 | Wölfel et al. (1994) | Melanoma | Melanocytes |
| | YMNGTMSQV | A2 | Wölfel et al. (1994) | Melanoma | Melanocytes |
| | [a] | A24 | [a] | Melanoma | Melanocytes |
| | [a] | B44 | [a] | Melanoma | Melanocytes |
| Melan-A/ MART-1 | AAGIGILTV | A2 | Kawakami et al. (1994b) | Melanoma | Melanocytes |
| Pmel 17/ gp100 | LLDGTATLRL | A2 | Kawakami et al. (1994b) | Melanoma | Melanocytes |
| | YLEPGPVTA | A2 | Cox et al. (1994) | Melanoma | Melanocytes |
| HER2/neu | IISAVVGIL | A2 | Yoshino et al. (1994) | Lung carcinoma | None |

[a] Manuscript in preparation or submitted for publication.

tially immunogenic tumor antigens sheds a new light on the prospective of adding immunotherapy to the repertoire of anticancer treatments (Table 5.2). Although the number of defined tumor antigens undoubtedly will continue to increase during the next years, what we have learned thus far has clear implications for developing new cancer immunotherapy protocols. Our comments will focus on therapeutic vaccination approaches, but they apply to adoptive immunotherapy as well.

It is now obvious that patients have to be selected for antitumor antigen immunization on the basis of the expression of the relevant antigen(s) by their tumor (Figure 5.5). It is reasonable to ascribe part of the failures in tumor immunotherapy to the previous impossibility of matching immunogens to patients. Even when autologous tumor cells were used, there was no way to ascertain whether or not a tumor antigen was expressed by these cells. Eligibility criteria should include HLA typing of the patient and analysis of expression by the tumor of the genes encoding defined antigens. This can be ascertained readily by reverse transcription and polymerase chain reaction (PCR) amplification using RNA

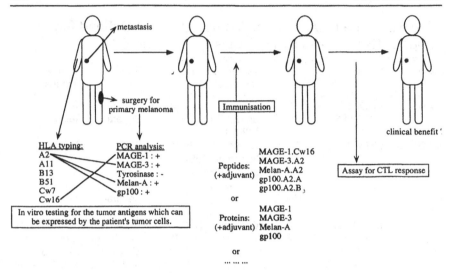

**Figure 5.5** Specific immunotherapy of cancer using several defined tumor antigens. Each line between an HLA allele and a gene coding for tumor antigens indicates the existence of one peptide–HLA combination that constitutes a defined tumor antigen recognized by CTL.

extracted from a small tumor sample frozen at the time the patient undergoes surgery. The PCR analysis is not necessary for the melanocytic differentiation antigens: they are expressed by virtually all melanoma samples. For antigens encoded by genes like MAGE, the PCR analysis is mandatory to assess the expression of the gene in a given sample. It is worth noting that, in melanoma and bladder tumors, MAGE genes are more often expressed by metastatic or advanced tumors than by primary tumors. This implies that a tumor scoring negative might prove to express the gene later on. It is very easy with PCR to assess the expression of several genes by the same tumor sample, each of them encoding a different antigen recognized by CTL on a given HLA class I molecule. As the number of defined antigens increases, the HLA type of the patient should indicate which genes have to be tested for, based on a list of the peptide–HLA combinations corresponding to defined tumor antigens. However, this way of typing for antigen expression suffers from several drawbacks. First, it is not quantitative. PCR analysis can be made quantitative but then loses its simplicity. Second, there is no information about the distribution of gene expression within the sample: the same result is obtained if a minority of cells express the gene at a high level or if all the cells express it somewhat less. Assessment of gene expression using in situ RT-PCR or in situ hybridization should avoid this problem. Finally, there is no information about the antigen itself: the peptide–HLA combination at the surface of the tumor cell. The simplest example is tumor cells which do not express the relevant HLA molecules but express very well the gene encoding the antigen.

With defined tumor antigens it should be possible to monitor in vitro the efficacy of the immunization procedures. CTL response seems to be the obvious parameter to monitor, but it is worth noting that no strong correlation has been established so far between tumor rejection and CTL responses in patients. The quantitative assessment of the CTL response against a tumor antigen is not an easy task. We set up limiting dilution conditions to evaluate the frequency of precursors of antitumor CTL (CTL-P) in the blood of melanoma patients (Coulie et al., 1992). This approach depended on autologous tumor cell lines to stimulate the CTL-P and such cell lines will not be available for most immunized patients. Pilot experiments indicated that it should be possible to do similar CTL-P evaluations against one peptide–HLA combination only, using peptide-pulsed cells to stimulate the CTL. In the presence of a large tumor burden in the vaccinated patient, an additional difficulty resides in the pattern of circulation of the activated antitumor lymphocytes. A majority of them may well reside in the tumor masses so that the fraction detectable in the blood may not be representative. Another possibility to follow the T cell immunization is PCR analysis for the T cell receptor (TCR) variable gene repertoire. This procedure can evaluate a T cell response irrespective of its effector mechanism: an increase in the number of CTL as well as of other types of T cells would be detected, but it requires a narrow TCR repertoire against a given antigen. This may prove to be the case for some antigens, but we feel that the diversity of the anti-MAGE-1–A1 TCR repertoire that we observed with the CTL of patient MZ2 suggests that it will not be the rule (Romero et al., manuscript in preparation). An in vivo assessment of immunity may be obtained by comparing delayed type hypersensitivity responses to inoculations of peptide or proteins before and after immunization.

## Modes of Immunization

There is a vast range of procedures that are proposed for T cell immunization. Which one of them will be optimal in cancer patients is totally unpredictable today. Immunizing with cells is a first possibility. Irradiated tumor cells have been inoculated into many cancer patients with no serious side effects. Allogenic cell lines are available that express several antigens but they will also induce an allogeneic response. Whether the latter will be a problem is a debatable point: in the murine model of CTL immunization against antigen P1A on mastocytoma P815, mice could be immunized with syngeneic cells expressing P1A, but not if the same cells expressed an allogeneic class I molecule by transfection (Uyttenhove, unpublished observations). The reason for this may be related to competition between the T cells at the site of immunization. An advantage of using cells is that they can easily be engineered to produce cytokines that play a role in the development of a CTL response, such as interleukin (IL)-1, IL-2, IL-6, IL-7, or IL-12 (see chapter 9). Expression of co-stimulatory molecules, such as B7, could also stimulate the differentiation and proliferation of specific CTL.

A second possibility is the inoculation with peptides or proteins, the latter being considerably more expensive to produce in quantity and quality suitable for human use. Peptides are easy to synthesize. In vivo they could be endocytosed by cells, associated with the relevant class I molecules and expressed at the cell surface. Alternatively, peptides may bind directly to a small fraction of empty class I molecules, which are already expressed at the surface of the cells. Whole proteins normally have to be endocytosed and digested into peptides, which are then presented by HLA molecules. Part of this could be done ex vivo: specialized antigen-presenting cells such as macrophages or dendritic cells can be isolated from the blood, pulsed in vitro or with peptide, and inoculated back into the patient. A more convenient approach is to inject patients with proteins or peptides mixed with adjuvants. Only a few of them are acceptable for human use and little is known about their efficacy when it comes to CTL responses because they have been mainly tested for antibody production. Proteins such as MAGE-1, MAGE-3, or tyrosinase have been shown to produce several peptides that are able to bind different MHC class I molecules. They can therefore be administered to many patients whose HLA molecules will make the choice of the adequate peptides to present to the T cells.

Recombinant constructs can also be used to immunize. Expression systems have been designed in several microorganisms for the purpose of vaccination: BCG (Stover et al., 1991; Yasutomi et al., 1993), *Salmonella* (Aggrawal et al., 1990; Flynn et al., 1990), vaccinia (Taylor et al., 1991, 1992), adenovirus (Rosenfeld et al., 1992), and retrovirus (Miller et al., 1983). Recombinant viruses or bacteria can be administered to the patients, or used in vitro to pulse antigen-presenting cells isolated from the blood. Inoculation of DNA encoding the antigen is yet another possibility (Ulmer et al., 1993).

If active immunization fails, an alternative approach is adoptive transfer of autologous T lymphocytes stimulated in vitro with the antigen (Rosenberg et al., 1986). Encouraging results were obtained with anti-cytomegalovirus CTL clones inoculated into bone-marrow recipients in whom they persisted and functioned for weeks or months (Riddell et al., 1992).

## Limitations

In the very near future, some cancer patients will enter immunotherapy protocols using some of the tumor antigens that we have described above. Foreseeable problems fall into two categories: in the induction of the CTL response, and in the capacity of these CTL to reject established tumors. As far as the induction phase of the response is concerned, there is an important difference between a tumor antigen against which a cancer patient has to be immunized and, for example, a viral antigen present in an antivirus vaccine. The immune system has been previously, and for a long period of time, exposed to antigen in the case of the former but not the latter. It is possible that a tumor antigen is initially ignored, for instance on a very small tumor, but eventually the number of tumor cells and the inflammatory reactions associated with tumor necrosis increase enormously the likelihood of contacts between tumor antigens and specific lymphocytes. It is possible that these contacts tolerize the antitumor T cells. These days immunologists have new ideas about immune tolerance (Matzinger, 1994). Basically, the emerging concept is that T cells can be properly activated only when encountering their antigen presented by specialized antigen-presenting cells. The latter express co-stimulatory molecules, such as B7, that are mandatory for T cell activation. A very limited number of cells are embodied with this capacity to co-stimulate T cells: dendritic cells, macrophages, and some B lymphocytes. If the antigen is presented by any other type of cells, not only is the T cell not properly activated, but this leads to its functional blockade (anergy) or to its apoptotic death. Though some pieces of the puzzle are still missing, more and more experiments have lent support to the model. It has obvious implications in tumor immunology. A tumor antigen presented by the tumor cells themselves, unable to provide the co-stimulus, may be tolerogenic for the specific T lymphocytes. This could explain why tumor cells can afford to express several tumor antigens without being rejected. It could also explain the reduced clonogenic potential observed with tumor-infiltrating lymphocytes compared to blood T cells (Miescher et al., 1987, 1988). Such tolerance could be even more pronounced in patients carrying a large residual tumor burden. Now that a few tumor antigens are identified it will be possible to verify whether or not antitumor T cells are present but tolerized in cancer patients.

Despite these potential problems we feel that it will be possible soon to generate antitumor CTL responses, at least in some patients. However, this does not mean yet that therapeutic successes will follow. A first problem could be the expression of the antigen in other cells than those of the tumor, resulting in autoimmunity. MAGE genes are expressed in testis, but in the absence of information about the type of cells within this organ that express those genes, it is difficult to discuss potential side effects of anti-MAGE immunizations. Melanocyte differentiation antigens could be more of a problem. Vitiligo is sometimes associated with melanoma and reported to be of good prognostic value (Nordlund et al., 1983; Bystryn et al., 1987). T cells specific for melanocytic differentiation antigens may have contributed to the destruction of melanocytes. These antigens are also present in the retina, brain, and inner ear, and postvaccine immunity might be much stronger than the spontaneous T cell responses observed in some patients with no symptoms of adverse effects. Clearly caution has to be exerted when manipulating immunogenic formulations of differentiation antigens.

The reverse situation is also a problem: many tumor cells may not express the antigen. A first reason is that the transcription of the relevant gene may simply be activated in some but not all tumor cells. In the absence of appropriate antibodies or in situ hybridization methods, no information is available about the potential heterogeneity of expression of tumor antigens like those encoded by the MAGE genes. A second reason is a decrease or absence of gene expression occurring spontaneously in a tumor cell and selected for by the immune response. The $E^-$ antigen-loss variant of melanoma MZ2-MEL, obtained by selection in vitro with an anti-MAGE-1.A1 CTL clone, had a deletion affecting gene MAGE-1 (van der Bruggen et al., 1991). In vitro, many melanoma cell lines lose their original pigmentation after a few weeks or months of culture, owing to loss of expression of one or several genes coding for the melanocyte-specific antigens (Brichard et al., 1993; Coulie et al., 1994). It is likely that similar types of antigen-loss variants will emerge in vivo as a result of selection with CTL. However, if CTL are raised simultaneously against several antigens on the same tumor cells, an escape variant would have to lose the expression of several independent genes. If we reason with data from the in vitro immunoselections where antigen-loss variants for a single gene are present at a frequency of about $10^{-7}$, one double-loss variant would be present among $10^{14}$ tumor cells, corresponding to 100 kg of tumor tissue!

However, tumors have a simpler way to escape: by down-regulating their expression of HLA molecules. This phenotype is fairly common for tumor cells (Lopez-Nevot et al., 1989; Momburg et al., 1989; Smith et al., 1989), and we have observed it several times as a result of immunoselections in vitro by CTL. Very often it is the loss of expression of one allele or one haplotype. Here also the multiantigenic vaccine should cope with

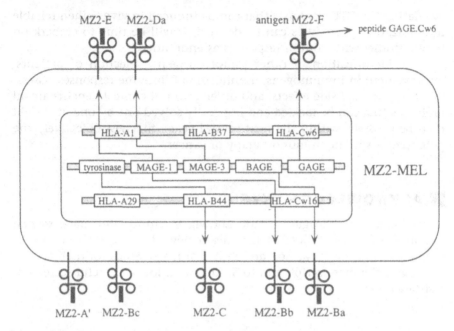

**Figure 5.6**  The multiple antigens recognized by autologous CTL clones on melanoma cells MZ2-MEL.

such cells, especially if the different antigens are presented by HLA molecules encoded by the two haplotypes of the patient (Figure 5.6). Another possibility is the inoculation of interferon-$\gamma$ (IFN-$\gamma$), which up-regulates the expression of MHC molecules. A much more serious situation is that of tumor cells having completely lost HLA class I expression, for instance, because of a defect in the $\beta_2$-microglobulin or TAP gene (Momberg & Koch, 1989; Cabrera et al., 1991; Bicknell, Rowan & Bodmer, 1994; Cromme et al., 1994). Perhaps such HLA-negative cells could be eliminated by NK cells, which appear to display specificity for cells that have lost expression of HLA class I molecules. Treatment with systemic IL-2, known for its strong capacity to activate NK cells, could help to deal with HLA-loss variants of the tumor.

# ■ CONCLUSION AND SUMMARY

Even though there is no direct evidence that CTL can play a general role in anticancer defense, there are to date very good candidates. Now that several antigens are defined, it is reasonable to test different vaccination protocols with these antigens and to compare their efficacies by evaluating the CTL responses that can be induced in vivo. When reliable immunization procedures can be defined, it will be time to embark on longer studies with clinical responses as endpoints.

The identification of other tumor antigens, selection of patients, improvement in immunogens, monitoring of immune responses, assessment of potential side effects, and observation of clinical benefits are all problems that can be tackled and hopefully solved one by one. It should then be possible, within the next several years, to assess objectively the potential of specific immunotherapy of cancer.

# ACKNOWLEDGMENTS

I thank my colleagues at the Ludwig Institute who made several unpublished results available for this review. I am grateful to Dr T. Gajewski, Professor P. Masson and Professor J. Van Snick for their critical reading of the manuscript, and to S. Khaoulali for her careful secretarial assistance.

## REFERENCES

Adema G.J., deBoer A.J., van't Hullenaar R., Denijn M., Ruiter D.J., Vogel A.M. & Figdor C.G. (1993) Melanocyte lineage-specific antigens recognized by monoclonal antibodies NKI-beteb, MHB-50, and HMB-45 are encoded by a single DNA. *American Journal of Pathology*, 269, 20126–33.

Adema G.J., de Boer A.J., Vogel A.M., Loenen W.A.M. & Figdor C.G. (1994) Molecular characterization of the melanocyte lineage-specific antigen gp100. *Journal of Biochemistry and Chemistry*, 269, 20126–33.

Aggarwal A., Kumar S., Jaffe R., Hone D., Gross M. & Sadoff J. (1990) Oral Salmonella: malaria circumsporozoite recombinants induce specific CD8+ cytotoxic T cells. *Journal of Experimental Medicine*, 172, 1083–90.

Anichini A., Fossati G. & Parmiani G. (1985) Clonal analysis of cytotoxic T-lymphocytes response to autologous human metastatic melanoma. *International Journal of Cancer*, 36, 683–9.

Anichini A., Maccalli, C., Mortarini R. et al. (1993) Melanoma cells and normal melanocytes share antigens recognized by HLA-A2-restricted cytotoxic T cell clones from melanoma patients. *Journal of Experimental Medicine*, 177, 989–8.

Bakker A.B.H., Schreurs M.W.J., de Boer A.J. et al. Melanocyte lineage-specific antigen gp100 is recognized by melanoma-derived tumor-infiltrating lymphocytes. *Journal of Experimental Medicine*, 179, 1005–9.

Barnd D.L., Kerr L.A., Metzgar R.S. & Finn O.J. (1988) Human tumor-specific cytotoxic T cell lines generated from tumor-draining lymph node infiltrate. *Transplantation Proceedings*, 20, 339–41.

Barnd D.L., Lan M.S., Metzgar R.S. & Finn O.J. (1989) Specific, major histocompatibility complex-unrestricted recognition of tumor-associated mucins by human cytotoxic T cells. *Proceedings of the National Academy of Sciences USA*, 86, 7159–63.

Bicknell D.C., Rowan A. & Bodmer W.F. (1994) $\beta_2$-microglobulin gene mutations: a study of established colorectal cell lines and fresh tumors. *Proceedings of the National Academy of Sciences USA*, 58, 177–210.

Boël P., Wildmann C., Sensi M.-L. et al. (1995). BAGE, a new gene encoding an antigen recognized on human melanomas by cytolytic T lymphocytes. *Immunity*, 2, 167–75.

Boon T. (1992) Toward a genetic analysis of tumor rejection antigens. *Advances in Cancer Research*, 58, 177–210.

Boon, T., De Plaen E., Lurquin C. et al. (1992) Identification of tumour rejection antigens recognized by T lymphocytes. *Cancer Surveys*, 13, 23–37.

Brasseur F., Marchand M., Vanwijck, R., et al. (1992) Human gene MAGE-1, which codes for a tumor rejection antigen, is expressed bo some breast tumors. *International Journal of Cancer*, 52, 839–41.

Brichard V., Van Pel A., Wölfel T., Wölfel C., De Plaen E., Lethé B., Coulie P. & Boon T. (1993) The tyrosinase gene codes for an antigen recognized by autologous cytolytic T lymphocytes on HLA-A2 melanomas. *Journal of Experimental Medicine*, 178, 489–95.

Bystryn J.-C., Darrell R., Friedman R.J. & Kopf A. (1987) Prognostic significance of hypopigmentation in malignant melanoma. *Archives of Dermatology*, 123, 1053–5.

Cabrera T., Concha A., Ruiz-Cabello F. & Carrido F. (1991). Loss of HLA heavy chain and $\beta_2$-microglobulin in HLA negative tumors. *Scandinavian Journal of Immunology*, 34, 147–52.

Celis E., Tsai V., Crimi C., DeMars R., Wentworth P.A., Chesnut R.W., Grey H.M., Sette A. & Serra H.M. (1994) Induction of anti-tumor cytotoxic T lymphocytes in normal humans using primary cultures and synthetic peptide epitopes. *Proceedings of the National Academy of Sciences USA*, 91, 2105–9.

Chambost H., Brasseur F., Coulie P. et al. A tumor-associated antigen expression in human haematological malignancies. *British Journal of Haematology*, 84, 524–6.

Chen W., Peace D.J., Rovira D.K., You S.-G. & Cheever M.A. (1992) T-cell immunity to the joining region of p210$^{BCR-ABL}$ protein. *Proceedings of the National Academy of Sciences USA*, 89, 1486–72.

Coulie P.G., Brichard V., Van Pel A. et al. (1994) A new gene coding for the differentiation antigen recognized by autologous cytolytic T lymphocytes on HLA-A2 melanomas. *Journal of Experimental Medicine*, 180, 35–42.

Coulie P., Lehmann F., Lethé B. et al. (1995) A mutated intron sequence codes for an antigenic peptide recognized by cytolytic T lymphocytes on a human melanoma. *Proceedings of the National Academy of Sciences USA*, 92, 7976–80.

Cox A.L., Skipper J., Chen Y. et al. (1994) Identification of a peptide recognized by five melanoma-specific human cytotoxic T cell lines. *Science*, 264, 716–19.

Cromme F.V., Airey J., Heemels M.-T. et al. (1994) Loss of transporter protein, encoded by the TAP-1 gene, is highly correlated with loss of HLA expression in cervical carcinomas. *Journal of Experimental Medicine*, 179, 335–40.

Crowley N.J., Slingluff C.L., Darrow T.L. & Seigler H.F. (1990) Generation of human autologous melanoma-specific cytotoxic T-cells using HLA-A2-matched allogeneic melanomas. *Cancer Rsearch*, 50, 492–8.

De Plaen E., Arden K., Traversari C. et al. (1994) Structure chromosomal localization and expression of twelve genes of the MAGE family. *Immunogenetics*, 40, 360–9.

De Plaen E., Lurquin C., Van Pel A. et al. (1988). Immunogenic (tum⁻) variants of mouse tumor P815: cloning of the gene of tum⁻ antigen P91A and identification of the tum⁻ mutation. *Proceedings of the National Academy of Sciences USA*, 85, 2274–8.

De Smet C., Lurquin C., Van der Bruggen P., De Plaen E., Brasseur F. & Boon T. (1994) Sequence and expression pattern of the human MAGE2 gene. *Immunogenetics*, **39**: 121–9.

Espevik T. & Nissen-Meyer J. (1986) A highly sensitive cell line, WEHI 164 clone 13, for measuring cytotoxic factor/tumor necrosis factor from human monocytes. *Journal of Immunological Methods*, **95**, 99–105.

Fisk B., Chesak B., Pollack M.S., Wharton J.T. & Ioannides C.G. (1994). Oligopeptide induction of a cytotoxic T lymphocyte response to HER-2/neu proto-oncogene in vitro. *Cell. Immunology*, **157**, 415–27.

Flynn J.L., Weiss W.R., Norris K.A., Seifert K.A., Seifert H.S., Kumar, S. & So M. (1990) Generation of a cytotoxic T-lymphocyte response using a Salmonella antigen-delivery system. *Molecular Microbiology*, **4**, 2111–8.

Fossum B., Gedde-Dahl T. III, Breivik J., Eriksen J.A., Spurkland A., Thorsby E. & Gaudernack G. (1994) p21-ras-peptide-specific T-cell responses in a patient with colorectal cancer. CD4$^+$ and CD8$^+$ T cells recognize a peptide corresponding to a common mutation (13Gly− >Asp). *International Journal of Cancer*, **56**, 40–5.

Fossum B., Olsen A.C., Thorsby E. & Gaudernack G. (1995) Cytotoxic T cells recognizing mutant p21 ras. CD8$^+$ T cells from a patient with colon carcinoma, specific for a p21 ras derived peptide carrying a 13Gly− >Asp mutation, are cytotoxic towards a carcinoma cell line harbouring the same mutation. *Cancer Immunol. Immunother.*, **42**, 165–72.

Gaugler B., Van den Eynde B., van der Bruggen P. et al. (1994) Human gene MAGE-3 codes for an antigen recognized on a melanoma by autologous cytolytic T lymphocytes. *Journal of Experimental Medicine*, **179**, 921–30.

Gavioli R., De Campos-Lima P.-O., Kurilla M.G., Kieff E. Klein G. & Masucci M.G. (1992) Recognition of the EBV encoded nuclear antigens EBNA-4 and EBNA-6 by HLA-A11-restricted cytotoxic T-lymphocytes. Implications for down-regulation of HLA-A11 in Burkitt's lymphoma. *Proceedings of the National Academy of Sciences USA*, **89**, 5862–6.

Gedde-Dahl T.I., Fossum B., Eriksen J.A., Thorsby E. & Gaudernack G. (1993) T cell clones specific for p21 ras-derived peptides: characterization of their fine specificity and HLA restriction. *European Journal of Immunology*, **23**, 754–60.

Gedde-Dahl T. III, Spurkland A., Fossum B., Wittinghofer A., Thorsby E. & Gaudernack G. (1994) T cell epitopes encompassing the mutational hot spot position of 61 of p21 ras. Promiscuity in ras peptide binding to HLA. *European Journal of Immunology*, **24**, 410–14.

Gendler S., Taylor-Papadimitriou J., Duhog T., Rothbard J. & Burchell J. (1988) A highly immunogenic region of a human polymorphic epithelial mucin expressed by carcinomas is made up of tandem repeats. *Journal of Biological Chemistry*, **263**, 12820–3.

Girling A., Bartkova J., Burchell J., Gendler S., Gillett C. & Taylor-Papadimitriou J. (1989) A core protein epitope of the polymorphic epithelian mucin detected by the monoclonal antibody SM-3 is selectively exposed in a range of primary carcinomas. *International Journal of Cancer*, **43**, 1073–6.

Hérin M., Lemoine C., Weynants P., Vessière F., Van Pel A., Knuth A., Devos R. & Boon, T. (1987) Production of stable cytolytic T-cell clones directed against autologous human melanoma. *International Journal of Cancer*, **39**, 390–6.

Hom S.S., Topalian S.L., Simonis T., Mancini M. & Rosenberg S.A. (1991) Common expression of melanoma tumor-associated antigens recognized by human tumor infiltrating lymphocytes: analysis by human lymphocyte antigen restriction. *Journal of Immunotherapy*, **10**, 153–64.

Houbiers J.G.A., Nijman H.W., van der Burg S.H. et al. (1993) In vitro induction of human cytotoxic T lymphocyte responses against peptides of mutant and wild-type p53. *European Journal of Immunology*, 23, 2071–7.

Ioannides C.G., Freedman R.S., Ionnides M.G., Fisk B. & O'Brian C.A. (1992) CTL clones isolated from ovarian tumor infiltrating lymphocytes can recognize peptides with sequences corresponding to the HER2/NEU gene product. *FASEB Journal* 6.

Ioannides C.G., Fisk B., Jerome K.R., Irimura T., Wharton J.T. & Finn O.J. 1(993) Cytotoxic T cells from ovarian malignant tumors can recognize polymorphic epithelial mucin core peptide. *Journal of Immunology*, 151, 3693–703.

Jacobson S., Reuben J.S., Streilen R.D. & Palker T.J. (1991) Induction of CD4⁺, human T lymphotropic virus type-1-specific cytotoxic T lymphocytes from patients with HAM/TSP. *Journal of Immunology*, 146, 1155–62.

Jerome K.R., Barnd D.L., Bendt K.M. et al. (1991) Cytotoxic T-lymphocytes derived from patients with breast adenocarcinoma recognize an epitope present on the protein core of a mucin molecule preferentially expressed by malignant cells. *Cancer Research*, 51, 2908–16.

Jerome K.R., Domenech N. & Finn O.J. (1993) Tumor-specific cytotoxic T cell clones from patients with breast and pancreatic adenocarcinoma recognize EBV-immortalized B cells transfected with polymorphic epithelial mucin cDNA. *Journal of Immunology*, 151, 1654–62.

Jung, S. & Schluesener, H.J. (1991) Human T lymphocytes recognize a peptide of single point-mutated, oncogenic ras proteins. *Journal of Experimental Medicine*, 173, 273–6.

Kannagi M., Sugamura K., Sato H., Okochi K., Uchino H. & Hinuma Y. (1983) Establishment of human cytotoxic T cell lines specific for human adult T cell leukemia virus-bearing cells. *Journal of Immunology*, 130, 2942–6.

Kast W.M., Brandt R.M.P., Drijfhout, J.W. & Meleif C.J.M. (1993) HLA-A2.1 restricted candidate CTL epitopes of human papillomavirus type 16 E6 and E7 proteins identified by using the processing defective human cell line T2. *Journal of Immunology*, 14, 115–20.

Kawakami Y., Eliyahu S., Delgado C.H. et al. (1994a) Cloning of the gene coding for a shared human melanoma antigen recognized by autologous T cells infiltrating into tumor. *Proceedings of the National Academy of Sciences USA*, 91, 3515–9.

Kawakami Y., Eliyahu S., Delgado C.H. et al. (1994b) Identification of a human melanoma antigen recognized by tumor-infiltrating lymphocytes associated with in vivo tumor rejection. *Proceedings of the National Academy of Sciences USA*, 91, 6458–62.

Kawakami Y., Eliyahu S., Sakaguchi K. et al. (1994c) Identification of the immunodominant peptides of the MART-A human melanoma antigen recognized by the majority of HLA-A2-restricted tumor infiltrating lymphocytes. *Journal of Experimental Medicine*, 180, 347–52.

Kawakami Y., Zakut R., Topalian, S.L., Stötter H. & Rosenberg S.A. (1992) Shared human melanoma antigens. Recognition by tumor-infiltrating lymphocytes in HLA-A2.1-transfected melanomas. *Journal of Immunology*, 148, 638–43.

Knuth A., Danowski B., Oettgen H.F. & Old L. (1984) T-cell mediated cytotoxicity against autologous malignant melanoma: analysis with interleukin-2-dependent T-cell cultures. *Proceedings of the National Academy of Sciences USA*, 81, 3511–5.

Kwon B.S., Chintamaneni C., Kozak C.A. et al. (1991) A melanocyte-specific gene, Pmel 17, maps near the silver coat color locus on mouse chromosome 10 and is a syntenic region on human chromosome 12. *Proceedings of the National Academy of Sciences USA*, 88, 9228–32.

Lehmann F., Marchand M., Hainaut P. et al. (1995). Differences in the antigens recognized by cytolytic T cells on two successive metastases of a melanoma patient are consistent with immune selection. *Eur. J. Immunol.*, **25**, 340–7.

Livingston P.O., Shiku H., Bean M.A., Pinsky C.M., Oettgen H.F. & Old L.J. (1979) Cell-mediated cytotoxicity for cultured autologous melanoma cells. *International Journal of Cancer*, **24**, 34–44.

Lopez-Nevot M.A., Esteban F., Ferron A. et al. (1989) HLA Class I gene expression on human primary tumours and autologous metastases: demonstration of selective losses of HLA antigens on colorectal, gastic and laryngeal carcinomas. *British Journal of Cancer*, **59**, 221–6.

Lurquin C., Van Pel A., Mariamé B. et al. (1989) Structure of the gene coding for tum-transplantation antigen P91A. A peptide encoded by the mutated exon is recognized with Ld by cytolytic T cells. *Cell*, **58**, 293–303.

Maruyama K., Usami M., Aizawa T. & Yoshikawa K. (1991) A novel brain-specific mRNA encoding nuclear protein (necdin) expressed in neurally differential embryonal carcinoma cells. *Biochemical and Biophysical Research Communications*, **178**, 291–6.

Matzinger P. (1994) Tolerance, danger, and the extended family. *Annual Review of Immunology*, **12**, 991–1045.

Miescher S., Stoeck M., Qiao L., Barras C., Barrelet L. & von Fliedner V. (1988) Proliferative and cytolytic potentials of purified human tumor infiltrating T lymphocytes. Impaired response to mitogen-driven stimulation despite T-cell receptor expression. *International Journal of Cancer*, **42**, 659–66.

Miescher S., Whiteside T.L., Moretta L. & von Fliedner V. (1987) Clonal and frequency analyses of tumor-infiltrating T lymphocytes from human solid tumors. *Journal of Immunology*, **138**, 4004-11.

Miller A.D., Jolly D.J., Friedmann T. & Verma I.M. (1983) A transmissible retrovirus expressing human hypoxanthine phosphoribosyltransferase (HPRT): gene transfer into cells obtained from humans deficient in HPRT. *Proceedings of the National Academy of Sciences USA*, **80**, 4709-13.

Mitsuya H., Matis L.A., Megson M., Bunn P.A., Murray C., Mann D.L., Gallo R.C. & Broder S. (1983) Generation of an HLA-restricted cytotoxic T cell line reactive against cultured tumor cells from a patient infected with human T cell leukemia/lymphoma virus. *Journal of Experimental Medicine*, **158**, 994–9.

Momburg F. & Koch S. (1989) Selective loss of $\beta^2$-microglobulin mRNA in human colon carcinoma. *Journal of Experimental Medicine*, **169**, 309-14.

Momburg, F., Ziegler A., Harpprecht J., Möler P., Moldenhauer G. & Hämmerling G.J. (1989) Selective loss of HLA-A or HLA-B antigen expression in colon carcinoma. *Journal of Immunology*, **142**, 352–8.

Mukherji B. & MacAlister T.J. (1983) Clonal analysis of cytotoxic T cell response against human melanoma. *Journal of Experimental Medicine*, **158**, 240–5.

Murray R.J., Kurilla M.G., Brooks J.M., Thomas W.A., Rowe M., Kieff E. & Rickinson A.B. (1992) Identification of target antigens for the human cytotoxic T cell response to Epstein–Barr virus (EBV): implications for the immune control of EBV-positive malignancies. *Journal of Experimental Medicine*, **176**, 157–68.

Nordlund J.J., Kirkwood J.M., Forget B.M., Milton G., Albert D.M. & Lerner A.B. (1983) Vitiligo in patients with metastatic melanoma: a good prognostic sign. *Journal of the American Academy of Dermatology*, **9**, 689–96.

Patard J.-J., Brasseur F., Gil-Diez S. et al. (1995) Expression of MAGE genes in transitional-cell carcinomas of the urinary bladder. *International Journal of Cancer*, **64**, 60-4.

Rickinson A.B., Murray R.J., Brooks J., Griffin H., Moss D.J. & Masucci M.G. (1992) T cell recognition of Epstein–Barr virus associated lymphomas. *Cancer Surveys*, **13**, 53–80.

Riddell S.R., Watanabe K.S., Goodrich J.M., Li C.R., Agha M.E. & Greenberg P.D. (1992) Restoration of viral immunity in immunodeficient humans by the adoptive transfer of T cell clones. *Science*, **257**, 238–41.

Rimoldi D., Romero P. & Carrel S. (1993) The human melanoma antigen-encoding gene MAGE-1 is expressed by other tumour cells of neuroectodermal origin such as glioblastomas and neuroblastoma. *International Journal of Cancer*, **54**, 527–8.

Robbins P.F., El-Gamil M., Kawakami Y. & Rosenberg S.A. (1994) Recognition of tyrosinase by tumor-infiltrating lymphocytes from a patient responding to immunotherapy. *Cancer Research*, **54**, 3124–6.

Rosenberg S.A., Spiess P. & Lafrenière R. (1986) A new approach to the adoptive immunotherapy of cancer with tumor-infiltrating lymphocytes. *Science*, **233**, 1318–21.

Rosenfeld M.A., Yoshimura K., Trapnell B.C. et al. (1992) In vivo transfer of the human cystic fibrosis transmembrane conductance regulator gene to the airway epithelium. *Cell*, **68**, 143–55.

Schendel D.J., Gansbacher B., Oberneder R. et al. (1993) Tumor-specific lysis of human renal cell carcinomas by tumor-infiltrating lymphocytes. *Journal of Immunology*, **151**, 4209–20.

Seed B. & Aruffo A. (1987) Molecular cloning of the CD2 antigen, the T-cell erythrocyte receptor, by a rapid immunoselection procedure. *Proceedings of the National Academy of Sciences USA*, **84**, 3365–9.

Sibille C., Chomez P., Wildmann C., Van Pel A., De Plaen, E., Maryanski J., de Bergeyck V. & Boon T. (1990) Structure of the gene of tum⁻ transplantation antigen P198: a point mutation generates a new antigenic peptide. *Journal of Experimental Medicine*, **172**, 35–45.

Slingluff C.L., Cox A.L., Stover J.M., Jr, Moore M.M., Hunt D.F. & Engelhard V.H. (1994) Cytotoxic T-lymphocyte response to autologous human squamous cell cancer of the lung: epitope reconstitution with peptides extracted from HLA-Aw68. *Cancer Research*, **54**, 2731–7.

Slovin S.F., Lackman R.D., Ferrone S., Kielly P.E. & Mastrangelo M.J. (1986) Cellular immune response to human sarcomas: cytotoxic T cell clones reactive with autologous sarcomas. I. Development, phenotype, and specificity. *Journal of Immunology*, **137**, 3042–8.

Smith M.E.F., Bodmer S.G., Kelly A.P., Trowsdale J., Kirkland S.C. & Bodmer W.F. (1989) Variation in HLA expression on tumors: an escape from immune response. *Cold Spring Harbor Symposia on Quantitative Biology*, **54**, 581–6.

Stover C.K., de la Cruz V.F., Fuerst T.R. et al. (1991) New use of BCG for recombinant vaccines. *Nature (London)*, **351**, 456–60.

Taylor J., Trimarchi C., Weinberg R., Languet B., Guillemin F., Desmettre P. & Paoletti E. (1991) Efficacy studied on a canarypox-rabies recombinant virus. *Vaccine*, **9**, 190–3.

Taylor J., Weinberg R., Tartaglia J. et al. (1992) Nonreplicating viral vectors as potential vaccines: recombinant canarypox virus expressing measles virus fusion (F) and hemagglutinin glycoproteins. *Virology*, **187**, 321–8.

Topalian S.L., Rivoltini L., Mancini M., Markus N.R., Robbins P.F., Kawakami Y. & Rosenberg S.A. (1994) Human CD4⁺ T cells specifically recognize a shared melanoma-associated antigen encoded by the tyrosinase gene. *Proceedings of the National Academy of Sciences USA*, **91**, 9461–5.

Traversari C., van der Bruggen P., Luescher I.F. et al. (1992a) A nonpeptide encoded by human gene MAGE-1 is recognized on HLA-A1 by cytolytic T lymphocytes directed against tumor antigen MZ2-E. *Journal of Experimental Medicine*, **176**, 1453–7.

Traversari C., van der Bruggen P., Van den Eynde B. et al. (1992b) Transfection and expression of a gene coding for a human melanoma antigen recognized by autologous cytolytic T lymphocytes. *Immunogenetics*, **35**, 145–52.

Ulmer J.B., Donnelly J.J., Parker S.E. (1993) Heterologous protection against influenza by injection of DNA encoding a viral protein. *Science*, **259**, 1745–9.

Uyttenhove C., Van Snick J. & Boon T. (1980) Immunogenic variants obtained by mutagenesis of mouse mastocytoma P815. I. Rejection by syngeneic mice. *Journal of Experimental Medicine*, **152**, 1175–83.

Van den Eynde B., Hainaut P., Hérin M. et al. (1989) Presence on a human melanoma of multiple antigens recognized by autologous CTL. *International Journal of Cancer*, **44**, 634–40.

Van den Eynde B., Peeters O., De Backer O. et al. (1995) A new family of genes coding for an antigen recognized by autologous cytolytic T lymphocytes on a human melanoma. *Journal of Experimental Medicine*, **182**, 689–98.

van der Bruggen P., Bastin J., Gajewski T. et al. (1994a) A peptide encoded by human gene MAGE-3 and presented by HLA-A2 induces cytolytic T lymphocytes that recognize tumor cells expressing MAGE-3. *European Journal of Immunology*, **24**, 3038–43.

van der Bruggen P., Traversari C., Chomez, P. et al. (1991) A gene encoding an antigen recognized by cytolytic T lymphocytes on a human melanoma. *Science*, **254**, 1643–7.

van der Bruggen P., Szikora J.-P., Boell P. et al. (1994b) Autologous cytolytic T lymphocytes recognize a MAGE-1 nonapeptide on melanomas expressing HLA-Cw* 1601. *European Journal of Immunology*, **24**, 2134–40.

Vanky F. & Klein E. (1982) Specificity of auto-tumor cytotoxicity exerted by fresh, activated and propagated human T lymphocytes. *International Journal of Cancer*, **29**, 547–53.

Viret C., Davodeau F., Guilloux Y., Bignon J.-D., Semana G., Breathnach R. & Jotereau F. (1993) Recognition of shared melanoma antigen by HLA-A2-restricted cytolytic T cell clones derived from human tumor-infiltrating lymphocytes. *European Journal of Immunology*, **23**, 141-6.

Vose B.M. & Bonnard G.D. (1982) Specific cytotoxicity against autologous tumour and proliferative responses of human lymphocytes grown in interleukin-2. *International Journal of Cancer*, **29**, 33-9.

Wölfel T., Hauer M., Klehmann E., Brichard V., Ackermann B., Knuth A., Boon T. & Meyer zum Büschenfelde K.-H. (1993c) Analysis of antigens recognized on human melanoma cells by A2-restricted cytolytic T lymphocytes (CTL). *International Journal of Cancer*, **55**, 237–44.

Wölfel T., Herr W., Coulie P., Schmitt U., Meyer zum Büschebnfelde K.-H. & Knith A. (1993b) Lysis of human panecreatic adenocarcinoma cells by autologous HLA-Class I-restricted cytolytic T-lymphocyte (CTL) clones. *International Journal of Cancer*, **54**, 636–44.

Wöolfel T., Klehmann E., Müller C., Schütt K.-H., Meyer zum Büschenfelde K.-H. & Knuth A. (1989). Lysis of human melanoma cells by autologous cytolytic T cell clones. Identification of human histocompatibility leukocyte antigen A2 as a restriction element for three different antigens. *Journal of Experimental Medicine*, **170**, 797–810.

Wölfel T., Van Pel A., Brichard V., Schneider J., Seliger B., Meyer zum Büschenfelde K.-H. and Boon T. (1994) Two tyrosine nonapeptides recognized on HLA-A2 melanomas by autologous cytolytic T lymphocytes. *European Journal of Immunology*, **24**, 759–64.

Yasumura S., Hirabayashi H., Schwartz D. R., Toso J. F., Johnson J. T., Herberman R. B. & Whiteside T. L. (1993) Human cytotoxic T-cell lines with restricted specificity for squamous cell carcinoma of the head and neck. *Cancer Research*, **53**, 1461–68.

Yasutomi Y., Koenig S., Haun S. S. et al. (1993) Immunization with recombinant BCG-SIV elicits SIV-specific cytotoxic T lymphocytes in rhesus monkeys. *Journal of Immunology*, **150**, 3101–7.

Yoshino I., Goedegenbuure P. S., Peoples G. E. et al. (1994) HER2/neu-derived peptides are shared antigens among human non-small cell lung cancer and ovarian cancer. *Cancer Research*, **54**, 3387–90.

# 6

## Peptide-specific Cytotoxic T Lymphocytes Directed Against Viral Oncogene Products

MARIET C.W. FELTKAMP, CORNELIS J.M. MELIEF
AND W. MARTIN KAST

## ■ INTRODUCTION

Despite the progress made in cancer treatment over the last few decades, specific treatment of malignant cells without affecting healthy tissue is still in its initial phase. An important step forward in this respect would be to take advantage of the tumor-bearing host's T cell immune response, which is highly specific by its nature. The capability of T cells to interfere with tumor development has been known for several years inasmuch as susceptibility to several cancer types is increased in individuals with impaired T cell responses. These observations suggest that T cell immunity impedes tumor development and, therefore, can be used as a tool to fight cancer. For that purpose it is necessary to identify tumor-specific structures (antigens) to direct immunotherapy against, and to activate those T cells that have the largest potential to destroy tumor cells upon recognition of a tumor-specific antigen.

Although both intracellular (DNA misreplication) and extracellular events (irradiation, mutagens) induce cancer, the direct cause of uncontrolled proliferation is DNA damage inside the tumor cell itself. Via transcription (DNA→mRNA) and translation (mRNA→protein), DNA damage (deletions, mutations, translocations) leads to changes within the proteins synthesized intracellularly, leading to synthesis of altered or new proteins as well as (increased) production of (formerly silent) proteins. All of these might serve as possible tumor-specific antigens. If specific immunotherapy of cancer is considered, therefore, the most rational approach is to activate those cells of the host immune system that attack autologous cells after recognizing specific antigens derived from within the tumor cells. In that perspective, activation of cytotoxic T lymphocytes (CTL) seems a likely choice, since they have the ability to kill target cells after specifically recognizing antigenic fragments of intracellular origin.

**126**

In theory, almost all intracellular proteins can serve as the source of antigens recognized by CTL. In general, however, immunologic tolerance exists for common self antigens. Therefore, tumor-specific antigens should be of foreign origin or of self origin with a limited distribution, either in time (for example, before T cells develop during embryogenesis) or in place (for example, tissue specific such that they are neglected by T cells). A desirable second category of CTL target tumor antigens would be those that are involved in the maintenance of the tumor cell transformed state. In that case, escape from CTL immunity by down-modulation of the tumor antigen would lead automatically to loss of tumor growth. Virus-encoded oncogene products (oncoproteins), being both foreign to the tumor-bearing host and involved in transformation, meet both requirements. The efficacy of CTL to deal with tumors expressing these model tumor-specific antigens can serve as an example for other tumor antigens.

In this review we will deal with several viral oncogene products and the CTL they induce. Examples will be given of the use of virus-encoded oncoproteins, and their respective CTL in vaccination and adoptive transfer studies. First of all we will outline how CTL function, what the antigens they recognize look like and how these antigenic fragments end up at the cell surface. While dealing with the different subjects, we will come across of some of the hurdles which have to be taken to make CTL-based specific anticancer immunotherapy successful and applicable in the human situation on a regular basis.

# ■ CYTOTOXIC T LYMPHOCYTES

## Generation and Maturation

T lymphocytes originate from pluripotent hematopoetic stem cells and are generated in the bone marrow. Subsequently, they migrate to the thymus for further maturation. Here they undergo specific gene rearrangements resulting in development of an enormous array of T cells (Shortman, 1992). Their difference in specificity is the result of expression of a unique T cell receptor (TCR), of which $\pm 10^{12}$ entities can possibly arise. Via positive selection, T cells are selected whose TCR interacts with self major histocompatibility complex (MHC) molecules (Von Boehmer, 1994). Composition and function of MHC molecules are explained below. Subsequently, positively selected T cells are subjected to negative selection resulting in deletion or inactivation (anergy) of those T cells that recognize self antigens presented by self MHC (Nossal, 1994). Finally, only T cells that, under physiological conditions, interact with self MHC molecules and do not recognize self antigens enter the periphery. In the thymus it is also decided which T cells become T helper lymphocytes ($T_H$, CD4$^+$) and which become CTL (CD8$^+$) (Von Boehmer, 1994).

## MHC Restriction and Antigen Recognition

The way in which CTL recognize antigen has gradually been solved over the last two decades. Along with this line of discovery comes the understanding that CTL are extremely well designed to defend the organism against intracellular 'pathogens.' It is a long-standing observation that CTL recognize antigen only in the context of specific MHC class I molecules (MHC restriction) (Zinkernagel and Doherty, 1974). MHC molecules come in two varieties, class I and class II, the first of which specifically interacts with the TCR expressed on CTL. MHC class I molecules are transmembrane glycoproteins present on the cell surface of almost every cell and consist of a heavy polypeptide chain noncovalently linked to a light chain ($\beta_2$-microglobulin) (Orr et al., 1979). The membrane distal part of the heavy chain consists of two extended $\alpha$-helices lying on a floor formed by a $\beta$-pleated sheet (Lopez de Castro et al., 1985). The genetic variation, especially within the $\alpha_1$ and $\alpha_2$ domains of the molecule, gives rise to a variety of MHC class I molecules [human leukocyte antigens (HLA) in humans, H-2 antigens in mice] which are uniquely combined in each individual. This MHC polymorphism is of importance to tumor immunologists for reasons to be discussed further. MHC class II molecules roughly show the same molecular composition and genetic variability as MHC class I molecules. (Brown et al., 1993). Their presence, however, is confined to the cell surface of specialized antigen-presenting cells (APC), such as dendritic cells, macrophages and B cells. Analogous to CTL and MHC class I, helper T cells ($T_H$) are restricted by MHC class II molecules.

The first crystallographic studies of an MHC class I molecule (HLA-A*0201) showed that a small cavity ('the groove') was present between the $\alpha$-helices in which a peptide was lying that was not part of the MHC class I molecule itself (Bjorkman et al., 1987a, 1987b). This finding almost coincided with observations done by Townsend and colleagues who showed that CTL recognized not only virus-infected cells but also non-infected cells expressing the same MHC class I molecules, loaded exogenously with a virus-encoded peptide (Townsend et al., 1986). These observations together led to the concept that MHC class I molecules bind peptides intracellularly and present them at the cell surface to encountering CTL. Both the research groups of Rammensee and Nathenson demonstrated that this was indeed the case. They showed that particular viral peptides recognized by specific CTL clones, when added exogenously to MHC class I-positive cells, could also be eluted out of the MHC class I molecules obtained from identical cells when these cells were infected with virus (Rötschke et al., 1990; Van Bleek & Nathanson 1990).

The unique molecular structure of the MHC class I $\alpha_1$- and $\alpha_2$-helices and the peptide in between is specifically recognized by the TCR (Jorgensen et al., 1992). Following specific recognition, signaling takes place within the CTL, which results in the release of permeabilizing agents by the CTL and, subsequently, target cell death (Kägi et al., 1994). In order to be activated at its first engagement with antigen, CTL require an additional (co-stimulatory) signal. This is provided by B7 molecules, exclusively present on specialized APC, that interact with CTLA-4 molecules present on the CTL (Chen et al., 1992a; Townsend & Alison, 1993). Furthermore, most CTL need interleukin-2 (IL-2) to proliferate. Further details on the interactions between CTL and target cells, the co-stimulatory and adhesion molecules involved, and the mechanisms by which target cell death is induced are beyond the scope of this review.

## Antigen Processing and Presentation

**MHC Class I** To comprehend the possibilities and restrictions of immunotherapy fully based on the action of tumor-specific CTL, it is important to know how antigenic peptides are processed and presented at the cell surface. MHC class I heavy and light chains are cotranslationally synthesized in the endoplasmatic reticulum (ER) lumen where they assemble to a heterodimer (Neefjes et al., 1993a). This heterodimer is unstable at physiological temperature (Ljunggren et al., 1990) and is retained in the ER via linkage to calnexin (Rajagopalan & Brenner, 1994). Only when a peptide is bound by the MHC class I heterodimer, a stable heterotrimeric complex is formed, which is disconnected from calnexin and transported to cell surface (Germain & Margulies, 1993; Neefjes & Momburg, 1993).

The supply of peptides in the ER is mainly controlled by the ER membrane-spanning transporters associated with antigen-processing (TAP) 1 and 2 (Powis et al., 1991; Kleijmeer et al., 1992; Neefjes & Momburg, 1993). They translocate peptides from the cytosol into the ER and thereby provide the MHC class I molecule with this third component (Van Kaer et al., 1992; Neefjes et al., 1993b). The peptides themselves are generated in the cytosol by protein degradation in a manner that is to some extent linked to the ubiquitin protein degradation pathway (Michalek et al., 1993). Involvement of proteasomes and their subunits LMP2 and 7 has been proposed, but several studies have reported recently that neither proteasomes nor the LMP2 and 7 subunits are essential for peptide processing (Arnold et al., 1992; Momburg et al., 1992). Recently evidence has emerged that members of the heat shock protein (HSP) family may also be involved in antigen processing (Udono & Srivastava, 1993). It is hypothesized that these nonpolymorphic proteins bind peptides in the cytosol and form a relay line by which the peptides are chaperoned towards TAP and MHC class I (Srivastava et al., 1994) (discussed in great detail in Chapter 13).

A second pathway to provide the ER with MHC class I presentable peptides is observed in the antigen-processing defective cell line T2. HLA-A*0201 molecules isolated from TAP-deficient T2 cells were shown to contain peptides derived from signal sequences cleaved from transmembrane proteins, which were cotranslationally shifted to the ER (Henderson et al., 1992; Hunt et al., 1992).

**MHC Class II**   In contrast to peptides presented by MHC class I molecules, MHC class II-bound peptides are derived from proteins synthesized outside the APC. Analogous to MHC class I molecules, class II molecules are also cotranslationally synthesized within the ER (Lotteau et al., 1990; Germain & Margulies, 1993; Neefjes & Momburg, 1993). However, here they are linked to the invariant chain (Ii), which prevents binding of peptides (Roche & Cresswell, 1990), and directs the complex towards a lysomsomal-like compartment (Peters et al., 1991; Anderson & Miller, 1992). Under influence of the low pH locally, the Ii is released allowing endocytosed protein degradation products, peptides, to bind within the antigen-presenting groove. Finally, the MHC class II–peptide complex is transported to the cell surface (Neefjes & Momburg, 1993) where they can interact with the TCR of encountering $T_H$ cells. In general this specific interaction does not lead to target cell death but results in release of cytokines, such as IL-2.

### Restrictions to MHC Class I-dependent Peptide Presentation

During protein degradation, peptide translocation and MHC class I complex formation, selection of peptides takes place that limits the number of MHC class I presentable peptides and thereby the number of potential CTL epitopes (Germain, 1994). An important observation in this respect was made by Rammensee and co-workers who took normal cells and isolated the MHC class I molecules thereof. Via acid treatment, the peptides present in the MHC class I molecules were eluted out of the antigen-presenting groove (Falk et al., 1991). Analyzing different MHC class I alleles, they found that naturally processed and presented MHC class I-bound peptides are restricted in size. The average peptide size appears to be 9±1 amino acids (Falk et al., 1991), which is confirmed by sequencing of some naturally processed peptides (Rötschke et al., 1990, 1991; Van Bleek & Nathanson, 1990). Furthermore, the eluted peptides applied to MHC class I allele-specific rules concerning amino acid (aa) composition. At certain aa positions within the peptide sequence ('anchor positions') only specific aa, which share features such as hydrophobicity or possession of a specific side chain (for example, aliphatic or aromatic) were found (Falk et al., 1991; Rötschke & Falk, 1991). Crystallographic studies showed later that these anchor positions correspond to MHC class I allele-specific pockets within the antigen-presenting groove (Madden et al., 1992; Matsumara et al., 1992). At these sites there is intense contact between peptide and MHC class I molecule.

The MHC class I allele-specific peptide size and sequence requirements, better known as MHC class I allele-specific peptide motifs, are of enormous importance to the MHC class I-bound peptide repertoire expressed at the cell surface. For several MHC class I alleles, specific peptide motifs have now been determined. Peptides that do not conform to these motifs are not (expected to be) presented at the cell surface, which implies a gross reduction of the number of peptides recognizable by CTL. An important implication thereof is that, because of MHC polymorphism, MHC class I-bound peptides will differ between individuals and, ultimately, that some (tumour-specific) proteins will be antigenic in some individuals as opposed to others. Of practical importance is that, on the basis of the MHC class I allele-specific peptide motifs, candidate CTL epitopes can now be predicted with success (Pamer, Harty & Bevan, 1991; Sijts et al., 1994). It is important to mention that most CTL epitopes identified so far comply with the MHC class I allele-specific peptide motifs (Rammensee, Falk & Rötschke, 1993), but that peptides that bind to MHC class I molecules and bear the motif are not necessarily naturally processed CTL epitopes (Feltkamp et al., 1994a). It should be kept in mind, however, that most motifs are not perfect (yet) and often need fine adjustments (Hunt et al., 1992; Ruppert et al., 1993).

Other levels of peptide selection are TAP-mediated peptide translocation and, possibly, protein degradation. All TAP alleles studied thus far transport peptides of 6–15 aa in length (Momburg et al., 1994a; Schumacher et al., 1994). They do not necessarily transport peptides of optimal length for MHC class I binding, since some CTL epitope-containing peptides are only efficiently transported by TAP as peptides somewhat longer than the optimal MHC class I-binding sequence (Neisig et al., 1995). TAP displays specificity towards the peptide C-terminal as residue, which serves as an anchor residue for many MHC class I alleles (Momburg et al., 1994b; Schumacher et al., 1994). TAP preference for particular C-terminal residues coincides with the peptide-binding specificity of the respective MHC class I allele. Since the genes encoding MHC class I, TAP1, TAP2 (and LMP2 and LMP7) all reside within the MHC complex, coevolution of peptide specificity seems a likely explanation for this finding (Momburg, Neefjes & Hämmerling, 1994c).

As discussed above, only a limited number of peptides is destined to be a CTL epitope. In general, this choice is dictated by three items: (1) the protein aa composition; (2) the MHC class I and TAP alleles involved; and (3) the CTL repertoire available. It is now up to the tumor immunologist to combine these three items in such a way that tumor antigens are identified that encode CTL epitopes useful for cancer therapy.

# ■ TUMOR-SPECIFIC ANTIGENS RECOGNIZABLE BY CTL

## In General

Based on the principles concerning the functioning of CTL and the origin of the peptides recognized, several tumor-specific antigens can now be considered, for instance, peptides derived from oncogene or (mutated) tumor suppressor gene products (Melief & Kast, 1993), as well as peptides derived from fusion proteins resulting from tumor-specific DNA translocation. Specific CTL have been described for all these cases, as well as for peptides derived from immunoglobulin idiotypes potentially relevant for treatment of B cell lymphoma (Finn, 1993). Of particular interest are the melanoma-specific antigens recognized by CTL (MAGE 1 and MAGE 3, tyrosinase, gp100 and MART 1; see Chapter 5). Although they appear tissue specific rather than tumor specific, they are expected to be of use in melanoma treatment (Pardoll, 1994). Other parts of this volume are completely dedicated to the tumor antigens just mentioned. The list of tumor-specific antigens is completed with the virus-encoded antigens expressed in virus-induced tumors.

## In Virus-induced Cancer

Viruses are believed to be involved in the development of about 15% of human cancers (Zur Hausen, 1991). Epstein–Barr virus (EBV) is associated with several lymphoma types, hepatitis B virus (HBV) with hepatocellular carcinoma, human papillomaviruses (HPV) with skin and anogenital cancer, and human T-lymphotropic virus type-1 (HTLV-1) with adult T cell leukemia (Klein, 1991; Masucci, 1993). Sometimes the human immunodeficiency virus (HIV) is added to this list. However, the tumors that occur in immunosuppressed HIV-infected individuals are often associated with a viral cause. This observation seems to underscore the importance of T cell immunosurveillance in prevention of (virus-induced) tumor formation rather than suggesting the oncogenicity of HIV itself.

Although in vitro studies have demonstrated that virus-encoded oncogene products induce cellular transformation, tumor-associated viruses are not regarded as the sole cause of transformation of the cells in which they reside. Still, they are obvious targets against which to direct CTL-mediated immunotherapy. The reasons for this (they are foreign to the tumor-bearing host, and involved in the transformed state of the tumor) were mentioned before. To achieve this goal, knowledge has to be gained about CTL that are specific for viral oncogene products, and their potential to prevent formation of virus-induced tumors and/or to eradicate established virus-induced tumors. To this end in vitro and in vivo animal models were developed, which have now shown the power of CTL-based specific immunotherapy against virus-induced tumors. The most relevant studies in this respect will now be discussed in detail, followed by an overview of what is known about CTL specific for viral oncogene products involved in human cancer. Finally, the prospects in human cancer of some of the methods successfully applied in mice will be discussed.

# ■ VIRAL ONCOGENE PRODUCT-SPECIFIC CTL IN MURINE TUMOR MODELS

The best studied in vitro and in vivo murine models of virus-induced tumors and their specific CTL relate to small DNA tumor viruses such as simian virus 40 (SV40), mouse polyomavirus (MPyV), human adenovirus, and HPV. All four express oncogene products that induce cellular transformation in vitro. Other well-studied virus-induced tumors are those induced by murine leukemia viruses. The oncogenicity of these retroviruses is often not the result of expression of virus-specific oncoproteins but rather of random integration of provirus DNA in the vicinity of cell regulatory genes. Therefore, we will mention these studies only if they add to the concepts distilled from the small DNA tumor virus models.

## Simian Virus 40

SV40 is a small DNA tumor virus, which was initially isolated from monkey kidney cell cultures. Although now pathogenic in monkeys, SV40 induces sarcomas in hamsters when administered neonatally (Schreier & Gruber, 1990). Its oncogenicity can be attributed to the large (T) and the small (t) tumor antigen, both encoded by the same gene via alternative splicing (Schreier & Gruber, 1990). Important aspects of the mechanism by which T induces cellular transformation have been unravelled recently and are shared with oncogene products of other small DNA tumor viruses (Phelps et al., 1988; Vousden & Jat, 1989; Levine, 1990; Mietz et al., 1992). T is able to bind the tumor suppressor gene products pRB and p53 (Weinberg, 1991), thereby hampering the interaction between these proteins and transcription factors such as E2F that regulate cell cycle-specific gene expression (Volgelstein & Kinzler, 1992).

By the 1970s it had already become clear that T is immunogenic in the sense that it harbored a tumor-specific transplantation antigen (TSTA) (Anderson et al., 1977; Chang et al., 1979; Vogelstein & Kinzler, 1992). In the late 1980s, Tevethia and co-workers identified T as the source of a number of CTL epitopes (Anderson et al., 1988; Tanaka et al., 1988). Via SV40 T deletion mutants, the origin of the CTL epitopes was mapped to four distinct antigenic sites (Tanaka et al., 1988), each of which could be reduced to a 10–15 aa-long peptide stretch (Deckhut, Lippolis & Tevethia, 1992). In that study no particular CTL epitope was immunodominant over the others. Only when cells were used for immunization that bear mutations in all four CTL epitope-encoding regions such that they were no longer seen by the epitope-specific CTL clones (Tanaka & Tevethia, 1988), CTL were isolated that specifically recognized a fifth epitope (Tanaka et al., 1989). This CTL epitope was termed 'immunorecessive,' since it does not seem to be immunogenic when the other CTL epitope-encoding regions are intact and expressed.

An important aspect of the research carried out by this group is that mutations within CTL epitope-encoding regions occur when transformed cells are grown in the presence of specific CTL clones. Under the continuous pressure of SV40 T-specific CTL clones, antigenic loss variants arose, which were no longer sensitive to lysis by the CTL clones (Tanaka & Tevethia, 1988). The mutations observed within the CTL epitope-encoding regions of the antigenic loss variants are such that the mutated antigenic peptides still bind with the same affinity to the relevant MHC class I molecule but do not trigger the CTL (Lill et al., 1992). Whether the latter is the result of loss of physical interaction between the MHC class I–peptide complex, and the TCR or abrogated signaling within the CTL after TCR engagement (T cell antagonism) is not known. An important question for tumor immunologists in this respect is whether virus-transformed tumor cells escape from CTL surveillance in vivo as frequently as in the just described situation in vitro.

## Mouse Polyomavirus

Unfortunately, the ability of the SV40 T-specific CTL clones to cope with an SV40-expressing tumor in vivo was never examined. Neither have T-derived CTL epitope-containing peptides been used for immunization purposes. A similar approach, however has been performed in an MPyV-induced murine tumor model. MPyV roughly has the same composition as SV40 and causes tumors in mice under certain conditions (Schreier & Gruber, 1990). Besides T and t, MPyV expresses also middle tumor antigen (MT), all three of which were identified as TSTA (Dalianis et al., 1982). Dalianis and colleagues showed that an MT-derived peptide could delay tumor formation following a challenge with MPyV-induced tumor cells in CBA mice (H-$2^k$) (Ramqvist et al., 1989). The tumor protective effect observed after peptide immunization was, however, less efficient than after immunization with whole MPyV. Later on they could repeat the decrease in tumor progression with a number of other MT- and LT-derived peptides in another mouse strain (C57BL/6 mice, H-$2^b$) (Reinholdsson-Ljunggren et al., 1992). The mechanism behind the anti-MPyV tumor effect seen after peptide immunization was not determined, although involvement of T cells is proposed. When the binding capacity to H-$2K^b$ and $D^b$ was analyzed, only a minority of the protective peptides bound to these MHC class I molecules (Reinholdsson et al., 1993). This result might imply that the protection seen cannot be accounted to the action of CTL. However, it should be noted that the peptides used were 15 aa or longer. Peptide–MHC class I binding could have been overlooked, since MHC class I molecules only bind peptides of optimal length 9±1 aa) with high affinity (Schumacher et al., 1991). Notably, strict peptide length is not required when CTL epitope-containing peptides are used in vivo for immunization (Kast, Brandt & Melief, 1993b).

## Human Adenovirus

In humans, adenoviruses (Ads) cause infection of the respiratory tract. However, in immunocompetent mice, some types (Ad12) are tumorigenic, whereas others (Ad5) are not. Adenoviruses express the oncogene products E1A and E1B, which induce cellular transformation in a manner similar to SV40 T (Phelps et al., 1988; Vousden & Jat, 1989; Levine, 1990). The difference in tumorigenicity between Ad5 and Ad12 is most likely the result of efficient CTL surveillance in the case of Ad5-transformed cells, which fails in the case Ad12-transformed cells (Bernards et al., 1983). The reason for CTL failure in the latter case most likely lies in the fact that Ad12, in contrast to Ad5, abrogates MHC class I expression by physical linkage to one of its components

(Schrier et al., 1983). Since MHC class I expression is a *conditio sine qua non* for CTL activation, Ad12-transformed cells can grow out without CTL interference. Down-regulation of MHC class I expression is a phenomenon seen in many advanced staged tumors and is one of the major problems that have to be faced when thinking of CTL-based cancer intervention (see below and Chapter 4).

The observation that the difference in tumorigenicity between Ad5- and Ad12-transformed cells could result from hampered functionality of MHC class I-restricted CTL brought us to study Ad-specific CTL responses in detail. For that purpose Ad5-transformed mouse embryo cells from C57BL/6 mice (H-2$^b$) were generated (Kast et al., 1989). As expected these cells were nontumorigenic in immunocompetent C57BL/6 mice whereas they form tumors in T cell-deficient C57BL/6 nude mice. When the Ad5-transformed cells were used to immunize immunocompetent C57BL/6 mice, CTL were raised that specifically lyse Ad5-transformed cells expressing the Ad5 E1A oncoprotein (Kast et al., 1989). The reactivity of these H-2D$^b$-restricted CTL is specifically directed towards the Ad5 E1A-encoded peptide 234-243 (SGPSNTPPEI) (Kast & Melief, 1991). To show that these Ad5-encoded peptide-specific CTL were responsible for abrogating the outgrowth of Ad5-transformed tumor cells, C57BL/6 nude mice were inoculated with Ad5-transformed tumor cells. When tumors had formed, the mice received intravenously $15 \times 10^6$ cultured Ad5 E1A-specific CTL. Two weeks later the treated animals were cured of their tumor burden, even in the case of large (1–2 cm$^3$) tumors (Kast et al., 1989). To obtain this result, it was obligatory to give the mice 10$^5$ units of recombinant interleukin-2 (rIL-2) at the same time as the transfer of CTL, underscoring the dependency on IL-2 of most CTL. Tumor protection was long-lasting inasmuch as a challenge with tumor cells after 3 months did not induce tumor formation provided that rIL-2 was given simultaneously (Kast et al., 1989). Recently we were able to repeat tumor eradication with two other CTL clones that specifically recognize an Ad5 E1B-encoded peptide (Toes et al., unpublished data). Overall, this study is one of the best examples in which the power of CTL in the defence against (virus-induced) cancer is illustrated, especially against established tumors.

### Friend's Murine Leukemia Virus

Another example of successful antitumor therapy via adoptive T cell transfer is seen in the case of Friend's murine leukemia virus (Friend MuLV)-induced leukemia (Melief, 1992). Besides CD8$^+$ CTL, CD4$^+$ T$_H$ cells are also employed in this model, all of which were generated by immunizing C57BL/6 mice with syngeneic Friend MuLV-induced tumor cells (FBL-3 cells) (Greenberg et al., 1988). Both T cell subsets are specifically directed against viral structural proteins encoded by the *gag* and *env* genes, which are not considered to be oncoproteins in the strict sense. Injected separately, T cell clones of both subsets were capable of curing disseminated disease (Klarnet et al., 1989). For the CD4$^+$ T cells this is remarkable, since FBL-3 tumor cells do not express MHC class II molecules. In this case, the tumoricidal effect is probably accounted for by macrophages, which become activated by interferon-$\gamma$ (IFN-$\gamma$) secreted by FBL-3-specific T$_H$ cells (Kern et al., 1986). One could envisage that the MHC class II-restricted T$_H$ cells start producing IFN-$\gamma$ following engagement with professional MHC class II-positive APC, which have processed and presented endocytosed FBL-3 tumor material. It is important to note that tumor eradication in this model is only achieved when the adoptive transfer is combined with simultaneous administration of cyclophosphamide. At the cyclophosphamide dose used, only a slight delay in FBL-3 tumor growth is seen. Of greater importance is probably the gross reduction in host's T cell numbers, some of which might suppress the action of the T cells transferred (Greenberg et al., 1988).

## Human Papillomavirus

To date over 70 HPV types have been isolated (De Villiers, 1989), all of which are epitheliotropic and replicate in differentiated keratinocytes at various anatomic sites. Several types are detected in benign lesions, such as the 'low-risk' HPV types 6 and 11 in genital warts and condylomata accuminata (De Villiers, 1989). 'High-risk' HPV types are found in malignancies, such as HPV16 and 18 in cervical cancer (Van den Brule et al., 1991), which is estimated to be the second most frequent cancer-related cause of death in women worldwide (Parkin, Pisani & Ferlay, 1993). One of the differences between 'low' and 'high-risk' HPV types is that the 'low-risk' HPV-encoded early proteins E6 and E7 do not bind, or bind only weakly the tumor suppressor gene products pRB and p53, whereas their 'high-risk' counterparts do bind these gene products (Scheffner et al., 1990; Crook, Tidy & Vousden, 1992). As a result, cell-cycle control mechanisms are deregulated (Weinberg, 1991; Vogelstein & Kinzler, 1992) and an important step in HPV16/18-induced cellular transformation is taken. Whether this mechanism is of great importance to cervical carcinogenesis in vivo is not yet settled. In any event, E6 and E7 are always found to be retained in cervical cancer cells, whereas expression of the other genes is often abrogated (Smotkin & Wettstein, 1986; Baker et al., 1987). Additionally, maintenance of the transformed state of cervical cancer-derived cell lines depends on intact E6 and E7 expression (Crook et al., 1989). For these reasons, tumor immunologists have focused their attention on these two oncoproteins. Since HPV16 also transforms rodent cells (Kanda et al., 1988; Storey et al., 1988), initial studies were carried out in mice, which offered the possibility of performing tumor vaccination and therapy studies in a syngeneic system.

It was Chen and colleagues who showed that HPV16 E7 codes for a tumor rejection antigen (Chen et al., 1991). They took mouse melanoma cells, which are tumorigenic in C57BL/6 mice, and transfected them with the HPV16 E7 gene. E7 transfection was also carried out in a nontumorigenic fibroblast cell line. This cell line was used to immunize mice, which were subsequently challenged with the E7-transfected melanoma cells. The immunized mice were now protected against tumor outgrowth of the E7-expressing melanoma cells. In vivo depletion of CD8$^+$ cells and not of CD4$^+$ cells completely abrogated tumor protection (Chen et al., 1991). A year later identical results were obtained in a similar setup with HPV16 E6, again pointing to CD8$^+$ CTL as the mediators of the tumor protection (Chen et al., 1992b). In both studies the epitopes against which the protective CTL responses were directed were not determined. It was Stauss and colleagues who identified the first HPV16 E6 and E7 encoded peptides that induce a CTL response in vitro (Stauss et al., 1992). The ability of these peptide-specific CTL to lyse HPV16-expressing tumor cells was not established.

At the same time in our own laboratory, we generated a tumorigenic HPV16-transformed cell line of C57BL/6 origin, called C3, against which CTL were raised (Feltkamp et al., 1993). In order to identify CTL epitopes expressed on C3 cells, we used a new strategy based on knowledge about peptides recognized by CTL. We generated a set of 240 peptides that covered the HPV16 E6 and E7 aa sequences completely. The peptides, 9 aa long and overlapping by 8 aa, were separately analyzed for their ability to bind to the MHC class I molecules expressed in cells of C57BL/6 origin, H-2K$^b$ and D$^b$. Finally, we ended up with six peptides that bound to K$^b$ and/or D$^b$ with high affinity, one of which (E7 49-57, RAHYNIVTF) was selected for the immunization of C57BL/6 mice (Feltkamp et al., 1993, 1994b). A subcutaneous (s.c.) injection of this peptide in incomplete Freund's adjuvant (IFA) resulted in the induction of CTL that specifically lysed E7 49–57-loaded syngeneic cells and, more importantly, HPV16-transformed C3 cells (Feltkamp et al., 1993). The ability of E7 49–57-specific cultured CTL to eradicate established C3 tumors in T cell-deficient nude C57BL/6 mice via adoptive transfer is under current investigation. At this point we would like to mention that the E7 49–57 peptide, although it binds to H-2D$^b$ with high affinity, only partially applies to the published D$^b$ allele-specific peptide motif (Falk et al., 1991; Feltkamp et al., 1993; Sadnikova et al., 1994). Therefore, it should be said that selection of candidate CTL epitope-bearing peptides on the basis of an MHC class I-specific peptide motif alone is not without risk.

With the identification of an HPV16-derived peptide that induces specific CTL in vivo, which lyse HPV16-transformed tumor cells, a potential specific antitumor vaccine was within reach. To that end immunocompetent C57BL/6 mice were immunized twice with 100 $\mu$g of the E7 49–57 peptide mixed with IFA. Two weeks later the mice were challenged with $5 \times 10^5$ C3 tumor cells, a dose that normally induces formation of a lethal tumor in 80% of the animals. In the vaccinated mice, however, less than 10% of the mice developed a tumor (Feltkamp et al., 1993). The ability of this peptide to induce eradication of established C3 tumors is under current investigation.

One of the striking observations in this model is that the E7 49–57 peptide is not recognized by CTL induced by immunization with C3 cells themselves (Feltkamp et al., 1993). This suggests that C3 cells express at least one other CTL epitope, which seems immunodominant over E7 49–57. Furthermore, our data show that a CTL epitope, which is not able to induce a CTL response (immunogenic) when presented on the tumor cell, is very well recognized (antigenic) on the same tumor cell by peptide-specific CTL induced otherwise. This information is of general importance, since most tumors occurring in humans are not immunogenic or are only weakly immunogenic (Koeppen et al., 1993).

## ■ VIRAL ONCOGENE PRODUCT-SPECIFIC CTL IN HUMAN CANCER

### Epstein–Barr Virus

EBV is associated with at least four types of lymphoma (immunoblastic B cell lymphoma, endemic Burkitt's lymphoma, nasopharyngeal lymphoma, and Hodgkin's lymphoma) (Masucci, 1993). The role of T cell surveillance in limiting the proliferative potential of EBV-infected cells is clearly illustrated by the development of EBV-positive immunoblastic B cell lymphomas in immunosuppressed individuals. CTL are believed to be the main effector cells in this context. Many EBV-encoded CTL epitopes have been described to date, which are recognized in the context of various MHC class I HLA alleles (Burrows et al., 1990; Gavioli et al., 1992, 1993; Khanna et al., 1992). Most CTL epitopes identified so far relate to the EBV nuclear antigens (EBNA) 3, 4 and 6, as well as to other EBNA and the latent membrane proteins (LMP) 1 and 2. LMP1 is considered an oncoprotein, since it transforms rodent cells in vitro (Moorthy & Thorley-Lawson, 1993), and induces hyperplasia in mice transgenic for the LMP1-encoding gene (Wilson et al., 1990). Against the other oncoprotein, EBNA-1, so far no specific CTL have been detected. Unfortunately, in many of the EBV-positive cancer types, this is the only EBV antigen expressed (Masucci, 1993). No attempts have been made so far to interfere with EBV-related disease in a way that relates to EBV-specific CTL or the peptide epitopes they recognize.

An interesting observation in terms of CTL surveillance and virus (-induced tumor) immune escape mechanisms was done by Masucci and Rickinson. They identified a CTL epitope in EBNA-4, which is recognized by CTL in an HLA-A*1101-restricted fashion (Gavioli et al., 1993). CTL specific for this particular epitope were tested for recognizing HLA-A*1101+ B cells immortalized with EBV isolates from different geographic regions. Strikingly, almost all isolates from New Guinea were insensitive to CTL lysis (De Campos-Lima et al., 1993). The molecular basis for this CTL insensitivity was a point mutation in the EBNA-4-encoding sequence, which changed the C-terminal peptide anchor residue lysine into a threonine. As a result, this peptide no longer binds to the HLA-A*1101 class I molecule, meaning most likely that it is not presented on EBV-infected EBNA-4 expressing B cells in vivo (De Campos-Lima et al., 1993). The reason for this EBV mutant to emerge in New Guinea lies probably in the fact the HLA-A*1101 MHC class I allele is very common in this part of the world. This finding indicates that HLA-restricted CTL responses can be of influence to the evolution of the pathogen and might also explain why some virus-induced tumors are restricted to specific regions.

## Hepatitis B Virus

Although most of the evidence for an association between HBV and hepatocellular carcinoma is of an epidemiological kind, there are now other reasons to believe that HBV is somehow involved in the transformation of long-term HBV-infected cells; for instance, in the development of tumors in nude mice inoculated with 3T3 cells expressing the HBV X gene (Shirakata et al., 1989), and of liver cancer in HBV X transgenic mice (Kim et al., 1991). Furthermore, the pre-S gene and the X gene are involved in transactivation. So far studies that analyse CTL responses against HBV have focused their attention on other HBV core antigens or on the HBV surface antigens. Chisari and colleagues have identified several naturally processed CTL epitopes (Bertoletti et al., 1991, 1993; Nayersina et al., 1993), such as the HLA-A*0201-restricted CTL epitope in the HBV nucleocapsid protein. This peptide is currently being used as part of a peptide-based therapeutic vaccine to induce HBV-specific CTL

(Vitiello et al., 1995). In another study performed recently by the same group, variants of CTL epitopes were described that act as TCR antagonists for HBV-specific CTL. It appeared that CTL that recognize the 'wild-type' epitope are inactivated (anergized) when a naturally occurring 'mutant' peptide, which has a slight change in its aa composition, is expressed on the same target cell (Bertoletti et al., 1994). These mutants are only seen in patients with CTL against the wild-type epitope, suggesting that they occur only under CTL pressure.

### Human T Lymphotropic Virus 1

HTLV-1 is a retrovirus associated with developments of adult T cell leukemia, which causes CD4$^+$ T cell proliferation in vitro. The transforming X-region of the virus encodes two proteins, Tax and Rex. The Tax protein, especially, is the source of well-characterized CTL epitopes that are recognized by CTL isolated from the peripheral blood of symptomatic as well as asymptomatic seropositive patients (Jacobson et al., 1990; Koenig et al., 1993). The role of these CTL in the immunopathology of HTLV-1-associated myelopathy is still a matter of debate (Parker et al., 1992; Kannagi et al., 1994). Studies which employ HTLV-1-specific CTL, or the epitopes they recognize, to interfere with HTLV-1-related disease have not yet been performed.

### Human Papillomavirus

As mentioned earlier, human papillomaviruses are involved in several human cancers of epithelial origin, such as cervical cancer. The HPV16-encoded oncogene products E6 and E7 are believed to be the most important viral proteins in terms of transformation (Vousden, 1993). Based on our findings in the HPV16 mouse tumor model (section IV E in Feltkamp et al., 1993), we started to identify E6- and E7-encoded candidate CTL epitopes by analysing their ability to be bound by human HLA class I molecules. Since we are now dealing with an MHC polymorphic outbred population and the final aim is to generate a CTL epitope-containing peptide vaccine applicable in as large as possible a population, we could not restrict ourselves to only two MHC class I alleles. Therefore, the set of 240 E6- and E7-derived overlapping peptides was tested for binding to five different MHC class I HLA-A alleles (A*0101, A*0201, A*0301, A*1101, and A*2401), which together cover a majority of all human races (Kast et al., 1994). Via two different peptide–MHC class I binding assays, several potential CTL epitopes have been identified (Kast et al., 1993a, 1994). As explained before, in order to be presented at the cell surface as a CTL epitope, peptides are subjected to selection criteria of which binding to

MHC class I is only one. For the HLA-A*0201 allele it was sorted out which of the A*0201-binding peptides are naturally presented on HPV16-expressing tumor cells. To that end, CTL clones were induced from HLA-A*0201$^+$ donor peripheral lymphocytes against each of the HLA-A*0201-binding peptides. Subsequently the CTL clones induced were analysed for their ability to lyse specifically HLA-A*0201$^+$ HPV16-expressing tumor cells. So far we have identified three naturally processed CTL epitopes (Ressing et al., unpublished data), two of which will be used in a phase I clinical trial to induce or boost HPV16 E7-specific CTL in cervical cancer patients.

HPV 6 and 11 are commonly found in benign proliferations such as genital and laryngeal warts (De Villiers, 1989), lesions which sometimes regress spontaneously and are relatively easy to monitor. For this reason, Davies and colleagues started looking at the presence of CTL epitopes on HPV6 and HPV11 E7. By using the lymphocytes of peripheral blood from healthy donors, which were stimulated in vitro with peptide-loaded dendritic cell-enriched autologous fractions from the same peripheral blood sample, CTL could be generated specific for a naturally processed HPV11 E7-encoded peptide (Tarpey et al., 1994). It will now be possible to analyse the natural CTL response against this peptide in patients with warts that spontaneously regressed.

# ■ PROSPECTS OF CTL-BASED IMMUNOTHERAPY AGAINST (VIRUS-INDUCED) CANCER IN HUMANS

The observations concerning impairment of virus-induced tumor formation in mice, either via adoptive CTL transfer or via CTL epitope-containing peptide vaccination, have opened up a whole new area of research. As discussed above, the first studies to identify CTL epitopes encoded by viral oncoproteins involved in human cancer are being undertaken. Several problems still have to be dealt with in order to make these approaches in the human situation just as successful as in the syngeneic mouse models. Recently, adoptive transfer of cytomegalovirus-specific CTL clones restored viral immunity in immunodeficient bone-marrow transplant recipients (Ridell et al., 1992). However, a crucial factor in the success of this experiment is probably the fact that the recipients were immunosuppressed. If they were not, because of MHC polymorphism, the transferred CTL would have been immediately rejected by the recipient's immune response against allo-antigens expressed on the T cells transferred. This means that, in order to make adoptive transfer applicable, either the cancer patient needs to be immunosuppressed (analogous to the Friend MuLV model), or autologous CTL have to be used. Another problem of adoptive transfer is that the antigen against which the tumor-specific CTL are directed has to be known. Only then can APC be generated which optimally stimulate CTL growth in vitro. For most cancers, however, tumor-specific antigens are not known to date. An alternative would be to use autologous or HLA-matched tumor cells as APC in vitro. Because of the reasons noted previously and the fact that propagation of large numbers of antigen-specific CTL is laborious and takes time, adoptive transfer of autologous tumor-specific CTL does not seem promising for large-scale use.

In contrast to adoptive transfer, peptide vaccination seems fast, cheap, and simple. Crucial for this approach is that more tumor-specific antigens have to be identified and peptide CTL epitopes derived thereof. One of the major drawbacks of peptide vaccination could be MHC polymorphism. To deal with this problem, it is necessary to identify several CTL epitopes on one tumor-specific protein that are recognized by CTL in the context of different MHC class I molecules. A well-chosen combination of peptides and MHC class I alleles could cover a large part of the population. The choice for peptides to use in such a vaccine may become less complicated if we learn more about HLA class I supertypes, such as recently found for HLA-A*0201-like molecules (A. Sette, personal communication). Still there is a fair risk that certain people cannot be immunized successfully against particular tumor antigens because they are nonresponders.

A way to overcome the need to identify CTL epitope-bearing peptides for all possible MHC class I haplotypes could be to immunize with whole protein instead of a peptide, and let the host immune response choose its own peptide(s) to mount a CTL response against. However, this approach often skews the response towards one single epitope, which increases the chance of antigen-loss variants occurring. An alternative would be to use heat shock proteins isolated from tumor cells, which carry all sorts of tumor cell-specific peptides (Srivastava et al., 1994). Because they are nonpolymorphic, these isolates could be used for vaccination of a heterogeneous population. Tumor protection induced in this way has already been shown to be successful in an animal model (Udono & Srivastava, 1993). Another great advantage of this approach would be that tumor-specific antigens do not need to be identified.

To date, most peptide vaccines in animals are administered in combination with an adjuvant, for example, IFA. They are expected to work as a depot allowing slow release of the immunogen. Furthermore, they are supposed to induce a local reaction, which provides the proper cytokine environment to attract the right APC for CTL induction. However, the sometimes mutilating inflammation reactions and the unknown long-term side effects of adjuvant use call for an alternative approach in humans. Animal models have now shown that peptides linked to a lipid tail and administered s.c. can induce similar responses as peptide given alone s.c. in IFA (Schild et al., 1991a, 1991b). In general, attention has also to be drawn to possible side effects of vaccinating with CTL epitope-bearing peptides, such as autoimmune reactions and induction of anergy.

A matter which is not carefully looked into is whether peptide vaccination also works in individuals (humans and mice) that already bear tumors. After all, many tumors develop in immunocompetent individuals, suggesting that CTL induction does not take place in the tumor-bearing individual or that the CTL induced are somehow abrogated in their function (Mizoguchi et al., 1992). Furthermore, we need to find answers to tumor immune escape mechanisms, such as down-regulation of MHC expression and the production of local immunosuppressive factors, such as transforming growth factor $\beta$. Therefore, it should be preferred to treat as small as possible tumor volumes, as in the case of minimal residual disease after debulking.

In the case of virus-induced cancers, it should be possible to interfere at an early stage before malignant transformation occurs. For instance, in the case of 'high-risk' HPV type-induced disease it is possible to detect early virus infection by analyzing cervical smears. Maybe at that early stage one should not monitor the disease further using expensive and laborious techniques, but start trying to induce HPV-specific CTL responses instead, by means of vaccination. At this stage the infected cells are supposedly (still) antigenic. Reassuring in this case is the observation that cervical dysplastic lesions often disappear after biopsies have been taken, suggesting that the local inflammation induced activates the immune system (compare with the adjuvant effect). Since we have the possibility to detect the disease so early, we should not wait for the disease to progress and lose its sensitivity for CTL by means of down-regulation of MHC class I expression (Connor & Stern, 1990; Cromme et al., 1994) or other immune escape mechanisms. In countries where cervical disease is not monitored, or even in general, it might be possible to immunize women before they become sexually active. Before entering this kind of program, more knowledge has to be obtained about the advantages and disadvantages of CTL epitope-containing peptide vaccinations in humans. Therefore, the studies that are now underway will be crucial for further development of CTL-based specific immunotherapy of cancer.

## REFERENCES

Anderson J.L., Martin R.G., Chang C., Mora P.T. & Livingston D.M. (1977) Nuclear preparations of SV40-transformed cells contain tumor-specific transplantation antigen activity. *Virology*, **76**, 420–6.

Anderson M.S. & Miller J. (1992) Invariant chain can function as a chaperone protein for MHC Class II molecules. *Proceedings of the National Academy of Sciences USA*, **89**, 2282–6.

Anderson R.W., Tevethia M.J., Kalderon D., Smith A.E. & Tevethia S.S. (1988) Fine mapping of two distinct sites on SV40 T antigen reactive with SV40 specific CTL clones using SV40 deletion mutants. *Journal of Virology*, **62**, 285–93.

Arnold D., Driscoll J., Androlewicz M., Hughes E., Cresswell P. & Spies T. (1992) Proteasome subunits encoded in the MHC are not generally required for the processing of peptides bound by MHC Class I molecules. *Nature (London)*, **360**, 171–4.

Baker C.J., Phelps W.C., Lindgren V., Braun M.J., Gonda M.A. & Howley P.M. (1987) Structural and transcriptional analysis of HPV 16 sequences in cervical carcinoma cell lines. *Journal of Virology*, **61**, 962–70.

Bernards R., Schrier P.I., Houweling A. et al. (1983) Tumorigenicity of cells transformed by adenovirus type 12 by evasion of T-cell immunity. *Nature (London)*, **305**, 776–9.

Bertoletti A., Chisari F.V., Penna A. et al. (1993) Definition of a minimal cytotoxic T cell epitope within the hepatitis B virus nucleocapsid protein. *Journal of Virology*, **67**, 2376–84.

Bertoletti A., Ferrari C., Fiaccadori F. et al. (1991) HLA Class I-restricted human cytotoxic T cells recognize endogenously synthesized hepatitis B virus nucleocapsid antigen. *Proceedings of the National Academy of Sciences USA*, **88**, 10445–50.

Bertoletti A., Sette A., Chisari F.V. et al. (1994) Natural variants of cytotoxic epitopes are T-cell receptor antagonists for antiviral cytotoxic T cells. *Nature (London)*, **369**, 407–10.

Bjorkman P.J., Saper M.A., Samraoui B., Bennett W.S., Strominger J.L. & Wiley D.C. (1987a) Structure of the human Class I histocompatibility antigen, HLA-A2. *Nature (London)*, **329**, 506–12.

Bjorkman P.J., Saper M.A., Samrauoi B., Benet W.S., Strominger J.L. & Wiley D.C. (1987b) The foreign antigen binding site and T cell recognition regions of Class I histocompatibility antigens. *Nature (London)*, **329**, 512–18.

Brown J.H., Jardetsky T.S., Gorga J.C. et al. (1993) Three dimensional structure of the human Class II histocompatibility antigen HLA-DR1. *Nature (London)*, **364**, 33–40.

Burrows S., Sculley T., Misko I., Schmidt C. & Moss D. (1990) An Epstein–Barr virus specific T cell epitope in EBNA-3. *Journal of Experimental Medicine*, **171**, 345–50.

Chang C., Martin R.G., Livingston D.M., Luborsky S.W., Hu C. & Mors P.T. (1979) Relation between T-antigen and tumor-specific transplantation antigen in SV40-transformed cells. *Journal of Virology*, **29**, 69–76.

Chen L., Ashe S., Brady W.A. et al. (1992a) Costimulation of antitumor immunity by the B7 counterreceptor for the T lymphocyte molecules CD28 and CTLA-4. *Cell*, **71**, 1093–102.

Chen L., Mizano M.T., Singhal M.C. et al. (1992b) Induction of cytotoxic T cells specific for a syngeneic tumor expressing the E6 oncoprotein of human Papillomavirus type 16. *Journal of Immunology*, **148**, 2617–21.

Chen L., Thomas E.K., Hu S.L., Hellström I. & Hellström K.E. (1991) Human Papillomavirus type 16 nucleoprotein E7 is a tumor rejection antigen. *Proceedings of the National Academy of Sciences USA*, **88**, 110–14.

Connor M.E. & Stern P.L. (1990) Loss of MHC Class I expression in cervical carcinomas. *International Journal of Cancer*, **46**, 1029–37.

Cromme F.V., Airey J., Heemels M.T. et al. (1994) Loss of transporter protein, encoded by the TAP-1 gene, is highly correlated with loss of HLA expression in cervical carcinomas. *Journal of Experimental Medicine*, **179**, 335–40.

Crook T., Morgenstern J.P., Crawford L. & Banks L. (1989) Continued expression of HPV16 E7 is required for maintenance of the transformed phenotype of cells co-transfected with HPV16 plus EJ ras. *EMBO Journal*, **8**, 513–20.

Crook T., Tidy J.A. & Vousden K.H. (1992) Degradation of p53 can be targeted by HPV E6 sequences distinct from those required for p53 binding and transactivation. *Cell*, **67**, 547–56.

Dalianis T., Magnussen G., Ito Y. & Klein G. (1982) Immunization against the polyoma virus induced tumor specific transplantation antigen by early region mutants of the virus. *Journal of Virology*, **43**, 772–77.

De Campos-Lima P.O., Gavioli R., Zhang Q.J. et al. (1993) HLA-A11 epitope loss isolates of EBV from a highly A11$^+$ population. *Science*, **260**, 98–100.

De Villiers E.M. (1989) Heterogeneity of the human Papillomavirus group. *Journal of Virology*, **63**, 4898–909

Deckhut A.M., Lippolis J.D. & Tevethia S.S. (1992) Comparative analysis of core amino acid residues of H-2D$^b$-restricted cytotoxic T-lymphocyte recognition epitopes in simian virus 40 T antigen. *Journal of Virology*, **66**, 440–7.

Falk K., Rötschke O., Stevenovic S., Jung G. & Rammensee H.-G. (1991) Allele-specific motifs revealed by sequencing of self-peptides eluted from MHC molecules. *Nature (London)*, **351**, 290–6.

Feltkamp M.C.W., Smits H.L., Vierboom M.P.M. et al. (1993) Vaccination with cytotoxic T lymphocyte epitope-containing peptide protects against a tumor induced by human Papillomavirus type 16-transformed cells. *European Journal of Immunology*, **23**, 2242–9.

Feltkamp M.C.W., Vierboom M.P.M., Ter Schegget J., Melief C.J.M. & Kast W.M. (1994b) Fine char .cterization of the HPV16 E7 49–57 tumor protective cytotoxic T cell epitope 'RAHYNIVTF.' In M.A. Stanley (ed.) *Immunology of human papillomaviruses*, pp. 275–281. New York, Plenum Press.

Feltkamp M.C.W., Vierboom M.P.M., Kast W.M. & Melief C.J.M. (1994a) Efficient MHC Class I–peptide binding is required but does not ensure MHC Class I-restricted immunogenicity. *Molecular Immunology*, **31**, 1391–1401.

Finn O. (1993) Tumor-rejection antigens recognized by T lymphocytes. *Current Opinion in Immunology*, **5**, 701–8.

Gavioli R., De Campos-Lima P.O., Kurrila M.G., Kieff E., Klein E. & Massuci M.G. (1992) Recognition of the EBV encoded nuclear antigens EBNA-4 and -6 by HLA-A11 restricted cytotoxic T cells. Implications for the down regulation of HLA-A11 in Burkitt's lymphoma. *Proceedings of the National Academy of Sciences USA*, **89**, 5862–6.

Gavioli R., Kurilla M., Po D.C.-L. et al. (1993) Multiple HLA-A11-restricted CTL epitopes of different immunogenicity in the EBV encoded nuclear antigen EBNA-4. *Journal of Virology*, **67**, 1572–8.

Germain R. & Margulies D.H. (1993) The biochemistry and cell biology of antigen processing and presentation. *Annual Review of Immunology*, **11**, 403–50.

Germain R.N. (1994) MHC-dependent antigen processing and peptide presentation: providing ligands for T lymphocyte activation. *Cell*, **76**, 287–99.

Greenberg P.D., Klarnet J.P., Kern D.E. & Cheever M.A. (1988) Therapy of disseminated tumours by adoptive transfer of specifically immune T-cells. *Progress in Experimental Tumor Research*, **32**, 104–27.

Henderson R.A., Michel H., Sakaguchi K. et al. (1992) HLA-A2.1 associated peptides from a mutant cell line: a second pathway of antigen presentation. *Science*, **255**, 1264–6.

Hunt D.F., Henderson R.A., Shabanowitz J. et al. (1992) Characterization of peptides bound to the Class I MHC molecule HLA-A2.1 by mass spectrometry. *Science*, **255**, 1261–3.

Jacobson S., Shida H., McFarlin D.E., Fauci A.S. & Koenig S. (1990) Circulating CD8+ cytotoxic T cells specific for HTLV-1 pX in patients with HTLV-1 associated neurological disease. *Nature (London)*, **348**, 245–8.

Jorgensen J.L., Esser U., Fazekas B., Reay P.A. & Davis M.M. (1992) Mapping T cell receptor contacts by variant peptide immunization of single strain transgenics. *Nature (London)*, **355**, 224–30.

Kägi D., Ledermann B., Bürki K. et al. (1994) Cytoxicity mediated by T cells and natural killer cells is greatly impaired in perforin-deficient mice. *Nature (London)*, **369**, 31–7.

Kanda T., Wanatabe S. & Yoshiike K. (1988) Immortalization of primary rat cells by HPV type 16 subgenomic DNA fragments controlled by the SV40 promotor. *Virology*, **165**, 321–5.

Kannagi M., Matsushita S., Shida H. & Harada S. (1994) Cytotoxic T cell response and expression of the target antigen in HTLV-1 infection. *Leukemia*, **8**, 54–9.

Kast W.M., Brandt R.M.P., Drijfhout J.W. & Melief C.J.M. (1993a) Human leukocyte antigen-A2.1 restricted candidate cytotoxic T lymphocyte epitopes of human Papillomavirus type 16 E6 and E7 proteins identified by using the processing-defective human cell line T2. *Journal of Immunotherapy*, **14**, 115–20.

Kast W.M., Brandt R.M.P. & Melief C.J.M. (1993b) Strict peptide length is not required for the induction of cytotoxic T lymphocyte-mediated antiviral protection by peptide vaccination. *European Journal of Immunology*, **23**, 1189–92.

Kast W.M., Brandt R.M.P., Sidney J. et al. (1994) Role of HLA-A motifs in identification of potential CTL epitopes in human Papillomavirus type 16 E6 and E7 proteins. *Journal of Immunology*, **152**, 3904–12.

Kast W.M. & Melief C.J.M. (1991) Fine peptide specificity of cytotoxic T lymphocytes against Adenovirus-induced tumours and peptide-MHC binding. *International Journal of Cancer*, **6** (Suppl.), 90–4.

Kast W.M., Offringa R., Peters P.J. et al. (1989) Eradication of Adenovirus E1-induced tumors by E1A-specific cytotoxic T lymphocytes. *Cell*, **59**, 603–14.

Kern D.E., Klarnet J.P., Jensen M.C.V. & Greenberg P.D. (1986) Requirement for recognition of Class II molecules and processed tumour antigen for optimal generation of syngeneic tumour-specific Class-I-restricted CTL. *Journal of Immunology*, **136**, 4303–10.

Khanna R., Borrows S., Kurilla M. et al. (1992) Localisation of EBV cytotoxic T cells epitopes using recombinant vaccinia: implications for vaccine development. *Journal of Experimental Medicine*, **176**, 169–76.

Kim C.M., Koike K., Saito I., Miyumura T. & Jay G. (1991) HBx gene of hepatitus B virus induces liver cancer in transgenic mice. *Nature (London)*, **351**, 317–20.

Klarnet J.P., Kern D.E., Okunu K., Holt C., Lilly F. & Greenberg P.D. (1989) FBL-reactive CD8+ cytotoxic and CD4+ helper T lymphocytes recognize distinct Friend leukemia virus-encoded antigens. *Journal of Experimental Medicine*, **169**, 457–67.

Kleijmeer M.J., Kelly A., Geuze H.J., Slot J.W., Townsend A. & Trowsdale J. (1992) Location of the MHC-encoded transporters in the enoplasmatic reticulum and cis-Golgi. *Nature (London)*, **357**, 342–4.

Klein G. (1991) Immunovirology of transforming viruses. *Current Opinion in Immunology*, 3, 665–73.

Koenig S., Woods R.M., Brewah Y.A. et al. (1993) Characterization of MHC Class I restricted CTL responses to tax in HTLV-1 infected patients with neurological disease. *Journal of Immunology*, 151, 3874–83.

Koeppen H., Acena M., Drolet A., Rowley D.A. & Schreiber H. (1993) Tumors with reduced expression of a cytotoxic T cell recognized antigen lack immunogenicity but retain sensitivity to lysis by cytoxtic T cells. *European Journal of Immunology*, 23, 2770–6.

Levine A.J. (1990) The p53 protein and its interaction with the oncogene products of the small DNA tumor viruses. *Virology*, 177, 419–26.

Lill N.L., Tevethia J., Hendrickson W.G. & Tevethia S.S. (1992) Cytotoxic T lymphocytes (CTL) against a transforming gene product select for transformed cells with point mutations within sequences encoding CTL recognition epitopes. *Journal of Experimental Medicine*, 176, 449–57.

Ljunggren H.-G., Stam N.J., Öhlen C. et al. (1990) Empty MHC Class I molecules come out in the cold. *Nature (London)*, 346, 476–80.

Lopez de Castro J.A., Barbosa J.A., Krangel M.S., Biro P.A. & Strominger J.L. (1985) Structural analysis of the functional sites of Class I HLA antigens. *Immunological Reviews*, 85, 149–68.

Lotteau V., Teyton L., Peleraux A. et al. (1990) Intracellular transport of MHC Class II molecules directed by the invariant chain. *Nature (London)*, 348, 600–5.

Madden D.R., Gorga J.C., Strominger J.L. & Wiley D.C. (1992) The three-dimensional structure of HLA-B27 at 2.1 Å resolution suggests a general mechanism for tight peptide binding to MHC. *Cell*, 70, 1035–48.

Masucci M.G. (1993) Viral immunopathology of human tumors. *Current Opinion in Immunology*, 5, 693–700.

Matsumara M., Fremont D.H., Peterson P.A. & Wilson I.A. (1992) Emerging principle for the recognition of peptide antigens by MHC Class I molecules. *Science*, 257, 927–34.

Melief C.J.M. (1992) Tumor eradication by adoptive transfer of cytotoxic T lymphocytes. *Advances in Cancer Research*, 58, 143–75.

Melief C.J.M. & Kast W.M. (1993) Potential immunogenicity of oncogene and tumor suppressor gene products. *Current Opinion in Immunology*, 5, 709–13.

Michalek M.T., Grant E.P., Gramm C., Goldberg A.L. & Rock K.L. (1993) A role for the ubiquitin-dependent proteolytic pathway in MHC Class I-restricted antigen presentation. *Nature (London)*, 363, 552–54.

Mietz J.A., Unger T., Huibregtse J.M. & Howley P.M. (1992) Transcriptional transactivation function of wild type p53 is inhibited by SV40 large T antigen and by HPV16 E6 oncoprotein. *EMBO Journal*, 11, 5013–20.

Mizoguchi H., O'Shea J.J., Longo D.L., Loeffler C.M., McVicar D.W. & Ochoa A.C. (1992) Alterations in the signal transduction molecules in T lymphocytes from tumor-bearing mice. *Science*, 258, 1795–8.

Momburg F., Neefjes J.J. & Hämmerling G.J. (1994c) Peptide selection MHC-encoded TAP transporters. *Current Opinion in Immunology*, 6, 32–7.

Momburg F., Ortiz-Navarette V., Neefjes J. et al. (1992) Proteasome subunits encoded by the MHC are not essential for antigen processing. *Nature (London)*, 360, 174–7.

Momburg F., Roelse J., Hämmerling G.J. & Neefjes J.J. (1994a) Peptide size selection by the MHC-encoded peptide transporter. *Journal of Experimental Medicine*, 179, 1613–23.

Momburg F.M., Roelse J., Howard G.W. et al. (1994b) Selectivity of MHC-encoded peptide transporters from human, mouse and rat. *Nature (London)*, 367, 648–52.

Moorthy R.K. & Thorley-Lawson D.A. (1993) All three domains of the EBV-encoded latent membrane protein LMP-1 are required for transformation of rat-1 fibroblasts. *Journal of Virology*, 67, 1638–46.

Nayersina R., Fowler P., Guihot G. et al. (1993) HLA-A2 restricted cytotoxic T lymphocyte responses to multiple hepatitis B surface antigen epitopes during hepatitis B virus infection. *Journal of Immunology*, 150, 4659–66.

Neefjes J.J., Hämmerling G.J. & Momburg F. (1993a) Folding and assembly of MHC Class I heterodimers in the endoplasmatic reticulum of intact cells precedes the binding of peptide. *Journal of Experimental Medicine*, 178, 1971–80.

Neefjes J.J. & Momburg F. (1993) Cell biology of antigen presentation. *Current Opinion in Immunology*, 5, 27–34.

Neefjes J.J., Momburg F. & Hämmerling G.J. (1993b) Selective and ATP-dependent translocation of peptides by the MHC-encoded transporter. *Science*, 261, 769–71.

Neisig A., Roelse J., Sijts E.J.A.M. et al. (1995) Major differences in TAP-dependent translocation of MHC Class I presentable peptides and the effect of flanking sequences. *Journal of Immunology*, 154, 1273–9.

Nossal G.J.V. (1994) Negative selection of lymphocytes. *Cell*, 76, 229–39.

Orr H.T., Lopez de Castro J.A., Lancet D.S. & Strominger J.L. (1979) Complete amino acid sequence of a papain-solubilized human histocompatibility antigen; HLA-B7.2 sequence determination and search for homologies. *Biochemistry*, 18, 5711–20.

Pamer E.G., Harty J.T. & Bevan M.J. (1991) Precise prediction of a dominant Class I MHC restricted epitope of Listeria monocytogenes. *Nature (London)*, 353, 852–5.

Pardoll D.M. (1994) A new look for the 1990s. *Nature (London)*, 369, 357–8.

Parker C.E., Daenke S., Nightingale S. & Bangham C.R. (1992) Activated, HTLV-1-specific CTL are found in healthy seropositives as well as in patients with tropical spastic paresis. *Virology*, 188, 628–36.

Parkin D.M., Pisani P. & Ferlay J. (1993) Estimates of the worldwide incidence of eighteen major cancers in 1985. *International Journal of Cancer*, 54, 594–606.

Peters P.J., Neefjes J.J., Orschot V., Ploegh H.L. & Geuze H.J. (1991) Segregation of MHC Class II molecules from MHC Class I molecules in the Golgi complex for transport to lysosomal compartments. *Nature (London)*, 349, 669–76.

Phelps W.C., Yee C.L., Münger K. & Howley P.M. (1988) The human papillomavirus type 16 E7 gene encodes transactivation and transformation functions similar to those of adenovirus. *Cell*, 53, 539–47.

Powis S.J., Townsend A.R.M., Deverson E.V. et al. (1991) Restoration of antigen presentation to the mutant cell line RMA-S by an MHC-linked transporter. *Nature (London)*, 354, 528–31.

Rajagopalan S. & Brenner M.B. (1994) Calnexin retains unassembled MHC Class I free heavy chains in the endoplasmic reticulum. *Journal of Experimental Medicine*, 180, 407–12.

Rammensee H.-G., Falk K. & Rötschke O. (1993) Peptides naturally presented by MHC Class I molecules. *Annual Review of Immunology*, 11, 213–44.

Ramqvist T., Reinholdsson G., Carlqvist M., Bergman T. & Dalianis T. (1989) A single peptide derived from the sequence common to polyoma small and middle T-antigen induces immunity against polyoma tumors. *Virology*, 172, 359–62.

Reinholdsson G., Franksson L., Dalianis T. & Ljunggren H.G. (1993) Identification of H-2K$^b$-, D$^b$-, and D$^d$-binding peptides derived from amino acid sequences of polyoma virus T antigens. *International Journal of Cancer*, **54**, 992–5.

Reinholdsson-Ljunggren G., Ramqvist T., Åhrlund-Richter L. & Dalianis T. (1992) Immunization against polyoma tumors with synthetic peptides derived from the sequences of middle- and large-T antigens. *International Journal of Cancer*, **50**, 142–6.

Ridell S.R., Wantabe K.S., Goodrich J.M., Li C.R., Agha M.E. & Greenberg P.D. (1992) Restoration of viral immunity in immunodeficient humans by the adoptive transfer of T cell clones. *Science*, **257**, 238–41.

Roche P.A. & Cresswell P. (1990) Invariant chain association with HLA-DR molecules inhibits immunogenic peptide binding. *Nature*, **345**, 615–8.

Rötschke O. & Falk K. (1991) Naturally-occurring peptide antigens derived from the MHC Class-I restricted processing pathway. *Immunology Today*, **12**, 447–55.

Rötschke O., Falk K., Deres K. et al. (1990) Isolation and analysis of naturally processed viral peptides as recognized by cytotoxic T cells. *Nature (London)*, **348**, 252–4.

Rötschke O., Falk K., Stevanovic S., Jung G., Walden P. & Rammensee H.-G. (1991) Exact prediction of a natural T cell epitope. *European Journal of Immunology*, **21**, 2891–4.

Ruppert J., Sidney J., Cells E., Kubo R.T., Grey H.M. & Sette A. (1993) Prominent role of secondary anchor residues in peptide binding to HLA-A2.1 molecules. *Cell*, **74**, 929–37.

Sadnikova E., Zhu X., Collins S. et al. (1994) Limitations of predictive motifs revealed by cytotoxic T lymphocyte epitope mapping of the human papillomavirus E7 protein. *International Immunology*, **6**, 289–96.

Scheffner M., Werness B., Huibregtse J.M., Levine A. & Howley P.M. (1990) The E6 oncoprotein encoded by HPV16 and 18 promotes degradation of p53. *Cell*, **63**, 1129–36.

Schild H., Deres K., Wiesmuller K.-H., Jung G. & Rammensee H.-G. (1991a) Efficiency of peptides and lipopeptides for in vivo priming virus-specific cytotoxic T cells. *European Journal of Immunology*, **21**, 2649–54.

Schild H., Norda M., Deres K. et al. (1991b) Fine specificity of cytotoxic T lymphocytes primed in vivo either with virus or synthetic lipopetide vaccine or primed in vitro with peptide. *Journal of Experimental Medicine*, **174**, 1665–8.

Schreier A.A. & Gruber J. (1990) Viral T-antigen interactions with cellular proto-oncogene and anti-oncogene products. *Journal of the National Cancer Institute*, **82**, 354–60.

Schrier P.I., Bernards R., Vaessen R., Houweling R.T.M.J. & Van der Eb A.J. (1983) Expression of Class I MHC antigens switched off by highly oncogenic adenovirus 12 in transformed rat cells. *Nature (London)*, **305**, 771–5.

Schumacher T.N.M., De Bruijn M.L.H., Vernie L.N. et al. (1991) Peptide selection by MHC Class I molecules. *Nature (London)*, **350**, 703–6.

Schumacher T.N.M., Kantesaria D.V., Heemels M.-T. et al. (1994) Peptide length and sequence specificity of the mouse TAP1/TAP2 translocator. *Journal of Experimental Medicine*, **179**, 533–40.

Shirakata Y., Kawada M., Fuyiki Y. et al. (1989) The X gene of HBV induces growth stimulation and tumorigenic transformation of mouse NIH3T3 cells. *Japanese Journal of Cancer Research*, **80**, 617–21.

Shortman K.D. (1992) Cellular aspects of early T cell development. *Current Opinion in Immunology*, **4**, 140–6.

Sijts E.J.A.M., Ossendorp F., Mengedé E.A.M., Van den Elsen P.J. & Melief C.J.M. (1994) An immunodominant MCF murine leukemia virus encoded CTL epitope identified by its MHC Class I-binding motif, explains MuLV type specificity of MCF-directed CTL. *Journal of Immunology*, **152**, 106–16.

Smotkin D. & Wettstein F.O. (1986) Transcription of HPV16 early genes in a cervical cancer and a cervical cancer derived cell line, and the identification of the E7 protein. *Proceedings of the National Academy of Sciences USA*, **83**, 4680–6.

Srivastava P.K., Udono H., Blanchere N.E. & Li Z. (1994) Heat shock proteins transfer peptides during processing and CTL priming. *Immunogenetics*, **39**, 93–8.

Stauss H.J., Davies H., Sadnikova E., Chain B., Horowitz N. & Sinclair C. (1992) Induction of cytotoxic T lymphocytes with peptides in vitro: identification of candidate T-cell epitopes in human Papillomavirus. *Proceedings of the National Academy of Sciences USA*, **89**, 7871–5.

Storey A., Pim D., Murray A., Osborn K., Banks L. & Crawford L. (1988) Comparison of the in vitro transforming activities of human papillomavirus types. *EMBO Journal*, **7**, 1815–20.

Tanaka Y., Anderson R.W., Lee Maloy W. & Tevethia S.S. (1989) Localization of an immunorecessive epitope on SV40 T antigen by H-2D$^b$-restricted cytotoxic T-lymphocyte clones and a synthetic peptide. *Virology*, **171**, 205–13.

Tanaka Y., Tevethia M.J., Kalderon D., Smith A.E. & Tevethia S.S. (1988) Clustering of antigenic sites recognized by CTL clones in the amino terminal half of SV40 T antigen. *Virology*, **162**, 427–34.

Tanaka Y. & Tevethia S.S. (1988) In vitro selection of SV40 T antigen epitope loss variants by site-specific cytotoxic T lymphocyte clones. *Journal of Immunology*, **140**, 4348–54.

Tarpey I., Stacey S., Hickling J. et al. (1994) Human cytotoxic T lymphocytes stimulated by endogeneously processed HPV11 E7 recognize a peptide containing a HLA-A2 (HLA-A*0201) motif. *Immunology*, **81**, 222–7.

Townsend A.R.M., Rothbard J., Gotch F.M. et al. (1986) The epitopes of Influenza Nucleoprotein recognized by cytotoxic T lymphocytes can be defined by short synthetic peptides. *Cell*, **44**, 959–68.

Townsend S.E. & Alison J.P. (1993) Tumor rejection after direct costimulation of CD8$^+$ T cells by B7-transfected melanoma cells. *Science*, **259**, 368–70.

Udono H. & Srivastava P.K. (1993) Heat shock protein 70-associated peptide elicit cancer-specific immunity. *Journal of Experimental Medicine*, **178**, 1391–6.

Van Bleek G.M. & Nathanson S.G. (1990) Isolation of an endogenously processed immunodominant viral peptide from the H-2K$^b$ molecule. *Nature (London)*, **348**, 213–26.

Van den Brule A.J.C., Walboomers J.M.M., Du Maine M., Kenemans P. & Meijer C.J.L.M. (1991) Difference in prevalence of HPV genotyes in cytomorphologically normal cervical smears is associated with a history of cervical intraepithelial neoplasia. *International Journal of Cancer*, **48**, 404–8.

Van Kaer L., Ashton-Rickardt P.G., Ploegh H.L. & Tonegawa S. (1992) TAP1 mutant mice are deficient in antigen presentation, surface Class I molecules, and CD4$^-$ 8$^+$ T cells. *Cell*, **71**, 1205–14.

Vitiello A., Ishioka G., Grey H.M. et al. (1995) Development of a lipopeptide-based therapeutic vaccine to treat chronic HBV infection: I. Induction of a primary CTL response in man. *Journal of Clinical Investigation*, **95**, 341–5.

Vogelstein B. & Kinzler R.W. (1992) p53 function and dysfunction. *Cell*, **70**, 523–6.

Von Boehmer H. (1994) Positive selection of lymphocytes. *Cell*, **76**, 219–28.

Vousden K. (1993) Interactions of human papillomavirus transforming proteins with the products of tumor suppressor genes. *FASEB Journal*, **7**, 872–9.

Vousden, K.H. & Jat P.S. (1989) Functional similarity between HPV16 E7, SV40 large T and adenovirus E1A proteins. *Oncogene*, **4**, 153–8.

Weinberg R.A. (1991) Tumor suppressor genes. *Science*, **254**, 1138–46.

Wilson J.B., Weinberg W., Johnson R., Yuspa S. & Levine A. (1990) Expression of the BNLF-1 oncogene of EBV in the skin of transgenic mice induces hyperplasia and aberrant expression of keratin 6. *Cell*, **61**, 1315–27.

Zinkernagel R.M. & Doherty P.C. (1974) Restriction of in vitro T cell mediated cytotoxicity in lymphocytic choriomeningitis within a syngeneic or allogeneic system. *Nature (London)*, **284**, 701–2.

Zur Hausen H. (1991) Viruses in human cancer. *Science*, **254**, 1167–72.

# 7

## Cellular Oncogenes for Tumour Immunity: Immunotherapy

### HANS J. STAUSS AND A. MARIA DAHL

## ■ INTRODUCTION

T lymphocyte responses against transformed cells can mediate tumour rejection in many experimental situations (Schreiber et al., 1988; Kast et al., 1989; Schreiber, 1992; Melief & Kast, 1993). The antigens recognized by tumour-specific T lymphocytes have remained elusive for a long time. The search for these antigens had initially focused on molecules expressed on the cell surface, since it seemed unlikely that T cells could recognize molecules that are expressed exclusively inside cells. The discovery of the mechanism of T cell recognition (Zinkernagel & Doherty, 1979; Townsend et al., 1986) and antigen presentation by MHC molecules (Bjorkman et al., 1987a, 1987b; Falk et al., 1991) has revolutionized the field of tumour immunology, because it became clear that T cells can recognize any cellular protein, including molecules present in the cytosol (Townsend et al., 1986; Townsend & Bodmer, 1989), the nucleus (Tevethia et al., 1983; O'Connell & Gooding, 1984) and even molecules whose expression is restricted to mitochondria (Fischer et al., 1991). There seems to be no intracellular hiding place for a protein to escape immune recognition. These findings have initiated a reevaluation of the immunogenicity of tumours, with the search for tumour antigens focusing on proteins that are expressed in cancers irrespective of the cellular compartment where they are located.

Two main groups of tumour antigens can be distinguished, with members of the first group being truly tumour specific, while members of the other group are also found in normal cells. Tumours associated with viral infection or mutational changes in cellular genes express tumour-specific antigens that are not found in normal cells. On the other hand, structurally unaltered proteins expressed at high levels in tumour cells can also be classified as tumour-associated antigens. The recently discovered human melanoma antigens belong to this latter group, and the demonstration of cytotoxic T lymphocytes (CTL) specific for these antigens shows that they can provoke immune responses (van der Bruggen et al., 1991; Brichard et al., 1993; Bakker et al., 1994; Coulie et al., 1994; Cox et al., 1994; Gaugler et al., 1994; Kawakami et al., 1994a). While most of the identified melanoma antigens represent tumour-associated differentiation antigens unrelated to transformation, there are also proteins encoded by cellular oncogenes whose overexpression is probably linked to transformation (Table 7.1). Since expression of these oncogene-encoded proteins may be required for acquisition and maintenance of a transformed phenotype, they represent promising targets for immune responses against cancers.

In this chapter, we will consider T helper ($T_H$) and CTL responses to both mutated and overexpressed proteins encoded by oncogenes. Immune responses to unaltered proteins may not violate the concept of self-tolerance, since distinct peptide epitopes may be involved in the establishment of self-tolerance and in the activation of autoreactive T lymphocytes. We will consider the likelihood that T cells may specifically recognize mutated oncogenic proteins. One prerequisite for T cell recognition of mutant proteins is that major histocompatibility complex (MHC) molecules display peptides containing mutated amino-acid residues. This, in turn, requires that appropriate peptides are produced by natural antigen processing and that peptides can bind to MHC molecules. Activation of $T_H$ and CTL by tumours in vivo is highly complex and may not occur at early stages of a neoplastic disease. Antigen-specific vaccination may establish T cell immunity, which may show prophylactic effects against development of overt neoplastic disease.

# ■ BENEFICIAL AUTOIMMUNITY AGAINST TRANSFORMED CELLS

Melanoma patients frequently contain CTL, which show lytic activity against autologous melanoma cells in vitro (Anichini, Fossati & Parmiani, 1985; De Vries & Spits, 1984; Herin et al., 1987). The first CTL-recognized target antigen to be identified was melanoma associated antigen 1 (MAGE1) (van der Bruggen et al., 1991), and the rapidly expanding family of CTL-recognized melanoma antigens now includes MAGE3, BAGE, GAGE, tyrosinase, MART1 (=melan A), gp100, and its splice variant pMe117 (Brichard et al., 1993; Bakker et al., 1994; Coulie et al., 1994; Cox et al., 1994; Gaugler et al., 1994; Kawakami et al., 1994a; and Chapter 5 in this volume). Significantly, all these antigens are encoded by structurally unaltered genes. Some of these genes (tyrosinase MART1, gp100, pMel17) encode differentiation antigens expressed in normal melanocytes, while the MAGE, BAGE, and GAGE genes are silent in melanocytes, and normally expressed only in cells of the central nervous system and testis. It appears that these self proteins do not induce T cell tolerance

Table 7.1. Overexpression of Oncogene-encoded Proteins in Human Tumours

| Protein | Normal function | Tumours known to express high levels of the protein |
|---|---|---|
| Cyclin D1 | Regulator of the G1-S transition via binding to cyclin dependent kinase | Breast cancer (approx. 20%) (Bartkova et al., 1994a; Buckley et al., 1993; Gillet et al., 1994; Keyomarsi et al., 1994) Colon cancer (20%) (Bartkova et al., 1994b) Some B cell lymphomas [up to 100% in mantle cell (centrocytic) lymphoma] (Jadayel et al., 1994; Rimokh et al., 1994; Yang et al., 1994) Thyroid cancer (parathyroid adenoma) (Motukura et al., 1991; Rosenberg et al., 1993) Liver cancer (11–13%) (Nishida et al., 1994; Zhang et al., 1993) Head and neck cancer (squamous cell carcinoma) (30–60%) (Jares et al., 1994; Lucas et al., 1994) |
| Cyclin E | Regulator of the G1-S transition via binding to cyclin-dependent kinase | Breast cancer (90%, nine patients studied) (Keyomarsi et al., 1994) |
| mdm2 | Nuclear phospho-protein. Inhibits the function of p53 by interaction with the protein | Sarcomas (30–36%) (Oliner et al., 1992; Leach et al., 1993; Cordon-Cardo et al., 1994) Leukaemia (between 42–73%) (Buesoramos et al., 1993) [breast cancer cell lines (Sheikh et al., 1993)] Gliomas (glioblastomas and anaplastic astrocytomas) (10–15%) (Reifenberger et al., 1994) |
| **Receptor tyrosine kinases** | | |
| Epidermal growth factor receptor | Receptor for the epidermal growth factor (TGF-$\alpha$) amphiregulin, heparin-binding EGF, viral growth factors, $\beta$-cellulin | Breast cancer (30–40%) (Perez et al., 1984; Ro et al., 1988; Sainsbury et al., 1987; Klijn & Foekens, 1990) Lung cancer (80%, one study with five patients) (Hunts et al., 1985) Gliomas (Libermann et al., 1985; Wong et al., 1987; Ekstrand et al., 1991) Bladder cancer (70%) (Sauter et al., 1994) Renal cell carcinoma (73%) (Weidner et al., 1990) Head and neck cancer (50% or more, depending on type) (Issing, Wurstrow & Heppt, 1993; Hunts et al., 1985) |
| erb B2 (Her-2/neu) | Receptor belonging to the same family as the EGFR receptor. Ligand not clearly identified | Breast cancer (26%) (Dawkins et al., 1993) Ovarian cancer (20–30%) (Slamon et al., 1989; Berchuck et al., 1990) Stomach cancer (overall 11%) Colorectal cancer (4%) Nonsmall-cell lung cancer (up to 30%) (Lofts & Gullick, 1991) |

*(continued)*

Table 7.1.    (contd.)

| Protein | Normal function | Tumours known to express high levels of the protein |
|---|---|---|
| erb B3 | Receptor belonging to the same family as the EGFR receptor. Ligand unknown | Breast cancer (10–30%) (Lemoine et al., 1992a; Gasparini et al., 1994) Colon cancer (Rajkumar et al., 1993) Cancer of the pancreas (35%) (Lemoine et al., 1992b) |
| Fibroblast growth factor receptor I | Receptor for acidic and basic fibroblast growth factor | Gliomas (100%, five cases) (Morrison et al., 1994; Ueba et al., 1994; Yamaguchi et al., 1994) Pancreatic cancer (adenocarcinoma) (100%, five cases) (Kobrin et al., 1993) Melamona (Natali et al., 1994) Breast cancer (10/82=12%) (Theillet et al., 1993) |
| Insulin-like growth factor-I receptor | Receptor for insulin-like growth factor I, a mitogen | Breast cancer (50–93%) (Foekens et al., 1989; Yee et al., 1989; Papa et al., 1993) Lung cancer (SCLC and squamous cancers) (Macaulay et al., 1988) |
| MET | Receptor for hepatocyte growth factor | Thyroid cancer (Di Renzo et al., 1991) Ovarian cancer (28%) (Di Renzo et al., 1994) |

**Nuclear oncogenes**

| | | |
|---|---|---|
| c-myc | Transcription factor | Breast cancer (6–57%) (Field & Spandidos, 1990) Small-cell lung cancer (20–30%) (Prins et al., 1993) Cervical cancer (30%) (Riou et al., Bourhis et al., 1987) Testicular cancer (Field & Spandidos, 1990) Colon cancer (Field & Spandidos, 1990) Head and neck cancer (Field & Spandidos, 1990) |
| N-myc | Transcription factor | Lung cancer (20%) (Nau et al., 1986) Neuroblastoma (20%) (Prins et al., 1993) |
| L-myc | Transcription factor | Lung cancer (Prins et al., 1993) |

**Proteins involved in the regulation of apoptosis**

| | | |
|---|---|---|
| WT p53 | Tumour suppressor protein, transcription factor can induce apoptosis in response to DNA damage | Gliomas (astrocytomas) (60–80%) (Lang et al., 1994) Head and neck cancer (34%) (Xu et al., 1994) Sarcoma (13/73=17%) (Cordon-Cardo et al., 1994) Acute myeloid leukaemia (69%) (Zhang et al., 1992) |
| bcl-2 | Inhibits apoptosis | Non-Hodgkin's lymphoma (40–80%) (Akagi, Kond & Yoshino, 1994) |

EGF, epidermal growth factor; EGFR, epidermal growth factor receptor; MET, a hepatocyte growth factor receptor.

and that exposure of the immune system to high antigen doses in melanoma patients leads to the stimulation of CTL responses. These CTL can be considered as effector cells of a beneficial autoimmunity against melanoma. Is beneficial autoimmunity a peculiarity of melanoma, or is it a more general principle that might involve immune responses to oncogene-encoded proteins that are expressed at high levels in tumours (Table 7.1)? Since proteins encoded by oncogenes are expressed in many normal tissues, this raises the further question as to whether immune responses against overexpressed antigens in tumour cells are compatible with immunological self-tolerance?

Oncogene products are attractive targets for beneficial autoimmunity because their overexpression may be required for initiation and maintenance of transformation, making it more difficult for tumours to escape immune recognition by down-regulating expression of these target antigens. As shown in Table 7.1, overexpression of cellular oncogenes has been demonstrated in a variety of human cancers. $T_H$ and CTL responses with apparent specificity for overexpressed ErbB2 have been observed in a few patients (see Table 7.3). If most of the known overexpressed oncogene products stimulate T cell responses, this would provide an opportunity for immunotherapy of many human tumours. As opposed to the restricted expression of melanoma antigens, most oncogene products listed in Table 7.1 are widely expressed in normal cells where they serve important regulatory functions. Thus T cell tolerance to these widely expressed proteins may be more profound than tolerance to melanoma antigens. At least two basic mechanisms establish self-tolerance in the T cell compartment. Firstly, expression of self antigens in the thymus usually induces central tolerance by clonal deletion of self-reactive T cells (Lo, 1992). In addition, there are also mechanisms to induce tolerance to self antigens, which are expressed in peripheral tissues only (Ferber et al., 1994; Schönrich et al., 1991, 1994). Several mechanisms have been described to establish peripheral tolerance including peripheral T cell deletion, induction of T cell anergy and down-regulation of T cell receptors (TCR) or T cell accessory molecules. Currently, there is little known about levels of self antigens required for induction of central and peripheral tolerance.

It is most likely that the well-documented phenomenon of immunodominance (Sercarz et al., 1993) not only applies to T cell responses to nonself antigens, but also to tolerance induction by self proteins. The functional units for T cell immunology are not intact proteins but protein-derived peptide fragments, which are presented by MHC molecules. Although one protein may give rise to several MHC/peptide complexes, not all of them are equally efficient in stimulating T lymphocytes. Frequently, T cell responses are directed against immunodominant peptides, whilst subdominant and cryptic peptides do not stimulate detectable responses (Sercarz et al., 1993). The implication for self tolerance is that it is most likely to be defined at the peptide level rather than the protein level. Immunodominant peptides may induce self tolerance, while subdominant and cryptic peptides probably fail to do so. Consequently, tolerance to self proteins may be rather patchy and involve only some immunodominant peptide epitopes but not subdominant peptides. Recent experiments with MHC class II-presented peptides have elegantly demonstrated that immunodominance applies to T cell repertoire selection and tolerance induction. Transgenic mice expressing the hepatitis B virus e antigen were tolerant to an immunodominant peptide epitope but still contained $T_H$ cells specific for a subdominant epitope in the e antigen (Milich et al., 1991). Immunization with peptides corresponding to the subdominant epitope resulted in activation of $T_H$ cells and in the production of 'autoantibodies' against the e antigen. In another study, hen egg lysozyme (HEL) containing well-defined MHC class II-presented dominant and subdominant peptide epitopes was used to generate transgenic mice (Cibotti et al., 1992; Cabaniols et al., 1994). Mice expressing approximately 10 ng/ml blood levels of HEL were tolerant to an immunodominant HEL peptide but still contained auto-reactive $T_H$ cells recognizing subdominant HEL peptides. Deletion of $T_H$ cells recognizing subdominant peptides occurred in transgenic mice expressing high levels of HEL. These experiments strongly imply that induction of self-tolerance requires a threshold concentration of MHC/peptide complexes, with peptides that are below this threshold failing to induce tolerance.

These observations are relevant for T cell responses against self proteins overexpressed in tumours. Responses against these proteins may be directed against subdominant and cryptic peptide epitopes, which did not establish self-tolerance. As a consequence of protein overexpression, subdominant peptides may pass the critical threshold from immunological ignorance to immunological attention, which may lead to activation of autoreactive T lymphocytes. Identification of subdominant peptide epitopes might provide a basis for vaccine-induced stimulation of beneficial autoimmunity against tumours. Although $T_H$ lymphocytes play an important role in the initiation of immune responses, CTL frequently show efficient tumour cell lysis in vitro (Schreiber et al., 1988) and can mediate tumour protection in experimental animals in vivo (Kast et al., 1989). Thus, the following discussion of subdominant peptide epitopes and induction of beneficial autoimmunity will focus on MHC class I-presented peptides.

Assuming that MHC class I-binding affinity is an important factor determining peptide immunogenicity, it is likely that immunodominant peptides bind strongly to class I molecules, while subdominant peptides bind weakly. Since class I binding can easily be measured with synthetic peptides in vitro, this provides an assay to tentatively group strong binding peptides as immunodominant, and weak binders as subdominant. Grouping based on MHC binding is certainly an oversimplification, because the number of MHC/peptide complexes produced in cells expressing relevant proteins endogenously does not only depend on peptide-binding affinities for class I molecules. Intracellular antigen-processing events such as cytosolic protein breakdown by proteasomes, peptide transport by heat shock proteins, and translocation into the endoplasmic reticulum (ER) by TAP (transporter associated with antigen processing) will affect the nature and amount of peptides available in the ER for class I binding (Monaco, 1992). Nevertheless, a grouping based on MHC-binding affinity may be useful because it predicts that candidate immunodominant peptides induce T cell tolerance while candidate subdominant peptides do not. This prediction can be tested experimentally by screening the T cell compartment for the presence of high- or low-avidity CTL. Peptides that induce self-tolerance would be expected to stimulate only low-avidity CTL, since high-avidity CTL have been removed from the T cell compartment during tolerance induction. In contrast, peptides that did not induce self-tolerance would be expected to stimulate high-avidity CTL. Among other factors, avidity is determined by the number of MHC/peptide complexes that are required to trigger CTL lysis. The number of MHC/peptide complexes can be estimated by measuring the threshold peptide concentrations required for CTL lysis and the threshold concentrations required for MHC binding. The ratio of these two concentrations [CTL recognition]/[MHC binding] can serve as a measure of the relative number of MHC/peptide complexes that are available for CTL recognition. The lower this ratio, the lower the number of available MHC/peptide complexes, indicating high CTL avidity.

Thus, this relatively simple experimental approach may provide a tool to identify peptide epitopes in oncogene products, which did not induce self-tolerance and are consequently targets for autoreactive CTL. As mentioned above, all melanoma antigens identified to date represent normal self proteins. Most of the CTL-recognized peptide epitopes identified in these proteins show weak MHC class I binding when compared with CTL epitopes derived from influenza virus (Cox et al., 1994, personal communication). Although this agrees with the hypothesis that weakly MHC binding, subdominant peptides are recognized by CTL against self proteins, more data are needed to confirm or discard this notion.

The beneficial nature of autoreactive CTL targeted against subdominant self epitopes needs to be assessed carefully in animal models. Beneficial autoimmunity against tumours might convert into detrimental autoimmune disease if stimulated autoreactive CTL attack normal tissues.

A relevant observation in this context is that the stimulation threshold to elicit CTL effector function is lower than the threshold for activation of naive CTL. Thus, it will be critical to determine that activated CTL do not lyse normal cells expressing physiological levels of protein but that CTL lysis is directed specifically against tumour cells with elevated levels of protein expression. The clinical observation that tumour regression in melanoma patients is sometimes associated with vitiligo suggests immune attack of normal melanocytes. The identification of several melanoma antigens and ongoing clinical trials of antigen-specific immunotherapy will help define conditions that lead to, or avoid destruction of normal melanocytes.

## ■ T CELL IMMUNITY AGAINST MUTATED ONCOGENE PRODUCTS

As shown in Table 7.2, a large number of proteins encoded by oncogenes or tumour-suppressor genes contain mutations that are not found in corresponding normal self proteins. Immune responses to mutant proteins are truly tumour-specific with little danger of causing damage to normal cells. In the case of oncogenes, mutations lead to acquisition of transforming activity and, in the case of tumour-suppressor genes, mutations can lead to a loss of suppressor activity as well as gain of transforming activity. In either case, the transformed phenotype of tumours may depend upon the function of the mutant proteins, which is one reason why they are attractive targets for antitumour T cell responses. Mutations can be subtle, involving only one amino acid residue in the entire protein as observed with *Ras*. Multiple amino-acid substitutions at various positions are frequently found in the p53 tumour-suppressor protein. Translocations can produce novel hybrid molecules like in the classical example of the bcr/abl fusion protein expressed in chronic myelogenous leukaemia. Finally, mutational frame shifts can generate a stretch of novel protein sequence as observed in the APC gene in colon cancer. T cell responses to mutant oncogene or tumour-suppressor gene products are expected to be exclusively tumour specific, provided that T cell recognition involves mutation-containing epitopes and not epitopes that are shared between normal and mutant proteins. Studies of mutant *Ras* proteins provided the first evidence in support of the concept of mutation-specific T lymphocyte responses. It was demonstrated that $CD4^+$ $T_H$ lymphocytes from human peripheral blood could be stimulated in vitro with synthetic peptides corresponding to amino acid 5–16 of *Ras* (Table 7.3). The stimulating Ras peptides contained a mutation at position twelve, and the responding $T_H$ lymphocytes specifically recognized mutant peptides but not peptides corresponding to the sequence of normal *Ras*.

Table 7.2.    Mutated Oncogenes Expressed in Human Tumours

| Protein | Mutation | Tumour type | Frequency of mutation |
|---|---|---|---|
| **Receptor tyrosine kinases** | | | |
| CSF-1 receptor (FMS) | (a) $Tyr_{969}$-Cys | (a) AML | (a) 6–12% (Ridge et al., 1990; Tobal et al., 1990) |
| | (b) $Tyr_{969}$-Cys | (b) MDS | (b) 9–12% (Ridge et al., 1990; Tobal et al., 1990) |
| RET | (a) $Met_{918}$-Thr | (a) MEN2B | (a) 100% (Carlson et al., 1994) |
| | (b) $Cys_{634}$ changes | (b) MEN2A and FMTC | (b) 80% (Mulligan et al., 1993; Xue et al., 1994) |
| EGFR | Deletion of bp 275–1075 (exon 2–7) | Gliomas | 10% ((Schlegel et al., 1994) |
| **Proteins involved in signal transduction** | | | |
| N-ras | $Gly_{12}$, $Gly_{13}$, or $Glu_{61}$ | (a) AML and other leukaemias (b) Melanoma (c) Thyroid cancer (d) Seminoma (e) Liver cancer (f) Lymphomas | Variable As many as 70% of AML (Bos, 1989) |
| K-ras | $Gly_{12}$, $Gly_{13}$, or $Glu_{61}$ | (a) Pancreatic cancer (b) Colon cancer (c) Thyroid cancer (d) Lung cancer (e) Seminoma | Variable As many as 80% of pancreatic cancers (Bos, 1989) |
| H-Ras | $Gly_{12}$, $Gly_{13}$, or $Glu_{61}$ | (a) Bladder cancer (b) Thyroid cancer (c) Renal cancer | 17% at most (Bos, 1989) |
| **Proteins involved in the regulation of apoptosis** | | | |
| p53 | More than 1,000 different mutations identified, 86% between codon 120 and 290. Mutations affecting $Arg_{175}$, $Arg_{248}$, and $Arg_{273}$ most common. | Most common: (a) Lung cancer (b) Breast cancer (c) Colon cancer (d) Cervical cancer (e) Lymphoma (f) Liver cancer | Overall 60% but variation dependent on type of cancer (Levine et al., 1994) |
| **Fusion proteins** | | | |
| $p210^{BCR-ABL}$ t(9,22) (q.34, q11) | c-abl exon 2–11 fused to bcl exon 1–3 or 1–2 | CML | 95% (Kagan, 1993) |

*(continued)*

Table 7.2.    (contd.)

| Protein | Mutation | Tumour type | Frequency of mutation |
|---|---|---|---|
| p185$^{BCR-ABL}$ t(9,22) (q34,q11) | c-abl exon 2–11 fused to bcl exon 1 | ALL | 10–15% (Kagan, 1993) |
| (a) PML-RARA | (a) RARA DNA and retinoic binding region fused to PML Zn finger domain | PML | 90% (Kagan, 1993) |
| (b) RARA-PML | (b) RARA transactive domains fused to PML | | |
| E2A-PBX1 | Replacement of DNA-binding domain of E2A with the DNA-binding domain of the PBX homeogene | (a) Pre-B cell leukaemias (b) Childhood acute leukaemias | (a) 30% (Kagan, 1993) (b) 6% (Kagan, 1993) |

CSF-1, colony-stimulating factor 1; FMS, CSF-1 receptor; AML, acute lymphoblastic leukaemia; MDS, myelodysplastic syndrome; RET, a receptor tyrosine kinase; MEN, multiple endocrine neoplasia; FMTC, familial medullary thyroid carcinoma; EGFR, epidermal growth factor receptor; CML, chronic myelocytic leukaemia; ALL, acute lymphoblastic leukaemia; RARA, retinoic acid receptor alpha; PML, promyelocytic leukaemia; PBX, A homeobox containing protein.

These responses were found in normal, cancer-free individuals who were unlikely to contain mutant *Ras*-specific memory T cells, suggesting that synthetic peptides stimulated naive T$_H$ lymphocytes in vitro. However, more recently a much higher precursor frequency of mutation-specific T$_H$ lymphocytes has been found in patients with mutant *Ras*-expressing cancers compared to tumour-free individuals, indicating activation of mutation-specific T$_H$ cells in vivo (Fossum et al., 1994). In one patient, the same group has also described HLA-B44-restricted CTL recognizing a Ras peptide containing a mutation at position 13 (Table 7.3).

Studies in murine models yielded similar results to those obtained in humans. T$_H$ cells specific for *Ras* mutations at position 12 and 13 have been demonstrated. These T$_H$ cells were specific for individual amino-acid substitutions at position 12, and did not recognise the wild-type residue or other mutant residues at this position (Peace et al., 1991). This indicates that, for possible vaccination approaches, it will be important to determine the type of *Ras* mutation present in patients and to administer a mutation-matched vaccine preparation. *Ras*-specific CTL have been demonstrated in mice immunized with recombinant vaccinia constructs, expressing a transforming N-*Ras* protein with a mutation at position 61 (Skipper & Stauss, 1993). Two CTL-recognized peptide epitopes were

## Table 7.3.   Human Immune Responses Against Oncogene-encoded Proteins

| Protein | Cellular responses | Humoral responses |
|---|---|---|
| **Overexpressed wild-type proteins** | | |
| ErbB2 (HER2/neu) | *Breast cancer:* Proliferative CD4$^+$ T cell response in one patient. Not seen in normal healthy individuals (Disis et al., 1994a) *Lung cancer* HLA-A2-restricted CTLs from TILs from lung cancer patients. Antigen shared with Her2/neu$^+$ ovarian tumour (Yoshino et al., 1994a) *Ovarian cancer:* HLA-A2-restricted CTLs from TILs from two ovarian cancer patients. Cytotoxicity correlates with levels of HER2/neu in target cell (Yoshino et al., 1994b) *Healthy individuals:* Peptide-specific CD8+HLA A2.1 restricted CTL responses generated from PBMC from healthy individuals (Disis et al., 1994b) | *Breast cancer:* 11/20 (55%) of breast cancer and normal healthy individuals (Disis et al., 1994a) |
| p53 | Peptide-specific CD8+ HLA A2.1 restricted CTL responses generated from PBMC from healthy individuals (Houbiers et al., 1993; Nijman et al., 1994) | Breast cancer (Angelopoulo et al., 1994; Crawford, Pim & Bulbrok, 1982; Davidoff, Iglehart & Marks, 1992; Schlichtholz et al., 1992; Lubin et al., 1993) Lung cancer (Winter et al., 1992; Lubin et al., 1993; Angelopoulo et al., 1994) Ovarian cancer (Labrecque et al., 1993; Lubin et al., 1993; Angelopoulo et al., 1994) Colon cancer (Angelopoulo et al., 1994) Bladder cancer (Lubin et al., 1993) Cancer of the pancreas (Angelopoulo et al., 1994; Laurentpuig et al., 1994) Prostate cancer (Lubin et al., 1993; Angelopoulo et al., 1993) |

*(continued)*

## Table 7.3.    (contd.)

| Protein | Cellular responses | Humoral responses |
|---------|-------------------|-------------------|
| p53 (contd.) | | Thyroid cancer (Lubin et al., 1993) Liver cancer (Lubin et al., 1993; Mueller et al., 1993) Multiple myeloma (Angelopoulo et al., 1994) Lymphoma ( Caron de Fromentel et al., 1987; Angelopoulo et al., 1994) |
| c-myc | | Colorectal cancer (Ben-Mahrez et al., 1990) |
| c-myb | | Breast cancer (Sorokine et al., 1991) |
| ras | *Colorectal adenocarcinoma*: CD8$^+$ and CD4$^+$ proliferative responses to K-Ras peptide (Gly$_{13}$-Asp) in one out of ten patients. Mutation not found in the tumour of the patient (Fossum et al., 1994) *Follicular thyroid carcinoma*: CD4$^+$ proliferative responses to Ras (Gln$_{61}$-Leu) in one out of 35 patients. Recognize processed protein (Gedde-Dahl et al., 1993; Geddedahl et al., 1994) *PBL from healthy individuals*: Peptide-specific CD4$^+$ proliferative responses to Ras (Gly$_{12}$-Val) in two individuals (Jung & Schluesener, 1991) Peptide-specific CD4$^+$ proliferative responses to Ras (Gly$_{12}$-Arg), Ras (Gly$_{12}$-Lys), Ras (Gly$_{13}$-Val) and Ras (Gly$_{12}$-Ala, Val, Cys, or Ser-) (Gedde-Dahl et al., 1992; Gedde-Dahl et al., 1993) | Colon cancer (Cheever et al., 1993) |

HER, human epidermal growth factor receptor; TIL, tumour-infiltrating lymphocyte; PBMC, peripheral blood mononuclear cells.

identified, one mutation-specific epitope corresponding to amino acids 60–67, and one epitope from amino acid 152–159 that was shared between mutant and normal *Ras* protein. Apparently, mice were not tolerant to this self sequence and overexpression of *Ras*, during immunization with recombinant vaccinia virus, stimulated not only CTL to a mutant epitope but also to an unaltered self epitope. Again, this observation has some implications for vaccination, namely that immunization with mutant proteins may activate both mutation-specific as well as autoreactive CTL. In the murine studies, induced CTL only recognized target cells overexpressing *Ras* and normal level of *Ras* expression were insufficient to elicit CTL lysis. In general, activation of autoreactive $T_H$ or CTL by vaccination is a possibility, and needs to be monitored carefully.

Mutations caused by chromosomal rearrangements can result in the production of fusion proteins, with the sequences surrounding the fusion generating novel peptide epitopes, which might be recognized by T cells. Using synthetic peptides corresponding to the fusion sequence of the *bcr/abl* protein, it was possible to raise peptide-specific $CD4^+$ $T_H$ cells from the peripheral blood of healthy individuals. Importantly, these peptide-specific $T_H$ cells were able to recognize leukaemic cells containing a *bcr/abl* translocation in an HLA-class II restriction fashion. A similar approach, based upon in vitro stimulation of peripheral blood lymphocytes with synthetic peptides corresponding to p53 sequences, was used to induce human HLA-A2-restricted CTL (Table 7.3). Although these CTL lysed target cells that had been coated with synthetic p53 peptides, they were unable to recognize cells expressing p53 endogenously. At least two explanations might account for this observation. The induced CTL may be of low avidity, recognizing high concentrations of synthetic peptides but not physiological concentrations of naturally produced peptides. Alternatively, it is possible that natural processing does not produce the p53 peptides used for CTL induction.

For possible immunotherapy it would be useful to estimate the likelihood that CTL can recognize mutations in oncogenic proteins. One requirement for CTL recognition is binding of mutation-containing peptides to MHC class I molecules. One can envision five possibilities for how mutations may affect MHC class I binding:

1. Mutations may create novel class I-binding sites, which were not present in peptides with the normal sequence.
2. The normal sequence may bind to class I and binding is not affected by the mutation.

3. Frameshift mutations and translocations may create novel class I-binding epitopes, which are not present in corresponding parental proteins.
4. The normal wild-type sequence may bind to class I and the mutation abolishes binding.
5. Neither peptides with the normal nor the mutant sequence can bind to class I molecules.

Only mutations falling into the first three categories can possibly induce CTL responses, while mutations falling into the last two categories are unlikely be recognized by CTL since they are not presented by MHC class I molecules. In Table 7.4 we have taken a simplistic approach to estimate the likelihood that point mutations in *Res* and the bcr/abl fusion proteins might be recognized by CTL. We have screened the mutant sequences for the presence of MHC class I-binding motifs for 17 HLA class I molecules. The underlying assumption that motif-containing peptides can bind to class I molecules may be true for many but certainly not for all peptides. A further limitation is the natural antigen processing may not generate appropriate motif-containing peptides, even if they bind to class I molecules. Taken these limitations into account, it is nevertheless fair to say that motif-containing peptides are more likely to be presented by MHC class I molecules and to be recognized by CTL than motif-negative peptides.

Interestingly, peptides corresponding to amino acids 8–16 of K-*Ras* and N-*Ras* have binding motifs for HLA-A3, HLA-A11, HLA-A31, and HLA-A68 class I molecules. Mutations at *Ras* positions 12 and 13 do not disrupt the class I-binding motifs of these mer *Ras* peptides. The mutations occur at peptide position P5 and P6, which are not involved in MHC class I binding, but may be available for CTL recognition. In the wild-type sequence, both position 12 and 13 are occupied by small glycine residues, which are replaced by rather large amino acids in some of the mutant proteins. Thus, provided that these *Ras* peptides are produced by natural processing and presented by MHC molecules, it is conceivable that CTL may be able to discriminate between normal and mutant peptides. In addition to the A3, A11, A31 motifs, which are found in wild-type and mutant *Ras* protein, there are also *Ras* mutations that create motifs that are not found in the wild-type sequence. For example, a mutation at position 12 of K-*Ras*, which replaces glycine for arginine, creates a binding motif for HLA-B27 (Table 7.4). Since this particular substitution is one of the more frequent K-Ras mutations found in solid tumours (up to 31% of solid tumours with a position 12 mutation have an arginine for glycine substitution), it might create a CTL epitope in B27-positive patients. It

**Table 7.4. MHC Class I-Binding Motifs in Human Mutant Oncogene Products**

| Oncogene[a] | Mutated sequence[b] | Frequency of listed mutation[c] | Human MHC class I-binding motif[c] |
|---|---|---|---|
| K-ras (12) | MTEYKLVVVGASGVGKSA LTIQ | 12% (colon) 43% (lung) 0–36% (pan) | HLA-A3, HLA-A11 HLA-A31, HLA-A6801 |
| K-ras (12) | MTEYKLVVVGACGVGKSA LTIQ | 12% (colon) | HLA-A3, HLA-A11 HLA-A31, HLA-A6801 |
| K-ras (12) | MTEYKLVVVGARGVGKSA LTIQ | 4–31% (pan) | HLA-A3, HLA-A11 HLA-A31, HLA-A6801 HLA-B2705 |
| K-ras (12) | MTEYKLVVVGADGVGKSA LTIQ | 16% (colon) 21% (lung) 28–31% (pan) 10% (AML/MDS) | HLA-A3, HLA-A11 HLA-A31, HLA-A6801 |
| K-ras (12) | MTEYKLVVVGAVGVGKSA LTIQ | 37% (colon) 29% (lung) 32–36% (pan) | HLA-A3, HLA-A11 HLA-A31, HLA-A6801 |
| K-ras (12) | MTEYKLVVVGAAGVGKSA LTIQ | 7% (colon) 7% (lung) 0–2% (pan) | HLA-A3, HLA-A11 HLA-A31, HLA-A6801 |
| K-ras (13) | MTEYKLVVVGAGDVGKSA LTIQ | 21% (colon) | HLA-A3, HLA-A11 HLA-A6801 |
| N-ras (12) | MTEYKLVVVGADGVGKSA LTIQ | 29% (AML) | HLA-A3, HLA-A11 HLA-A31, HLA-A6801 |

(continued)

## Table 7.4. (contd.)

| Oncogene[a] | Mutated sequence[b] | Frequency of listed mutation[c] | Human MHC class I-binding motif[d] |
|---|---|---|---|
| N-ras (13) | MTEYKLVVVGAGVVGKSA LTIQ | 9% (AML/MDS) | HLA-A0201<br>HLA-A3, HLA-A11<br>HLA-A31, HLA-A6801 |
| N-ras (61) | CLLDILDTAGREEYSAMRD Q | 13% (AML) | HLA-A3, HLA-A11<br>HLA-B2705 |
| N-ras (61) | CLLDILDTAGKEEYSAMRD Q | Neuroblastoma<br>Melanoma<br>Fibrosarcoma | HLA-A3<br>HAL-A11 |
| BCR-ABL | (a) (bcr econ 3 spliced to abl exon 2)<br>HSATGFKQSSKALQRPVAS DFE<br>(b) (Alternative splicing of bcr exon 2 to abl exon 2;<br>(Shtivelman et al., 1986))<br>HSIPLTINKEKALQRPVASD FE | 95% (of all cases)<br>CML | (a) HLA-A3, HLA-A11<br>HLA-A24, HLA-A6801<br>HLA-Cw0401<br>(b) HLA-A11, HLA-A31<br>HLA-A6801<br>HLA B8 |
| BCR-ABL | bcr exon 1 fused to abl exon 2 (Shtivelman et al., 1986; Clark et al. 1988)<br>DGEGAFHGDAEALQRPVAS DFE | 10–15% (of all cases) ALL | HLA-A3, HLA-A11<br>HLA-A24<br>HLA-Cw0401 |

[a] Ocogenes listed are with mutant residues shown in parenthesis.
[b] The deduced amino-acid sequences of mutated regions of human oncogenic proteins are shown. Mutated amino acids or the amino acids representing break points in fusion proteins are in bold and underlined.
[c] The percentage of the listed mutations of the total number of mutations found at that amino-acid residue is shown.
[d] HLA motifs which bind the oncogene sequence, novel motifs are underlined.

would be interesting to know whether B27 individuals have a lower incidence of solid tumours with a glycine to arginine mutations of K-*Ras*. As shown in Table 7.4, mutations at position 13 and 6 of N-*Ras* also create MHC-binding motifs for the human class I molecules A2, A3, A11, and B27. Since these mutations are found in patients with AML it would be interesting to investigate whether HLA-A2, A3, A11, and B27-positive individuals show any protection against acute myeloblastic leukaemia (AML) containing these N-*Ras* mutations.

Analysis of *bcr/abl* fusion proteins yielded interesting results. The Philadelphia chromosome translocation found in CML patients results in a *bcr/abl* hybrid gene from which two alternatively spliced transcripts are produced, which encode for two distinct fusion proteins (Shtvelman et al., 1986). As shown in Table 7.4, one of these fusion proteins contains five novel MHC class I-binding motifs, while the other fusion protein contains four novel motifs. Similarly, the *bcr/abl* translocation found in acute lymphoblastic leukaemia (ALL) patients encodes a fusion protein, which contains four novel MHC class I-binding motifs. To date, no bcr/abl specific CTL have been reported. To address the possible significance of the MHC class I-binding motifs found in *bcr/abl* fusion proteins, experimental and statistical analysis of CML and ALL patients might provide useful information. Experimentally, it might be possible to demonstrate CTL responses in patients expressing the HLA class I alleles listed in Table 7.4, and statistical analysis might reveal a possible tumour-protective effect of these class I alleles.

Comparison of the MHC motif analysis of point mutations in Ras and the bcr/abl translocation suggests that the latter are more likely to produce candidate MHC class I-binding epitopes. Furthermore, the class I epitopes in bcr/abl fusion proteins are novel, and no corresponding wild-type epitopes are present in the parental proteins. Consequently, CTL recognition of candidate bcr/abl peptides will always be mutation specific, since no corresponding wild-type peptides are presented. In contrast, the majority of candidate MHC-binding epitopes found in point mutant Ras proteins are also present in normal wild-type Ras. CTL recognition of Ras peptides, therefore, is only mutation specific if stimulated CTL can discriminate between mutant and wild-type peptides.

Interestingly, there is experimental evidence that point mutations in cellular proteins can be recognized by tumour-specific CTL. The murine mastocytoma P815 was mutagenized and variants were selected that induced strong immune responses in syngeneic mice resulting in tumour rejection. Rejection correlated with the induction of CTL, which specifically recognised the mutagenized variant but not the parental tumour. Identification of the CTL-recognized target epitope revealed that it was a peptide containing a point mutation (Lurquin et al., 1989; Szikora,

Vanpel & Boon, 1993). This point mutation allowed MHC class I binding of the mutant sequence, while peptides with the normal sequence did not bind. Whether this is an exceptional case or whether mutant human oncogenes might serve as targets for CTL-mediated tumour destruction remains to be determined.

## ■ NATURAL ANTIGEN PROCESSING AND CTL EPITOPE SELECTION

MHC class I binding is not the only prerequisite for the generation of CTL-recognizable epitopes. Another important, perhaps more complex essential function is that appropriate peptides are produced by natural processing and delivered into the ER, where they can bind to MHC molecules (Monaco, 1992). Any changes in the mechanism of intracellular peptide production and transport may affect the types of MHC-presented peptides and consequently the immunogenicity of cells. Indeed, changes in intracellular peptide transport have been described in human cancers. Cancer cells were shown to down-regulate expression of TAP transporter proteins, which are required for ER delivery of peptides (Cromme et al., 1994). Insufficient amounts of class I-binding peptides in the ER resulted in inefficient MHC assembly and in reduced cell-surface expression of class I molecules. Thus, it appears that down-regulation of TAP may be a mechanism by which cancers try to evade CTL recognition.

It is also possible that changes in intracellular antigen processing can render cancer cells more immunogenic, although direct experimental evidence is sparse. As described in Chapter 13 of this volume, heat shock proteins (HSPs) isolated from transformed cells can bind peptides, which can induce tumour-specific CTL immunity. Purified HSP/peptide complexes from transformed cells but not from normal cells were capable of inducing CTL-mediated tumour immunity in mice (Udono and Srivastava, 1994). Immunization with HSP after ATP-stimulated peptide dissociation had no tumour-protective effects, indicating the essential role of HSP-bound peptides in the induction of tumour-specific CTL. The origin of the protective peptides is currently unknown. HSPs represent a large family of proteins, which show a high degree of conservations between species, as far apart as bacteria and humans. Although traditionally defined as proteins induced by heat, irradiation, and other types of stress, some HSPs are also constitutively expressed. Taking the evidence that HSPs may be involved in intracellular peptide processing, transport, and binding to class I molecules (Srivastava et al., 1994), it is conceivable that abnormal HSP expression in transformed cells may change the profile of MHC-presented peptides.

Changes in cellular protein breakdown are another possible mechanism by which transforming proteins might indirectly affect the set of MHC class I presented peptides. For example, the transforming activity of the E6 protein of HPV is dependent on its ability to neutralize the function of the cellular tumour suppressor proteins p53. E6 can bind to p53 and trigger its rapid degradation via ubiquitin-dependent protein breakdown. The rapid ubiquitin degradation could change both the quantity and quality of p53-derived peptides. As a consequence, the concentration and/or nature of MHC/p53 peptide complexes may be different in HPV-transformed and normal cells.

## A Bottleneck: Primary Stimulation of T Cell Responses

An important question is, whether MHC class I presentation of peptides derived from mutant or overexpressed normal cellular oncogenes is sufficient to induce antitumour CTL in vivo. Efficient CTL stimulation usually requires collaboration between CTL precursors and cytokine-producing $T_H$ cells. Generation of antitumour CTL may be different because many tumours are MHC class II negative and consequently do not display ligands recognized by $T_H$ cells. A possible solution to this dilemma was suggested in murine experiments analysing the immunogenicity of tumour cells transfected with various cytokine genes. When gene-transfected tumour cells were injected into mice, they were more immunogenic than untransfected cells and efficiently stimulated a tumour-protective T cell immunity (Pardoll, 1993). Surprisingly, histological examination revealed that the host cells invading the site of tumour injection were mostly macrophages and mononuclear cells other than CD4 and CD8 T cells. Nevertheless, T cell priming did occur, since memory T cells protected the mice against subsequent tumour injections. The interpretation of these experiments was that the site of primary tumour growth is not the same as the site of primary activation of T cell responses, which is thought to occur in regional draining lymph nodes. A proposed mechanism is that professional antigen presenting cells (APC), such as dendritic cells and activated macrophages, invade sites of local tumour growth and become exposed to tumour antigens. Antigen-loaded APC then migrate to draining lymph nodes where they either deliver antigen to resident APC, or present antigen directly to CD4[+] and CD8[+] T lymphocytes. Thus, in the local microenvironment of lymph nodes, activated $T_H$ cells would provide helper cytokines that are important for efficient activation of CTL precursors. The concept of antigen transfer from the site of tumour growth to lymph nodes is easily understood for MHC class II-presented antigens. Shed tumour antigen or antigen released from dying tumour cells may be endocytosed by APC, and processed and presented in the context of MHC class II molecules. However, in most APC, endocytosed antigen is not effectively processed for MHC class I presentation. It is therefore difficult to see how class I-presented tumour antigens can be transferred to local lymph nodes.

One possibility is migration of tumour cells to local nodes, although this is thought to occur only at late and not at early stages of tumour development. Another possibility is that locally growing tumours might shed MHC/peptide complexes, which can be reprocessed and presented by APC in the draining nodes. Possible mechanisms for transfer of class I-presented antigens includes shedding of class I/peptide complexes from tumour cells and presentation of these complexes by APC in lymph nodes. There is indeed experimental evidence that a subpopulation of APC might be specialized in processing of endocytosed antigens for MHC class I presentation (Huang et al., 1994). Such APC might be able to process proteins released from tumour cells or to process shed MHC/peptide complexes. The APC, which is presenting class I-restricted tumour antigens, would presumably be susceptible to lysis by activated effector CTL. Whether APC lysis in regional lymph nodes does indeed occur is not known. An alternative possibility is that only primary activation of CD4 cells occurs in regional nodes and that CD8 priming occurs at the tumour site. Activated antigen-specific $T_H$ cells may recirculate and home at sites of tumour growth, where they are efficiently stimulated by local MHC class II-positive APC presenting tumour antigens. These antigen-experienced $T_H$ cells would presumably produce sufficient helper cytokines for activation of CTL precursors. In this case, the CTL precursors would recognize class I/peptide complexes displayed by tumour cells and no antigen transfer to professional APC would be required. Also, APC would not become potential targets for lysis by activated CTL. The enhanced immunogenicity of B7 transfected tumour cells (Li et al., 1994) is more easily explained by direct tumour recognition during CTL priming than by indirect antigen presentation by professional APC.

It is clear from these considerations that the mechanisms by which developing tumours might activate T lymphocyte responses in vivo is far from understood. To date, all studies demonstrating tumour-specific T cell responses in melanoma and renal cancer patients were done at an advanced stage of the neoplastic disease. Whether tumour-specific immune responses represent a late phenomenon in cancer patients or whether they can be detected at early stages of the disease is clearly an important question that needs to be addressed in future studies. Indeed, it is possible that natural tumour history might favour induction of immunological unresponsiveness at early stages of the disease. The clonal origin of cancers indicates that one cell usually acquires a fully transformed phenotype, endowing it with unlimited proliferative capacity resulting in uncontrolled growth and tumour formation. Thus, the amount of tumour antigens is initially very small and restricted to one or a few cells, and gradually antigen dose increases during tumour progression. This is somewhat reminiscent of the experimental conditions that induce low-dose tolerance. In these experiments it has been shown that injection of mice with low doses of antigen can induce antigen-specific tolerance, suggesting that activation of primary immune responses is antigen dose dependent with suboptimal doses having adverse effects. This antigen dose dependence may enable the T cell compartment to efficiently perform its most important role, which is to combat viral infections. Since viral infections usually involve large numbers of infected cells producing abundant viral antigens, this may provide conditions that favour rapid activation of T cell responses. In contrast, the T cell compartment might be ill adapted to generate immunity to low doses of tumour antigens, which gradually increase over the course of many months and probably years.

Inadequate T cell function has been observed in a murine tumour model. CTL from tumour-bearing mice showed impaired cytotoxic function and decreased expression of tumour necrosis factor alpha and granzyme B genes (Mizoguchi et al., 1992). This hyporesponsiveness correlated with a change of the molecular composition of the CD3 components of the T cell antigen receptor complex. The CD3 $\zeta$-chains were replaced in T cells from tumour-bearing mice with $\gamma$-chains of the Fc-$\varepsilon$ receptor. A similar observation has been made recently in T cells from colon cancer patients (personal communication). At present the significance of these intriguing findings are unclear, but the possibility that this molecular change might be linked to T cell paralysis and that it might be induced by soluble factors secreted from tumour cells is being investigated.

## Bypassing the Bottleneck by Vaccination

Active vaccination may overcome possible inadequate T cell stimulation by naturally developing cancers and may prevent occurrence of hyporesponsive T cells. Vaccine preparations administered in a way that leads to T cell activation may generate a population of memory CD4 and CD8 cells, which may locate to sites of tumour growth to generate recall responses that may result in tumour elimination. Vaccination trails to stimulate immunity against transforming proteins in humans will commence in the near future. Several groups are preparing protocols to induce immunity against the transforming proteins E6 and E7 of human papilloma virus type 16 (see Chapter 6). This includes immunization with recombinant vaccinia virus expressing E6 and E7, immunization with E7 protein, and also immunization with HLA-A2 binding peptides derived from E7. Vaccination trials to immunize against Ras mutations will also start soon in patients with tumours harbouring mutant Ras. The Ras trials are based on the observation that patients contain CD4 and CD8 T lymphocytes, which showed specificity for point mutations of position 12 and 13 of Ras. Accordingly, synthetic peptides containing these mutations will be used as vaccines. These trials with E6, E7, and Ras will be done in patients with endstage disease to establish vaccine safety. The therapeutic and immune stimulating effects might be small in this patient group. These vaccines are possibly most promising at the early stage of disease or, indeed, as prophylactic vaccines. The goal of vaccination would be to establish a memory T cell population, which can eliminate small numbers of transformed cells.

Vaccination procedures more suitable for immunotherapy have been tested in melanoma patients. Injection of autologous T cells into melanoma patients after in vitro expansion with IL-2 showed good therapeutic effects in some cases. The identification of CTL recognized melanoma antigens may allow in vitro generation of antigen-specific CTL lines and clones, which may be more efficient than IL-2 expanded T cell populations of unknown antigen specificity. The feasibility of in vitro expansion of antigen-specific CTL and their in vivo efficiency has been demonstrated in the bone-marrow transplant patients (Riddell et al., 1992). In these immunosuppressed patients, infection by cytomegalovirus (CMV) frequently has a negative effect on the clinical outcome of bone-marrow transplantation. Donor-derived CMV-specific CTL were expanded to large numbers in vitro and protected against CMV infection when given to transplant recipients. Accordingly, the identification of T cell epitopes in normal or mutant oncogenic proteins would open the possibility of generating specific T cells lines in vitro, which might be useful for immunotherapy of cancer patients. The advantage of in vitro-generated T cell populations is that their specificity can be determined before they are given back to patients and that patients are not exposed to any vaccine preparation. There will always be considerable safety concern with vaccines containing oncogenic proteins or corresponding genes. Vaccination with recombinant viral vectors or intramuscular DNA injection, or injection of recombinant proteins might be unacceptable, although these procedures have been shown to efficiently stimulate T cell responses. A relatively safe vaccine, which is used in some of the trials described above, consists of synthetic peptides corresponding to sequences in oncogenic proteins. The drawback is that different peptides bind to different MHC molecules, which means that a peptide vaccine will be restricted to individuals expressing appropriate MHC molecules.

# ■ SUMMARY AND CONCLUSIONS

In this article we have discussed the immunobiology of mutated oncogenes and overexpressed normal oncogene products. We have focused on CTL immunity, because the majority of oncogenic proteins are expressed inside tumour cells and are not easily accessible for recognition by $T_H$ lymphocytes and antibodies. Nevertheless, antibodies to these intracellular proteins have been described in cancer patients and their titre frequently correlates with severity of disease (Table 7.3). It is possible that these antibody responses are triggered by proteins released from established tumour masses, possibly involving release from necrotic tumour areas. Generally, antibodies may be useful to monitor the state, severity, and progression of the malignant disease.

Similarly, $T_H$ responses to intracellular tumour proteins have been observed as exemplified by responses to mutant *Ras* protein. In addition, specific *Ras* mutations can also be recognized by CTL. The in vivo conditions that lead to activation of these T cell responses, and that allow collaboration between $T_H$ cells and CTL precursors are not yet clear. Also, it is currently unclear whether certain types of human cancers are more immunogenic than others, with melanoma and colon cancer possibly representing strongly and weakly immunogenic tumours. Independent of the ability to induce immune responses, even weakly immunogenic cancers might be susceptible to attack by established effector T lymphocytes.

Identification of tumour antigens that are recognized by $T_H$ and CTL will provide a basis for development of antigen-specific vaccines. Such vaccines may contain $T_H$ and CTL recognized epitopes identified in mutant or overexpressed oncogenic proteins. The critical event of T cell activation may be achieved by controlled vaccination, and consequently become independent of the immunogenicity of in vivo growing tumours. Perhaps more importantly, vaccination at early stages of the neoplastic disease or even prophylactically, may allow immune attack of small numbers of transformed cells. Efficient, early immune attack might decrease the likelihood of appearance of tumour cell variants, which escape immune recognition.

Immune targeting of overexpressed unaltered self proteins is currently pioneered in trials with melanoma patients. Investigations in the near future will reveal whether overexpressed normal oncogene products can serve as targets to induce beneficial autoimmunity against tumours. It might be possible to identify epitopes in these self proteins, which do not induce tolerance and are therefore capable of stimulating autoreactive T cells. The specificity of such T cells will be defined by the antigen dose required to stimulate T cell effector function. Tumour specificity might be observed if levels of over expression are sufficient to stimulate effector function, while physiological levels of protein expression in normal cells are insufficient. For this approach it may be desirable to choose proteins that show large differences in their expression levels in tumours and normal cells, since this might provide a wide window of specificity for T cell responses.

Truly tumour-specific vaccination may be achievable by targeting mutant oncogene products. Since mutant oncogenic proteins are only expressed in tumour cells, CTL specific for these proteins would not attack normal cells. However, the restrictions imposed by natural CTL epitope selection may prevent generation of mutation-specific responses. Such responses depend upon production of mutation-containing peptides in the cytosol of tumour cells, transport of these peptides into the lumen of the ER, and efficient peptide binding to MHC class I molecules. Since MHC class I-bound peptides generally contain allele-specific binding motifs, screening mutant oncogenic proteins for such motifs may be useful to identify candidate CTL epitopes. Analysis of 11 *Ras* proteins with distinct point mutations shows that each mutant epitope contains class I-binding motifs for at least two out of seventeen human HLA class I alleles. There is no point mutation in *Ras* that does not contain a binding motif for any of the seventeen HLA-class I alleles that were included in this analysis. The results obtained with three distinct *bcr/abl* fusion proteins that are frequently found in patients with CML and ALL are even more striking. The fusion region of each of these proteins contains binding motifs for at least four of the seventeen tested HLA class I alleles. Together, it appears that MHC class I molecules are well adapted to present protein sequences altered by mutations to the CTL compartment. However, since a limited number of six class I alleles is generally expressed in man, it is likely that, within a given patient, some oncogene mutations may not contain appropriate motifs for binding to one of the six MHC alleles. Nevertheless, in the future it might be rewarding to undertake an MHC allele guided search for oncogene-specific CTL responses in patients and to exploit identified CTL epitopes for tumour immunotherapy.

**REFERENCES**

Akagi T., Kondo E. & Yoshino T. (1994) Expression of bcl-2 protein and bcl-2 messenger-RNA in normal and neoplastic lymphoid-tissues. *Leukemia and Lymphoma*, **13**, 81–7.
Angelopoulo K., Diamandis E.P., Sutherland D.J.A., Kellen J.A. & Bunting P.S. (1994) Prevalence of serum antibodies against the p53 tumor suppressor gene protein in various cancers. *International Journal of Cancer*, **58**, 480–7.

Anichini A., Fossati G. & Parmiani G. (1985) Clonal analysis of cytotoxic T-lymphocyte response to autologous human metastatic melanoma. *International Journal of Cancer*, **35**, 683–9.

Bakker A., Schreurs M., Deboer A.J. et al. (1994) Melanocyte lineage-specific antigen gp100 is recognized by melanoma-derived tumor-infiltrating lymphocytes. *Journal of Experimental Medicine*, **179**, 1005–9.

Bartkova J., Lukas J., Müller H., Lützhöft D., Strauss M. & Bartek M. (1994a) Cyclin D1 protein expression and function in human breast cancer. *International Journal of Cancer*, **57**, 353–61.

Bartkova J., Lukas J., Strauss M. & Bartek J. (1994b) The Prad-1/cyclin D1 oncogene product accumulates aberrantly in a subset of colorectal carcinomas. *International Journal of Cancer*, **58**, 568–73.

Ben-Mahrez K., Sorokine I., Thierry D. et al. (1990) Circulating antibodies against c-myc oncogene product in sera of colorectal-cancer patients. *International Journal of Cancer*, **46**, 35–8.

Berchuck A., Kamel A., Whitaker R. et al. (1990) Overexpression of HER-2/neu is associated with poor survival in advanced epithelial ovarian cancer. *Cancer Research*, **50**, 4087–91.

Bjorkman P.J., Saper M.A., Samraoui B. et al. (1987a) The foreign antigen binding site and T cell recognition regions of Class I histocompatibility antigens. *Nature (London)*, **329**, 512–8.

Bjorkman P.J., Saper M.A., Samraoui B. et al. (1987b) Structure of the human Class I histocompatibility antigen, HLA-A2. *Nature (London)*, **329**, 506–12.

Bos J.L. (1989) ras oncogenes in human cancer: a review. *Cancer Research*, **49**, 4982–9.

Bourhis J., Le M.G., Barrois M. et al. (1990) Prognostic value of c-myc proto-oncogene overexpression in early invasive carcinoma of the cervix. *Journal of Clinical Oncology*, **8**, 1789–96.

Brichard V., Van Pel A., Wölfel T. et al. (1993) The tyrosinase gene codes for an antigen recognized by autologous cytolytic T lymphocytes on HLA-A2 melanoma. *Journal of Experimental Medicine*, **178**, 489–95.

Buckley M.F., Sweeney K.J.E., Hamilton J.A. et al. (1993) Expression and amplification of cyclin genes in human breast cancer. *Oncogene*, **8**, 2127–33.

Buesoramos C.E., Yang Y., Deleon E., McCown P., Stass S.A. & Albitar M. (1993) The human mdm-2 oncogene is overexpressed in leukemias. *Blood*, **82**, 2617–23.

Cabaniols J.-P., Cibotti R., Kourilsky P., Kosmatopoulos K. & Kannellopoulos J.M. (1994) Dose-dependent T cell tolerance to an immunodominant self peptide. *European Journal of Immunology*, **24**, 1743–9.

Carlson K.M., Dou S.S., Chi D. et al. (1994) Single mis-sense mutation in the tyrosine kinase catalytic domain of the ret protooncogene is associated with multiple endocrine neoplasis type 2b. *Proceedings of the National Academy of Sciences USA*, **91**, 1579–83.

Caron de Fromentel C., May-Levin F., Mouriesse H. et al. (1987) Presence of circulating antibodies against cellular protein p53 in a notable proportion of children with B cell lymphoma. *International Journal of Cancer*, **39**, 185–9.

Cheever M.A., Chen W., Disis M.L., Takahashi M. & Peace D.J. (1993) T-cell immunity to oncogenic proteins including mutated ras and chimeric bcr-abl. *Annals of the New York Academy of Sciences*, **690**, 101–12.

Cibotti R., Kanellopoulos J.M., Cabaniols J.P. et al. (1992) Tolerance to a self-protein involves its immunodominant but does not involve its subdominant determinants. *Proceedings of the National Academy of Sciences USA*, **89**, 416–20.

Clark S.S., McLaughlin J., Timmons M. et al. (1988) Expression of a distinctive bcr-abl oncogene in Ph[1]-Positive Acute lymphocytic leukemia. *Science*, 239, 775–7.

Cordon-Cardo C., Latres E., Drobnjak M. et al. (1994) Molecular abnormalities of mdm2 and p53 genes in adult soft tissue sarcomas. *Cancer Research*, 54, 794–9.

Coulie P.G., Brichard V., Vanpel A. et al. (1994) A new gene coding for a differentiation antigen recognized by autologous cytolytic T-lymphocytes on HLA-A2 melanomas. *Journal of Experimental Medicine*, 180, 35–42.

Cox A.L., Skipper J., Chen T. et al. (1994) Identification of a peptide recognized by five melanoma-specific human cytotoxic T cell lines. *Sciences*, 264, 716–19.

Crawford L.W., Pim D.C. & Bulbrrok R.D. (1982) Detection of antibodies against the cellular protein p53 in sera from patients with breast cancer. *International Journal of Cancer*, 30, 403–8.

Cromme F.V., Vanbommel P.F.J., Walboomers J.M.M. et al. (1994) Differences in MHC and TAP-1 expression in cervical-cancer lymph-node metastases as compared with the primary tumors. *British Journal of Cancer*, 69, 1176–81.

Davidoff A.M., Iglehart J.D. & Marks J.R. (1992) Immune response to p53 is dependent upon p53/HSP70. *Proceedings of the National Academy of Sciences USA*, 89, 3439–42.

Dawkins H.J.S., Robbins P.D., Smith K.L. et al. (1993) What's new in breast cancer? Molecular perspectives of cancer development and the role of the oncogene c-erbB-2 in prognosis and disease. *Pathology Research and Practice*, 189, 1233–52.

De Vries J. & Spits H. (1984) Clones human cytotoxic T lymphocyte (CTL) lines reactive with autologous melanoma cells. *Journal of Immunology*, 132, 510–19.

Di Renzo M.F., Narsimham R.P., Olivero et al. (1991) Expression of the Met/HGF receptor in normal and neoplastic human tissues. *Oncogene*, 6, 1977–2003.

Di Renzo M.F., Olivero M., Katsaros D. et al. (1994) Overexpression of the MET/HGF receptor in ovarian cancer. *Oncogene*, 58, 658–62.

Disis M.L., Calenoff E., McLaughlin G. et al. (1994a) Existent T-cell and antibody immunity to HER-2 neu protein in patients with breast-cancer. *Cancer Research*, 54, 16–20.

Disis M.L., Smith J.W., Murphy A.E., Chen W. & Cheever M.A. (1994b) In-vitro generation of human cytolytic T-cells specific for peptides derived from the HER-2/neu protooncogene protein. *Cancer Research*, 54, 1071–6.

Ekstrand A.J., James C.D., Cavenee W.K., Seliger B., Pettersson R.F. & Collins V.P. (1991) Genes for epidermal growth factor receptor, transforming growth factor α, and epidermal growth factor and their expression in human gliomas in vivo. *Cancer Research*, 51, 2164–72.

Falk K. & Rötzschke O. (1993) Consensus motifs and peptide ligands of MHC Class I molecules. *Seminars in Immunology*, 5, 81–94.

Falk K., Rötszchke O., Grahovac B. et al. (1993) Allele-specific peptide ligand motifs of HLA-C molecules. *Proceedings of the National Academy of Sciences USA*, 90, 12005–9.

Falk K., Rötzschke O., Stevanovic S., Jung G. & Rammensee H.-G. (1991) Allele-specific motifs revealed by sequencing of self-peptides eluted from MHC molecules. *Nature (London)*, 351, 290–6.

Ferber I., Schönrich G., Schenkel J., Mellor A.L., Hämmerling G.J. & Arnold B. (1994) Levels of peripheral T cell tolerance induced by different doses of tolerogen. *Science*, 263, 674–6.

Field J.K. & Spandidos D.A. (1990) The role of ras and myc oncogenes in human solid tumours and their relevance in diagnosis and prognosis. *Anticancer Research*, 10, 1–22.

Fischer L.K., Hermel E., Loveland B.E. & Wang C.R. (1991) Maternally transmitted antigen of mice: a model transplantation antigen. *Annual Review of Immunology,* 9, 351–71.

Foekens J.A., Portengen H., Janssen M. & Klijn J.G. (1989) Insulin-like growth factor-I receptors and insulin-like growth factor-I-like activity in human primary breast cancer. *Cancer,* 63, 2139–47.

Fossum B., Breivik J., Meling G.I. et al. (1994) A K-ras 13Gly-Asp mutation is recognized by HLA-DQ7 restricted T cells in a patient with colorectal cancer. Modifying effect of DQ7 on established cancers harbouring this mutation? *International Journal of Cancer,* 58, 506–11.

Fossum B., Geddedahl T., Breivik et al. (1994) P21-ras-peptide-specific T-cell responses in a patient with colorectal-cancer – CD4(+) and CD8(+) T-cells recognize a peptide corresponding to a common mutation (13 gly-]asp). *International Journal of Cancer,* 56, 40–5.

Gasparini G., Gullick W.J., Maluta S. et al. (1994) c-erbB3 and c-erB2 gene expression in node-negative breast carcinomas. *Cancer,* 30A, 16–22.

Gaugler B., Van den Eynde B., van der Bruggen P. et al. (1994) Human gene MAGE-3 codes for an antigen recognized on a melanoma by autologous cytolytic T lymphocytes. *Journal of Experimental Medicine,* 179, 921–30.

Gedde-Dahl T. III, Amund Eriksen J., Thorsby E. & Gaudernack G. (1992) T-Cell responses against products of oncogenes: generation and characterization of human T-cell cones specific for p21 Ras-derived synthetic peptides. *Human Immunology,* 33, 266–74.

Gedde-Dahl T. III, Fossum B., Eriksen J.A., Thorsby E. & Gaudernack G. (1993) T cell clones specific for p21 ras-derived peptides: characterization of their fine specificity and HLA restriction. *European Journal of Immunology,* 23, 754–60.

Gedde-Dahl T., Spurkland A., Fossum B. et al. (1994) T-cell epitopes encompassing the mutational hot-spot position-61 of p21 ras – promiscuity in ras peptide binding to hla. *European Journal of Immunology,* 24, 410–14.

Gillet C., Fantl V., Smith R. et al. (1994) Amplification and overexpression of cyclin D1 in breast cancer detected by immunohistochemical staining. *Oncogene,* 54, 1812–17.

Herin M., Lemoine C., Weynants P. et al. (1987) Production of stable cytolytic T-cell clones directed against autologous human melanoma. *International Journal of Cancer,* 39, 390–6.

Houbiers J.G.A., Nijman H.W., van der Burg S.H. et al. (1993) In vitro induction of human cytotoxic T lymphocyte responses against peptides of mutant and wild-type p53. *European Journal of Immunology,* 23, 2072–7.

Huang A.Y.C., Golumbek P., Ahmadzaheh M., Jaffee E., Pardoll D. & Levitsky H. (1994) Role of bone marrow-derived cells in presenting MHC Class I-restricted tumor antigens. *Science,* 264, 961–5.

Hunts J., Ueds M., Ozawa S. et al. (1985) Hyperproduction and gene amplification of the epidermal growth factors receptor in squamous cell carcinomas. *Japanese Journal of Cancer Research,* 76, 663–6.

Issing W.J., Wustrow T.P.U. & Heppt W.J. (1993) Oncogenes related to head and neck cancer. *Anticancer Research,* 13, 2541–52.

Jadayel D., Matutes E., Dyer M.J.S. et al. (1994) Splenic lymphoma with villous lymphoctyes – analysis of bcl-1 rearrangements and expression of the cyclin d1 gene. *Blood,* 83, 3664–71.

Jares P., Fernandez P.L., Campo E., Nadal A. et al. (1994) Prad-1 cyclin d1 gene amplification correlates with messenger-RNA overexpression and tumor progression in human laryngeal carcinomas. *Cancer Research*, **54**, 4813–17.

Jung S. & Schluesener H.J. (1991) Human T lymphocytes recognize a peptide of single point-mutated, oncogenic ras proteins. *Journal of Experimental Medicine*, **173**, 273–6.

Kagan J. (1993) Molecular biology of chromosomal aberrations in leukemia/lymphoma. *Hematologic Pathology*, **7**, 159–201.

Kast W.M., Offringa R., Peters P.J. et al. (1989) Eradication of adenovirus E1-induced tumours by E1A-specific cytotoxic T lymphocytes. *Cell*, **59**, 603–14.

Kawakami Y., Eliyahu S., Delgado C.H. et al. (1994) Cloning of the gene coding for a shared human-melanoma antigen recognized by autologous T-cells infiltrating into tumor. *Proceedings of the National Academy of Sciences USA*, **91**, 3515–19.

Kawakami Y., Eliyahu S., Sakaguhi et al. (1994) Identification of the immunodominant peptides of the MART-1 human melanoma antigen recognized by the majority of HLA-A2-restricted tumour infiltrating lymphocytes. *Journal of Experimental Medicine*, **180**, 347–52.

Keyomarsi K., O'Leary N., Molnar G., Lees E., Fingert H.J. & Pardee A.B. (1994) Cyclin E, a potential prognostic marker for breast cancer. *Cancer Research*, **54**, 380–5.

Klijn J.G.M. & Foekens J.A. (1990) Epidermal growth factor receptors (EGFR) in breast cancer. *Annals of Oncology*, **1**, 231–5.

Kobrin M.S., Yamanaka Y., Friess H., Lopez M.E. & Korc M. (1993) Aberrant expression of type I fibroblast growth factor receptor in human pancreatic adenocarcinomas. *Cancer Research*, **53**, 4741–4.

Kubo R.T., Sette A., Grey H.M. et al. (1994) Definition of specific peptide motifs for 4 major hla-a alleles. **152**, 3913–24.

Labrecque S., Noar N., Thomsom D. & Matlashewski G. (1993) Analysis of the anti-p53 antibody response in cancer patients. *Cancer Research*, **53**, 3468–71.

Lang F.F., Miller D.C., Pisharody S., Koslow M. & Newcomb E.W. (1994) High frequency of p53 protein accumulation without p53 gene mutation in human juvenile pilocytic, low grade and anaplastic astrocytomas. *Oncogene*, **9**, 949–54.

Laurentpuig P., Lubin R., Semhounducloux S. et al. (1994) Antibodies against p53 protein in sera of patients with benign or malignant pancreatic and biliary diseases. *Gastroenterology*, **106**, A407.

Leach F.S., Tokino T., Meltzer P. et al. (1993) p53 mutation and mdm2 amplification in human soft tissue sarcomas. *Cancer Research*, **53**, 2231–4.

Lemoine N.R., Barnes D.M., Hollywood D.P. et al. (1992a) Expression of the ERBB3 gene product in breast cancer. *British Journal of Cancer*, **66**, 1116–21.

Lemoine N.R., Lobresco M., Leung H. et al. (1992b) The erbB3 gene in pancreatic cancer. *Journal of Pathology*, **168**, 269–73.

Levine A.J., Perry M.E., Chang A., Silver A., Dittmer D., Wu M. & Welsh D. (1994) The 1993 Walter Hubert Lecture: the role of the p53 tumour-suppressor gene in tumorigenesis. *British Journal of Cancer*, **69**, 409–16.

Li Y.W., McGowan P., Hellstrom I., Hellstrom K.E. & Chen L.P. (1994) Costimulation of tumor-reactive CD4+ and CD8+ T-lymphocytes by B7, a natural ligand for CD28, can be used to treat established mouse melanoma. *Journal of Immunology*, **153**, 421–8.

Libermann T.A., Nusbaum H.R., Razon N. et al. (1985) Amplification, enhanced expression and possible rearrangement of EGF receptor gene in primary human brain tumours of glial origin. *Nature (London)*, **313**, 144–7.

Lo D. (1992) T-cell tolerance. *Current Opinion in Immunology*, **4**, 711–15.

Lofts F.J. & Gullick W.J. (1991) In Lippman M.E. & Dickson R.B. (eds) *Genes, oncogenes and hormones: Advances in cellular and molecular biology of breast cancer*, pp. 161–179. Boston, Kluwer Academic Publishers.

Lubin R., Schlichtholz B., Bengoufa D. et al. (1993) Analysis of p53 antibodies in patients with various cancers define B-cell epitopes of human p53 – distribution on primary structure and exposure on protein surface. *Cancer Research*, **53**, 5872–6.

Lucas J.M., Mountain R.E., Gramza A.W., Schuller D.E., Wilkie N.M. & Lang J.C. (1994) Expression of cyclin d1 in squamous-cell carcinomas of the head and neck. *International Journal of Oncology*, **5**, 469–72.

Lurquin C., Van Pel A., Mariamé B. et al. (1989) Structure of the gene of Tum⁻ transplantation antigen P91A: the mutated exon encodes a peptide recognized with $L^d$ by tytoytic T cells. *Cell*, **58**, 293–303.

Macaulay V.M., Everard M.J., Teale J.D. et al. (1988) Autocrine function for insulin-like growth factor I in human small cell lung cancer cell lines and fresh tumor cells. *Cancer Research*, **50**, 2511.

Melief C.J.M. & Kast W.M. (1993) Potential immunogenicity of oncogene and tumour suppressor gene products. *Current Opinion in Immunology*, **5**, 709–13.

Milich D.R., McLachlan A., Raney A.K. et al. (1991) Autoantibody production in hepatitis B e antigen transgenic mice elicited with a self T-cell peptide and inhibited with nonself peptides. *Proceedings of the National Academy of Sciences USA*, **88**, 4348–52.

Mizoguchi H., O'Shea J., Longo D.L., Loeffler C.M., McVicar D.W. & Ochoa A.C. (1992) Alterations in signal transduction molecules in T lymphocytes from tumour-bearing mice. *Science*, **258**, 1795–7.

Monaco J.J. (1992) A molecular model of MHC class-I-restricted antigen processing. *Immunology Today*, **13**, 173–9.

Morrison R.S., Yamaguchi F., Saya H. et al. (1994) Basic fibroblast growth-factor and fibroblast growth-factor receptor-i are implicated in the growth of human astrocytomas. *Journal of Neurooncology*, **18**, 207–16.

Motukura T., Bloom T., Kim H.G. et al. (1991) A novel cyclin encoded by a bcl1-linked candidate oncogene. *Nature (London)*, **350**, 512–15.

Mueller M., Meyer M., Volkmann M., Rath U., Kommerell B. & Gallet P.R. (1993) Anti-p53 serum antibodies in patients with hepatocellular-carcinoma and gi-tract tumours – clinical relevance and diagnostic usefulness. *Hepatology*, **18**, 559–65.

Mulligan L.M., Kwok J.B.J., Healey C.S. et al. (1993) Germ-line mutations of the RET proto-oncogene in multiple endocrine neoplasis type 2A. *Nature (London)*, **363**, 458–60.

Natali P.G., Nicotra M.R., Digiesi G. et al. (1994) Expression of gp185(her-2) in human cutaneous melanoma – implications for experimental immunotherapeutics. *International Journal of Cancer*, **56**, 341–6.

Nau M.M., Brooks B.J., Carney D.N. et al. (1986) Human small cell lung cancers show amplification and expression of the N-myc gene. *Proceedings of the National Academy of Sciences USA*, **83**, 1092–6.

Nijman H.W., Vanderburg S.H., Vierboom M.P.M. et al. (1994) P53, a potential target for tumor-directed T-cells. *Immunology Letters*, **40**, 171–8.

Nishida N., Fukuda Y., Komeda T. et al. (1994) Amplification and overexpression of the cyclin d1 gene in aggressive human hepatocellular-carcinoma. *Cancer Research*, **54**, 3107–10.

O'Connell K.A. & Gooding L.R. (1984) Cloned cytotoxic T lymphocytes recognise cells expressing discrete fragments of the SV40 tumour antigen. *Journal of Immunology*, **132**, 953–8.

Oliner J.D., Kinzler K.W., Meltzer P.S., George D.L. & Vogelstein B. (1992) Amplification of a gene encoding a p53-associated protein in human sarcomas. *Nature (London)*, **358**, 80–3.

Papa V., Gliozzo B., Clark G.M. et al. (1993) Insulin-like growth factor-I receptors are overexpressed and predict a low risk in human breast cancer. *Cancer Research*, **53**, 3736–40.

Pardoll D.M. (1993) New strategies for enhancing the immunogenecity of tumors. *Current Opinion in Immunology*, **5**, 719–25.

Peace D.J., Chen W., Nelson H. & Cheever M.A. (1991) T cell recognition of transforming proteins encoded by mutated ras proto-oncogenes. *Journal of Immunology*, **146**, 2059–65.

Perez R., Pascual M., Macias A. & Lage A. (1984) Epidermal growth factor receptors in human breast cancer. *Breast Cancer Research and Treatment*, **4**, 189–93.

Prins J. De V.E. & Mulder N.H. (1993) The myc family of oncogenes and their presence and importance in small-cell lung carcinoma and other tumour types. *Anticancer Research*, **13**, 1373–85.

Rajkumar T., Gooden C.S.R., Lemoine N.R. & Gullick W.J. (1993) Expression of the c-erbB3 protein in gastrointestinal tract tumours determined by monoclonal antibody RTJ1. *Journal of Pathology*, **170**, 271–8.

Reifenberger G., Reifenberger J., Ichimura K., Meltzer P.S. & Collins V.P. (1994) Amplification of multiple genes from chromosomal region 12q13-14 in human malignant gliomas: preliminary mapping of the amplicons shows preferential involvement of cdk4, sas and mdm2. *Cancer Research*, **54**, 4299–303.

Riddell S.R., Watanabe K.S., Goodrich J.M., Li C.R., Agha M.E. & Greenberg P.D. (1992) Restoration of viral immunity in immunodeficient humans by the adoptive transfer to T cell clones [see comments]. *Science*, **257**, 238–41.

Ridge S.A., Worwood M., Oscier D., Jacobs A. & Padua R.A. (1990) FMS mutations in myelodysplastic, leukemic, and normal subjects. *Proceedings of the National Academy of Science USA*, **87**, 1377–80.

Rimokh R., Berger F., Bastard C. et al. (1994) Rearrangement of ccnd1 (bcl1/prad1) 3' untranslated region in mantle-cell lymphomas and t(11q13)-associated leukemias. *Blood*, **83**, 3689–96.

Riou G., Le M.G., Doussal V.L., Barrouis M., George M. & Haie C. (1987) C-myc proto-oncogene expression and prognosis in early carcinoma of the uterine cervic. *Lancet*, **1**, 761–3.

Ro J., North S.M., Gallick G.E., Hortobaggy G.N., Gutterman J.U. & Blick M. (1988) Amplified and overexpressed epidermal growth factor receptor gene in uncultured primary human breast carcinoma. *Cancer Research*, **48**, 161–4.

Rosenberg C.L., Motokura T., Kronenberg H.M. & Arnold A. (1993) Coding sequence of the overexpressed transcript of the putative oncogene PRAD1/cyclin D1 in two primary human tumors. *Oncogene*, **8**, 519–21.

Sainsbury J.R., Farndon J.R., Needman G.K., Malcolm A.J. & Harris A.L. (1987) Epidermal-growth factor receptor status as predictor of early recurrence of and death from breast cancer. *Lancet*, **1**, 1398–402.

Sauter G., Haley J., Chew K. et al. (1994) Epidermal growth factor receptor expression is associated with rapid tumour proliferation in bladder cancer. *International Journal of Cancer*, **57**, 508–14.

Schlegel J., Merdes A., Stumm G. et al. (1994) Amplification of the epidermal-growth-factor receptor gene correlates with different growth behaviour in human glioblastoma. *International Journal of Cancer*, **56**, 72–7.

Schlichtholz B., Legros Y., Gillet D. et al. (1992) The immune response to p53 in breast cancer patients is directed against immunodominant epitopes unrelated to the mutational hot spot. *Cancer Research*, 52, 6380–4.

Schönrich G., Alferink J., Klevenz A. et al. (1994) Tolerance induction as a multistep process. *European Journal of Immunology*, 24, 285–93.

Schönrich G., Kalinke U., Momburg F. et al. (1991) Down-regulation of T cell receptors on self-reactive T cells as a novel mechanism for extrathymic tolerance induction. *Cell*, 65, 293–304.

Schreiber H., Ward P. L., Rowley D.A. & Stauss H.J. (1988) Unique tumor-specific antigens. *Annual Review of Immunology*, 6, 465–83.

Sercarz E.E., Lehmann P.V., Ametani A., Benichou G., Miller A. & Moudgil K. (1993) Dominance and crypticity of T cell antigenic determinants. *Annual Review of Immunology*, 11, 729–66.

Sheikh M.S., Shao Z.M., Hussain A. & Fontana J.A. (1993) The p53-binding protein mdm2 gene is differentially expressed in human breast-carcinoma. *Cancer Research*, 53, 3226–8.

Shtivelman E., Lifshitz B., Gale R.P., Roe B.A. & Cannani E. (1986) Alternative splicing of RNAs transcribed from the human abl gene and from the bcr-abl fused gene. *Cell*, 47, 277–84.

Skipper J. & Stauss H.J. (1993) Identification of two cytotoxic T lymphocyte-recognised epitopes in the Ras protein. *Journal of Experimental Medicine*, 177, 1493–8.

Slamon D.J., Godolphin W., Jones L.A. et al. (1989) Studies of the HER-2/neu proto-oncogene in human breast and ovarian cancer. *Science*, 244, 707–12.

Sorokine I., Ben-Mahrez K., Bracone A. et al. (1991) Presence of circulating anti c-myb oncogene product antibodies in human sera. *International Journal of Cancer*, 47, 665–9.

Srivastava P.K., Udono H., Blachere N.E. & Li Z. (1994) Heat shock proteins transfer peptides during antigen processing and CTL priming. *Immunogenetics*, 39, 93–8.

Szikora J.P., Vanpel A. & Boon T. (1993) Tum⁻ mutation p35b generates the mhc-binding site of a new antigenic peptide. *Immunogenetics*, 37, 135–8.

Tevethia S.S., Tevethia M.J., Lewis A.J., Reddy V.B. & Weissman S.M. (1983) Biology of Simian Virus 40 transplantation antigen (TrAg). IX. Analysis of TrAg in mouse cells synthesizing truncated SV40 large T antigen. *Virology*, 128, 319–30.

Theillet C., Adelaide J., Louason G. et al. (1993) FGFRI and PLAT genes and DNA amplification at 8p12 in breast and ovarian cancer. *Genes Chromosomes and Cancer*, 7, 219–26.

Tobal K., Paglucia A., Bhatt B., Bailey N., Layton D.M. & Mufti G.J. (1990) Mutation of the human FMS gene (M-CSF receptor) in myelodysplastic syndromes and acute myeloid leukemia. *Leukemia*, 4, 486–9.

Townsend A. & Bodmer H. (1989) Antigen recognition by Class I-restricted T lymphocytes. *Annual Review of Immunology*, 7, 601–24.

Townsend A.R., Rothbard J., Gotch F.M. et al. (1986) The epitopes of influenza nucleoprotein recognized by cytotoxic T lymphocytes can be defined with short synthetic peptides. *Cell*, 44, 959–68.

Udono H. & Srivastava P.K. (1994) Comparison of tumor-specific immunogenicities of stress-induced proteins gp96, hsp90, and hsp70. *Journal of Immunology*, 152, 5398–403.

Ueba T., Takahashi J.A., Fukomoto M. et al. (1994) Expression of fibroblast growth factor receptor-1 in human glioma and meningioma tissues. *Neurosurgery*, 34, 221–6.

Urban J.L. & Schreiber H. (1992) Tumour antigens. *Annual Review of Immunology*, **10**, 617–44.

van der Bruggen P., Traversari C., Chomez P. et al. (1991) A gene encoding an antigen recognized by cytolytic T lymphocytes on a human melanoma. *Science*, **254**, 1643–7.

Weidner U., Peter S., Strohmeyer T. et al. (1990) Inverse relationship of epidermal growth factor receptor and HER-2/neu gene expression in human renal cell carcinoma. *Cancer Research*, **50**, 4504–9.

Winter S.F., Minna J.D., Johnson, B.E. et al. (1992) Development of antibodies against p53 in lung cancer patients appear to be dependent on the type of p53 mutation. *Cancer Research*, **52**, 4168–74.

Wong A.J., Bigner S.H., Bigner D.D. et al. (1987) Increased expression of the epidermal growth factor receptor gene in malignant gliomas is invariably associated with gene amplification. *Proceedings of the National Academy of Sciences USA*, **84**, 6899–903.

Xu L., Chen Y.T., Huvos A.G. et al. (1994) Overexpression of p53 protein in squamous-cell carcinomas of head and neck without apparent gene-mutations. *Diagnostic and Molecular Pathology*, **3**, 83–92.

Xue F., Yu H., Maurer L.H. et al. (1994) Germline RET mutations in MEN2A and FMTC and their detection by simple DNA diagnostic tests. *Human Molecular Genetics*, **3**, 635–8.

Yamaguchi F., Saya G., Bruner J.M. & Morrison R.S. (1994) Differential expression of two fibroblast growth factor receptor genes is associated with malignant progression in human astrocytomas. *Proceedings of the National Academy of Sciences USA*, **91**, 484–8.

Yang W.-I., Zukerberg L.R., Motokura T., Arnold A. & Harris N.L. (1994) Cyclin D1 (Bcl-1, PRAD1) protein expression in low-grade B cell lymphomas and reactive hyperplasia. *American Journal of Pathology*, **145**, 86–96.

Yee D., Paik S., Lebovic G.S., Marcus R.R., Favoni R.E. & Cullen K.J. (1989) Analysis of insulin-like growth factor-I gene expression in malignancy: evidence for a paracrine role in human breast cancer. *Molecular Endocrinology*, **3**, 509–17.

Yoshino I., Goedegebuure P.S., Peoples G.E. et al. (1994a) Her2/neu-derived peptides are shared antigens among human nonsmall cell lung-cancer and ovarian-cancer. *Cancer Research*, **54**, 3387–90.

Yoshino I., Peoples G.E., Goedegeburre P.S., Maziarz R. & Eberlein T.J. (1994b) Association of HER2/neu expression with sensitivity to tumour-specific CTL in human ovarian cancer. *Journal of Immunology*, **152**, 2393–400.

Zhang W., Hu G., Estey E., Hester J. & Deisseroth A. (1992) Altered conformation of the p53 protein in myeloid leukemia cells and mitogen-stimulated normal blood cells. *Oncogene*, **7**, 1645–7.

Zhang Y.-J., Jiang W., Chen C.-J. et al. (1993) Amplification and overexpression of cyclin D1 in human hepatocellular carcinoma. *Biochemical and Biophysical Research Communications*, **196**, 1010–16.

Zinkernagel R.M. & Doherty P.C. (1979) MHC-restricted cytotoxic T cells: studies on the biological role of polymorphic transplantation antigens determining T cell restriction-specificity, function and responsiveness. *Advances in Immunology*, **27**, 51–177.

# 8

# Co-stimulatory Molecules and their Role in Tumour Immunity

A. G. DALGLEISH

## ◼ INTRODUCTION

The concept of stimulating the immune system to reject established tumours has been the goal of many cancer researchers over the years. Other chapters in this volume review a number of strategies whereby this might ultimately be achieved. Some of them mention the possibility of using co-stimulatory molecules as a means to achieving this goal. The importance of co-stimulatory molecules in tumour immunology has only been recognized in the last few years. The discovery of specific molecules involved in this process has allowed a more thorough understanding of antigen presentation as well as an insight into the potential importance of these molecules in the induction and, *ipso facto*, avoidance of anti-tumour immune responses.

The role of antigen presentation by the major histocompatibility complex (MHC) or the human leukocyte antigens (HLA) in humans to the T cell receptor has been known for some time, although the low affinity of the interaction and the variability of the outcome have been poorly understood. It is clear that signalling through the T cell receptor itself is insufficient to induce proliferation of T helper cells and optimal interleukin-2 (IL-2) production.

There would appear to be at least three stages in delivering a satisfactory signal. The first is the 'interaction' of the adhesion molecules, as blockade of these using antibodies inhibits a primary immune response. The second is the recognition of MHC plus peptide by the TCR with subsequent signalling. The third is co-stimulation, the absence of which not only results in the failure of proliferation but the induction of anergy.

The existence of apparent anergy to tumours, which can be broken by tumour cell vaccination strategies, highlights the importance of co-stimulation in tumour immunology. Moreover, a number of receptor–ligand pairs and cytokines can impart a co-stimulus to antigen-specific stimulation. These induce the adhesion molecules ICAM (intracellular adhesion molecule)-1, LFA (lymphocyte function-associated antigen)-1,

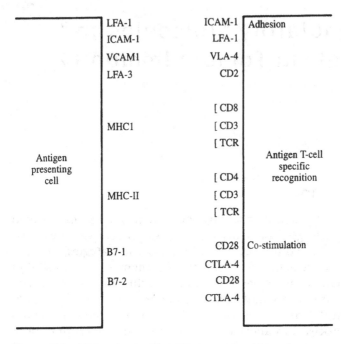

**Figure 8.1** Molecules involved in the recognition of tumour antigens.

LFA3-CD (cluster determinant) 2, as well as the more recently recognized B7 (B7-1) (CD80) and B7-2 (CD86) and the CD28/CTLA-4 (cytotoxic T lymphocyte antigen) 4 interaction. Others include CD40-CD40L, CD5-CD72, and CD24-CD24L (Figure 8.1).

These different pathways do not all 'signal' the same outcome, for instance, B7-1 stimulation and not ICAM-1 or LFA-3 co-stimulation results in proliferation of the T cell and the prevention of allo-antigen-specific anergy, which appears to be dependent on the synthesis of sufficient IL-2 (Table 8.1).

## ■ B7 AND CD28

The discovery of the co-stimulatory pathways confirms the importance of the two signal lymphocyte models initially proposed for B cells (by Bretcher & Cohn, 1970) and for other antigen-specific lymphocytes (Janeway, 1989; Swartz, 1989). One of the most important co-stimulators or secondary receptors B7 (not to be confused with HLA-B7) was found to be preferentially expressed on activated B cells and the antigen-presenting cells (APCs) (Freeman et al., 1989; Razi-Wolf et al., 1993). It was found

Table 8.1.    Outcome of T Cell Stimulation with and without
Additional Pathways

| Signalling | TCR activation | Proliferation | IL-2 accumulation | Prevention of anergy |
|---|---|---|---|---|
| TCR | + | – | – | – |
| TCR + CD28 | + | + | + | + |
| TCR + LFA-1 | + | + | –(+) | – |
| TCR + CD2 or CD25 | + | + | –(+) | – |
| TCR + IL-4R (interleukin 4 receptor) | + | + | + | + |

to bind to CD28 and CTLA-4 molecules on lymphocytes (Linsley et al., 1990, 1991). The importance of this interaction was shown by several workers who demonstrated that it was required for proliferation of both murine and human CD4+ cells, and that blocking co-stimulation by B7 suppresses humoral responses and makes long-term acceptance of tissue xenografts possible (Linsley et al., 1992a,b; Lenschow et al., 1992).

There are two major family members of B7: B7-1 and B7-2 and now designated CD80 for B7-1 and CD86 for B7-2. Both are members of the immunoglubin gene superfamily. B7-1 was identified with two antibodies and classified as CD80 (Freeman et al., 1989). The second member, B7-2, is assigned to the CD86 cluster and has only 25(PER) amino-acid identity with B7-1. However, both are low-affinity receptors for CD28 and high-affinity receptors for CTLA-4 (Linsley & Ledbetter, 1993). The main difference between the two is that, in contrast to the short cytoplasmic domain of B7-1, B7-2 has a long domain containing three potential sites for phosphorylation by protein kinase C (PKC), which could suggest that this component is involved in transmitting functional signals (Azuma et al., 1992a,b; Freeman et al., 1993a, 1993b).

B7-1 has been shown to be constitutively expressed in dendritic cells (Young et al., 1992; Larsen et al., 1994). However others have shown that dendritic cells need to be activated before they express B7-1, and hence it is induced as opposed to being constitutively expressed (Hart et al., 1993). B7-2 is constitutively expressed on monocytes but is also induced in the majority of APCs following the appropriate stimulus. Interestingly, B7-2 is induced more rapidly than B7-1 on both human and murine APCs. More recently, indirect evidence for a third B7-like molecule has been reported. It is defined by a monoclonal BB1 (Augustin et al., 1993; Boussiotis et al.,

1993a,b; Nickoloff et al., 1993) and is expressed on keratinocytes, which have no message for B7-1 or B7-2.

B7-1 and B7-2 both interact with CD28, and signal via the T cell receptor. CD28 is expressed on resting lymphocytes (95% CD4+ve and 50% of CD8+ve) and expression increases following activation (June et al., 1994). CTLA-4 also interacts with B7-1 and B7-2, although it is only 31% similar to CD28 at the amino-acid level. Furthermore, it is not expressed on resting T cells and requires the cells to be activated for it to be induced (Herper et al., 1991; Freeman et al., 1993; Gross et al., 1992; Linsley et al., 1992b). The CTLA-4 cytoplasmic domain is highly conserved amongst species (human, mouse, and chicken) and hence suggests a vital signalling function.

## ■ CD28/CTLA-4 SIGNALLING

Following T cell receptor (TCR)-mediated signalling, CD28 stimulation results in increased IL-2 mRNA and T cell proliferation as well as up-regulation of the CD40 ligand (de Boer et al., 1993). Other cytokines in addition to IL-2 are induced (June et al., 1994). CD28 signalling results in the increased phosphorylation of cellular substrates in activated T cells. Phosphorylated cytoplasmic CD28 can bind and activate phosphoinositide 3 (P13)-kinase (Nunes et al., 1993, Ward et al., 1993; Hutchcroft & Bierer, 1994; Rudd et al., 1994; Truitt, Hicks & Imboden, 1994).

In spite of containing a motif that predicts binding to P13-kinase, there is no evidence so far that a co-stimulatory signal is delivered by CTLA-4 in spite of the higher binding affinity and cross species conservation. In experiments using CD28/CTLA-4 cytoplasmic tail/CD8 fusion molecules expressed in T cells, cross linking only results in the CD28 containing constructs (Stein et al., 1994). However, CTLA-4 may only transmit signals in the presence of CD28 (Linsley et al., 1992a,b). More recently it has been proposed that CTLA-4 may induce an inhibitory signal, which may be antigen specific via a different CTLA-4 counter receptor.

One way to determine the importance of specific signalling pathways in determining function is to prepare 'knock-out' mice, which cannot express the protein of the chosen 'knock-out' gene. However, these models may be surprisingly misleading with the often predicted deficits, merely attenuated in these mice. It would appear that the recruitment of redundant pathways may explain some of these findings. In the case of CD28 knock-out mice, although IL-2 secretion and T cell proliferation is reduced in response to mitogens, cytolytic activity appears to be normal (Shahinian et al., 1993). CTLA-4 knock-out mice have not been developed at the time of writing.

## Antigen-specific Unresponsiveness: Implications for Tumour Immunology

The single most important thing about the B7-CD28 pathways as compared to other co-stimulatory ligands pairs is its role in the prevention and hence, *ipso facto*, induction of anergy. This can be demonstrated using antibodies to CD28 or cells transfected with MHC with or without B7-1. Absence of B7-CD28 signalling clearly results in anergy in both self and allo-antigen-specific systems (Gimmi et al., 1993; Boussiotis et al., 1993a, 1994). Interestingly, CTLA-4 Ig is to the most effective blocker of the B7-CD28 pathway.

The interplay between B7-1 and B7-2 would appear to be mainly temporal in that B7-2 is the quickest to initiate an immune response, and B7-1 amplifies the immune response at later times. The role of other cytokines in the co-stimulatory process has already been mentioned. It is worth noting that some cytokines such as interleukin-10 (IL-10) can down-regulate or prevent the expression of B7 on APCs and hence induce anergy (Ding et al., 1993). In addition to the obvious implications for tumour immunology reviewed here, the co-stimulatory pathways present an ideal handle by which to induce tolerance of transplanted organs. In addition, inappropriate expression of co-stimulatory molecules could interfere with peripheral tolerance and inhibit anergy, which could then result in autoimmunity. This has been shown in a transgenic mouse model of diabetes (Harlem et al., 1994). Where organ rejection and autoimmunity can be prevented or treated by inhibiting the B7-CD28 pathway (with CTLA-4 Ig!), the fight against cancer requires the opposite as the goal, that is, rejection of the transplant (tumour) and the induction of autoimmunity, that is, the self-antigens on the tumour.

The absence of a co-stimulatory molecule in the presentation of tumour-specific or associated antigens would from the foregoing not only result in the absence of a suitable proliferative response, but also induce anergy. This could explain why tumour cells are not rejected by immune surveillance and why tumour vaccine protocols can induce immune responses that can see the parental tumour. A number of studies have shown that tumour cells transfected with MHC class I or cytokine genes, and then given as a vaccine can induce a strong enough immune response to reject a challenge with the untransfected parental cells. In some cases, immune response is effective enough to induce the regression of an established tumour. This approach has been used to demonstrate the importance of the B7-CD28 pathway in tumour recognition and rejection.

B-7 transfected into certain tumour cell lines leads to rejection of the tumour cell inoculum and the induction of an immune response, which is able to eliminate a challenge with even untransfected cells of the parent tumour line.

Chen et al. (1993) were able to demonstrate in the E7L3/K1735 murine melanoma model that B7+ cells were able to induce a response against established micrometastases, which indicates that the B7 molecule was able to reverse a state of anergy or that the cytotoxic T lymphocytes (CTL) were not anergic. The immune responses were antigen and MHC specific, and mediated through CD8+ cells (and not CD4 or NK cells). The fact that B7 expression is not required in target cells suggests that the antitumour effect is induced by enhancing the cytolytic effector stage. However, it is important to point out that, in these experiments, only strong tumour antigens and not nonimmunogenic antigens were rejected, and that only B7+ micrometastases could be 'cured' by inducing tumour immunity.

It is possible that tumours can actively reanergise the immune response to their own antigens. Support for this comes from the demonstration by Becker et al. (1993) that a B7−ve melanoma is able to induce unresponsiveness in an autologous CD4+ clone.

Dohring et al. (1994) have extended these observations into human tumour cells of melanoma, ovarian cancer, and myelomonolytic leukaemia origin. Those expressing B7+ (introduced using a retroviral vector) were able to stimulate strong proliferative and cytotoxic responses in allogenic T cells in vitro. The effector CTL were able to recognize both transfected and untransfected tumour cells, as found in murine models in vivo. Similar experiments using B7 transfectants of colorectal tumour lines have failed to show enhanced immunogenicity for T cell proliferative and cytotoxic responses to allo-antigens (Browning, personal communication), emphasizing that, as with the animal models, the co-stimulatory effects of B7 in human tumour cells are not universal with regard to tumour type. Additionally B7+ cells were able to induce cytotoxic responses by both CD4- and CD8-depleted T cells, suggesting that B7 is able to induce a cytotoxic response in the absence of CD4 and other APCs.

If the B7-CD28 pathway is important in vitro, then this would be expected to be reflected in vivo. Using malignant melanoma, Hersey, Smith & Thomas (1994) examined the expression of B7 by FACS analysis of surface expression and by mRNA by polymerase chain reaction (PCR) analysis. PCR detected B7 mRNA in 50% (three of six) melanoma cell lines and 42% (eight of nineteen) cultures of metastatic melanoma. Using the BB1 antibody of FACS analysis, low levels of expression were seen in three of the ten melanoma cell cultures that were B7+ by PCR analysis. In two of the six cell lines tested, the expression could be increased by culture in granulocyte–macrophage colony-stimulating factor (GM-CSF), IL-2, interferon-$\gamma$ (IFN-$\gamma$), and IFN-$\alpha$2. Expression was sought and not demonstrated in eleven primary and nine metastatic melanoma tissue sections indicating that the B7-CD28 pathway is down-regulated or absent in vivo in human melanoma.

## ■ B7-CD28 AND THE POTENTIAL TREATMENT OF HUMAN CANCER

At the time of writing, it is not yet known whether expression of B7-1 or B7-2 (or B7-3!) will induce rejection of human melanoma in vivo. A number of approaches are being considered if initial attempts at this approach (which is inherently practical) is disappointing. One is to complement or supplement the transfected tumour cell lines being used as vaccines. This could be with the addition of other genes such as HLA or cytokines transfected into the cells, or by the addition of exogenous cytokines. Moreover, the mechanism of delivery and the use of adjuvants will also be crucial to all vaccination procedures mentioned in this book.

Much has been written about the tendency of certain cytokines to be expressed and together to be associated with particular types of immune response. Two major cytokine groupings are recognized; T helper 1 and T helper 2 ($T_{H1}$ and $T_{H2}$). $T_{H1}$ cytokines include IFN-$\gamma$ and IL-2, and are involved in inducing cell-mediated immunity (delayed-type hypersensitivity, cytotoxic T-cell induction). $T_{H2}$ cytokines include IL-4, IL-5, and IL-6, and are involved in mainly humoral mediated immunity. Two more recent cytokines appear to enhance the overall activities of these responses. $T_{H1}$ responses are enhanced by IL-12 and $T_{H2}$ responses are enhanced by IL-10. As IL-10 down-regulates co-stimulatory molecules, it may be that IL-12 enhances co-stimulatory pathways.

Two studies suggest that this is the case: Murphy et al. (1994) report that B7 and IL-12 cooperate in the induction of proliferation of mouse T helper clones and their resultant production of IFN-$\gamma$. The APCs used were L cells, which were transfected with FcR+ with or without B7+. $T_{H1}$ cells in the absence of IL-12 did not proliferate in response to stimulation with the APCs plus anti-CD3 monoclonal antibody. However, the addition of IL-12 resulted in a very pronounced proliferation of T cells and IFN-$\gamma$ production. In contrast, naive T cells proliferated well to stimulation in the absence of IL-12. The anti-$T_{H1}$ activity of IL-10 is probably due to its ability to inhibit the APC function of splenic and peripheral blood monocytes, and macrophages by inhibiting to the co-stimulatory pathways. However, IL-12 is shown in this system to overcome this defect. Similar findings are reported by Kubin et al. (1994) who show, in addition, that the combination of CD28 and IL-12 signalling is resistant to cyclosporin

A, and is largely independent of exogenous IL-2. Although the combination is most efficient at inducing IFN-$\gamma$, (TNF-$\alpha$) and GM-CSF production is also observed.

The combination effect is also seen when used to inhibit the B7-CD28 signalling system. Neither B7 antibody nor cyclosporin A by themselves inhibit a primary mixed lymphocyte reaction of freshly isolated human T cells towards a human B cell line. However, when used together, they are able to induce nonresponsiveness of allo-antigen-specific CTL precursors, while preserving reactivity to a third-party stimulator (van Good et al., 1994). The implications of these observations will inevitably lead to relevant combinatory studies against human tumours.

Another approach is to target tumour cells in vivo with vectors that will be able to deliver and express B7-1 and B7-2 on the surface of tumour tissue. This will require a specific tissue promoter (for example, tyrosinase in melanoma) to express the gene when it is in the right cell as well as an effective promoter has already been used to carry in enzymes for converting prodrugs to toxic analogues. Retroviral vectors are said not to be able to replicate to sufficiently enough titres for purposes of delivering such genes to the majority of tumour cells. However, having said this it would appear that an effective bystander effect (where uninfected cells are also killed) means that only about 50% of tumour cells need to be infected for complete resolutions in murine systems in vivo. Vaccinia viruses constructs, which result in a rapid and efficient expression of both B7-1 and B7-2 (greater than 97% of cells at 4 hours) have been developed in murine systems, and lead to the rejection of weakly syngeneic tumours when infected with vectors that enable these molecules to be expressed, in immunocompetent hosts.

## ■ MHC CLASS II AND TUMOUR ANTIGEN RECOGNITION

Although some of the studies report that CD4 help can be bypassed, most of then clearly show that it is the afferent arm of the immune system that is defective as opposed to the effector arm. If this was not the case, the 'vaccination' strategies discussed elsewhere in this book would not be expected to work. It is therefore perhaps surprising that more emphasis has not been placed on MHC class II expression. Indeed, several animal studies have shown that, when tumours are transfected with MHC class II, they can induce an effective antitumour response, which can prevent a challenge with parental or wild-type cells from taking (Chen et al., 1993; Ostrand-Rosenberg et al., 1991). This may explain the apparent relative immunogenocity of melanoma as opposed to most other spontaneous malignancies, as a reasonable proportion of melanomas express MHC class II, while the majority of spontaneously arising tumour types do not. Perhaps the reason why class II molecules have not been as popular as other molecules or cytokines is that they can occasionally make the tumour more aggressive. Based on current experience with co-stimulatory molecules, it is likely that this could occur when MHC class II is expressed in a tumour cell that is devoid of any co-stimulatory molecules, which would therefore induce anergy. The importance of signalling in this interaction is highlighted by the demonstration that MHC class II molecules with truncated cytoplasmic tails do not induce antitumour immunity against murine sarcoma cells. However, this can be overcome by supertransfecting with B7-1. Therefore, CD4+ T cell activation in this system appears to require the delivery of both an antigen-specific signal via the class II heterodimer and a co-stimulatory signal via B7 (Ostrand-Rosenberg et al., 1991; Baskar et al., 1993).

It would appear from these and other experiments that MHC class II-expressing tumour cells function as APCs for tumour peptides. However, class II molecules usually present exogenous and not endogenous peptides, and would not be expected to present endogenous peptides. The reason why tumour cells may, in fact, present their own peptides on class II may be that the invariant chain (Ii) prevents the interaction with endogenous peptides, and (Ii) would appear to be absent in tumour cells. When tumour cells are transfected with Ii they are no longer immunogenic in autologous mice (Clements et al., 1992). The ability of MHC class II to present tumour antigens in vitro has been shown in vitro using a lysozyme antigen to antigen-specific T cell hybridomers (Chen, Ullrich and Anathaswarmy, 1994).

## ■ THE ROLE OF CD40 AND GP39 THE CD40 LIGAND IN CO-STIMULATION

The CD40 ligand (gp39) is present on T helper cells and binds to CD40 on B cells. The CD40 antigen is a molecule with homology to the nerve growth factor receptor and tumour necrosis factor family of molecules. The CD40 'pathway' is intrinsically linked to the process of T cell activation and plays a vital role as a co-stimulus in signalling B cells (Lane et al., 1992; Roy et al., 1993).

The CD40L (gp39) expressed on activated helper cells triggers B cell cycling by binding to CD40. The efficiency of this triggering is associated with the increasing density of the CD40L on the T cell surface (Armitage et al., 1992; Noelle et al., 1992; Castle et al., 1993). The expression and function of CD40L and B7 are very interdependent during antigen-specific immune responses. Antibodies that block CD4, LFA-1, and

MHC class II prevent antigen-induced expression of CD40L, whereas anti-CD3 induces CD40L expression demonstrating that CD40L is induced after TCR signalling. Although antibodies to B7-1 or B7-2 do not interfere with CD40L expression, the converse is true, in that antibodies to CD40L inhibit the B7-1 and B7-2 up-regulation with complete inhibition being associated with antibodies to CD40L and IL-4. However, ligation of CD28 and CTA4 with B7 expressed on fibroblasts is reported by de Boer et al. (1993) to enhance expression of CD40L suggesting a close interdependency between B7 and CD40L.

The outcome of CD40 signalling would appear to depend on the type of B cell being triggered. Vastly different outcomes from proliferation to apoptosis induction can be induced depending on the activation state of the cell. The signalling pathways of CD40 are not fully elucidated and a review is beyond the scope of this chapter. However, it is worth noting that CD40 appears to be coupled to a protein tyrosine kinase (PTK) pathway and that CD40L expression uses a different pathway from anti-Ig-mediated activation.

Blockade of the CD40L prevents primary and secondary immune responses to thymus-dependent antigens, and hence is essential to the development of B cell immunity. In addition, it can inhibit the expression of B7-1 and B7-2, and, therefore, can induce long-term tolerance (Durie et al., 1994). Studies of graft-versus-host disease (GVHD) mice have shown that anti-CD40L antibody results in the prevention of allo-reactive cytotoxic lymphocytes and hence anti-CD40L is a potential treatment for preventing GVHD (Kennedy et al., 1994). The ability of the CD40 pathway to operate as a co-signal either directly or indirectly suggests that this ligand might be of use in antitumour strategies. However, to date there have been no reports. It may be of use in cases where B7 fails to co-stimulate when expressed in tumour cells.

## ■ OTHER MOLECULES WITH CO-STIMULATORY ROLE

There are a number of other molecules that have been shown to be associated with a co-stimulatory role in certain similarities. For instance, whereas B7 is involved in stimulating memory (CD45RO+) but not naive cells, CD27, which is another member of the NGFR (nerve growth factor receptor) TNF receptor family, interacts with CD70 and is associated with activation of naive T cells (CD45RA+). Cross linking of CD27 and CD27/CD70 interaction leads to the preferential proliferation of CD45RA-positive T cells in the presence of suboptimal dose of PHA (phytohaemagglutinin), PMA (phorbol myristate acetate), anti-CD2, or anti-CD3 (Kobata et al., 1994). The potential importance of this interaction with regard to tumour immunology is not yet known.

Other molecules that can modulate antigen-receptor signalling include CD22 and CD19 (which interacts with CD21). CD22 is involved in positive B cell receptor signalling whereas the CD19/CD21 complex abrogates B cell receptor signalling. CD23 is involved in coupling to cAMP on resting cells and phospholipase C (PLC) in activated cells. CD38 interacts with surface immunoglobulin, and is involved in rescuing activated B cells from apoptosis and interacts with IL-4 in providing co-stimulatory or antagonistic signals to B cells, depending on their state of activation (Harnett, 1994). The importance of cytokines in providing co-stimuli such as IL-4 and IL-7 should not be overlooked, and the synergistic importance of the IL-12 and B7 pathway has already been noted.

# ■ CONCLUSIONS

Although only the B7/CD28-CTLA-4 pathway has been shown so far to have a major impact on tumour immunology and hence to be a contender for therapeutic intervention, there are a number of other pathways that might also be important in some if not all tumours, which might be exploitable as either immunotherapeutic or direct 'gene therapy' strategies.

### REFERENCES

Armitage R.J., Fanslow W.C., Stockbine L. et al. (1992) Molecular and biological characterisation of a murine ligand and CD40. *Nature (London)*, **357**, 80–2.
Augustin M., Dietrich A., Niedner R. et al. (1993) Phorbol-12-myristate 1-acetate-treated human-keratinocytes express B7-like molecules that serve a co-stimulatory role in T-cell activation. *Journal of Invertigative Dermatology*, **100**, 275–81.
Azuma M., Ito D., Yagita H., Okumura K., Phillips J.H., Lanier L.L. & Somoza, C. (1993a) B70 antigen is a second ligand for CTLA-4 and CD28. *Nature (London)*, **366**, 76–9.
Azuma M., Yssel H., Phillips J.H., Spits H. & Lanier L.L. (1993b). Functional expression of B7/BB1 on activated T lymphocytes. *Journal of Experimental Medicine*, **177**, 845–50.
Baskar S., Ostrand-Rosenberg S., Habavi N., Nadler L.M., Freeman G.J. & Glimcher L.H. (1993) Constitutive expression of B7 restores immunology of tumour cells expressing truncated major histocompatibility complex Class II molecules. *Proceedings of the National Academy of Sciences USA*, **90**, 5687–90.
Becker J.C., Brablets T., Czerny C., Teermeer C. & Brocker E.B. (1993) Tumour escape mechanisms from immunosurveillance in a specific MHC-restricted CD4+ human T-cell clone by the autologous MHC Class II+ melonoma. *International Immunology*, **5**, 1501–8.
Boussiotis V.A., Freeman G.J., Gray G., Gribben J. & Nadler L.M. (1993) B7 but not ICAM-1 co-stimulation prevents the induction of human alloantigen specific tolerance: *Journal of Experimental Medicine*, **178**, 1753–63.

Boussiotis V.A., Freeman G.J., Gribben J.G., Daley, G. & Nadler L.M., (1993) Activated human B lymphocytes express three CTLA-4 binding counter-receptors which co-stimulate T-cell activation. *Proceedings of the National Academy of Sciences USA*, **90**, 11059–63.

Boussiotis V.A., Freeman J.G., Griffin J.D., Gray G.S., Gribben G. & Nadler L.M. (in press) CD2 is involved in maintenance and reversal of human alloantigen-specific clonal anergy. *Proceedings of the National Academy of Sciences USA*.

Bretscher P. & Cohn M. (1970) A theory of self-nonself discrimination. *Science*, **169**, 1042–9.

Castle B.E., Kishimoto K., Stearns C., Brown M.L. & Kehry M.R. (1993) Regulation of expression of the ligand for CD40 on T-helper lymphocytes. *Journal of Immunology*, **151**, 1777–88.

Chen P. & Anathaswamy H. (1993) Rejection of K1735 murine melanoma in syngeneic hosts requires expression of MHC Class I antigens and either Class II antigens or IL-2. *Journal of Immunology*, **151**, 55.

Chen P., Ullrich S. & Anathaswamy H. (1994) Presentation of endogenous tumour antigens to CD4+ T lymphocytes by murine melanoma cells transfected with major histocompatibility complex Class II genes. *Journal of Leukocyte Biology*, **564**, 469–74.

Clements V., Baskar S., Armstrong T., Ostrand-Rosenberg S. (1992) Invariant chain alters the malignant phenotype of MHC Class II$^+$ tumour cells. *Journal of Immunology*, **149**, 2391–6.

De Boer M., Kasran M., Kwekkeboom J., Walter H., Vandenberghe P. & Ceuppens J.L. (1993) Ligation with B7 with CD28/CTLA-4 on T-cells results in CD40 ligand expression, IL-4 secretion and efficient help for antibody production by B cells. *European Journal of Immunology*, **23**, 3120–5.

Ding L., Linsley P.S., Huang L.Y., Germain R.N. & Shevach E.M. (1993) IL-10 inhibits macrophage co-stimulatory activity by selectively inhibiting the up-regulation of B7 expression. *Journal of Immunology*, **151**, 1224–34.

Dohring C., Angman L., Spagnoli G. & Lanzavecchia A. (1994) T helper and accessory cell independent cytotoxic responses to human tumour cells transferred with a B7 retroviral vector. *International Journal of Cancer*, **57**, 754–9.

Durie F.H., Foy T.M., Masters S.R., Laman J.D. & Noelle R.J. (1994) The role of CD40 in the regulation of humoral and cell-mediated immunity. *Immunology Today*, **15**, 406–10.

Freeman G.J. Borriello F., Hodes R.J. et al. (1993b) Uncovering of functional alternative CTLA-4 counter-receptor in B7-difficient mice. *Science*, **262**, 907–9.

Freeman G.J., Freedman A.S., Segil J.M., Lee G., Whitman J.F. & Nadler L.M. (1989) B7, a new member of the Ig superfamily with unique expression on activated and neo-plastic B cells. *Journal of Immunology*, **143**, 2714–22.

Freeman G.J., Gribben J.G., Boussiotis V.A. et al. (1993a) Cloning of B7-2: a CTLA-4 counter-receptor that co-stimulates human T-cell proliferation. *Science*, **262**, 909–11.

Freeman G.J., Lombard D.B., Gimmi C.D. et al. (1992) CTLA-4 and CD28 mRNAa are co-expressed in most activated T-cells after activation: expression of CTLA-4 and CD28 mRNA does not correlate with the pattern of lymphokine production. *Journal of Immunology*, **149**, 3795–801.

Gimmi C.D., Freeman G.J., Gribben J.G., Gray G. & Nadler L.M. (1993) Human T-cell clonal anergy is induced by antigen presentation in the absence of B7 co-stimulation. *Proceedings of the National Academy of Sciences USA*, **90**, 6586–6590.

Gross J.A., Callas E. & Allison J.P. (1992) Identification and distribution of the co-stimulatory receptor CD28 in the mouse. *Journal of Immunology*, **149**, 380–8.

Harlan D.M., Hengartner H., Huang M.L. et al. (1994) Transgenic mice expressing both B7 and viral glycoprotein on pancreatic β cells along with glycoprotein-specific transgenic T-cells develop diabetes due to a breakdown of T-lymphocytes unresponsiveness. *Proceedings of the National Academy of Sciences USA*, **91**, 3137–41.

Harnett M.M. (1994) Antigen receptor signalling: from the membrane to the nucleus. *Immunology Today*, **19**, 1–2.

Harper K., Balzano C., Rouvier E., Mattei M.G. Luciani M.F. & Goldstein P. (1991) CTLA-4 and CD28 activated lymphocyte molecules are closely related in both mouse and human as to sequence, message, expression, gene structure and chromosomal location. *Journal of Immunology*, **147**, 1037–44.

Hart D.N., Starling G.C., Calder V.L. & Fernando N.S. (1993) B7/BB-1 is a leucocyte differentiation antigen on human dendritic cells induced by activation. *Immunology*, **79**, 616–20.

Hersey P., Si Z., Smith M.J. & Thomas W.D. (1994) Expression of the costimulatory molecule B7 on melanoma cells. *International Journal of Cancer*, **58**, 527–32.

Hutchcroft J.E., & Bierer B.E. (1994) Activation-dependent phosphorylation of the T-lymphocyte surface receptor CD28 and associated proteins. *Proceedings of the National Academy of Sciences USA*, **91**, 3260–4.

Janeway C.A. (1989) The role of CD4 in T cell activation accessory molecule or co-receptor. *Immunulogy Today*, **10**, 234–8.

June C.H., Bluestone J.A., Nadler L.M. & Thompson C.B. (1994) The B7 and CD28 receptor families. *Immunology Today*, **15**, 321–31.

Kennedy M.K., Mohler K.M., Shanebeck K.D. et al. (1994) Induction of B cell co-stimulatory function by recombinant murine CD40 ligand. *European Journal of Immunology*, **24**, 116–23.

Kobata T., Agematsu K., Kameoka J., Schlossman S.F. & Morimoto C. (1994) CD27 is a signal-transducing molecule involved in $CD45RA^+$ naive T-cell costimulation. *Journal of Immunology*, **12**, 5422–5432.

Kubin M., Karmoun M. & Trinchieri G. (1994) Interleukin 12 synergizes with B7/CD28 interaction in unduting efficient proliferation and cytokine production of human T-cells. *Journal of Experimental Medicine*, **180**, 211–22.

Lane, P., Traunecker A., Hubele S., Inui S., Lanzavecchia A. & Gray D. (1992) Activated human T-cells express a ligand for the human B cell-associated antigen CD40 which participates in T-cell dependent activation of B lymphocytes. *European Journal of Immunology*, **22**, 2573–8.

Larsen C.P., Ritchie S.C., Hendrix R. et al. (1994) Regulation of immuno-stimulatory function and co-stimulatory molecule (B7-1 and B7-2) expression on murine dendritic cells. *Journal of Immunology*, **152**, 5208–19.

Lenschow D.J., Zeng Y., Thistlehwaite J.R. et al. (1992) Long-term survival of xeno-geneic pancreatic islet grafts induced by CTLA-4Ig. *Science*, **257**, 789–92.

Linsley P.S., Brady W., Vries M., Gromairehs, Damle N.K., Ledbetter J. A. (1991) CTLA-4 is a second receptor for the B cell activation antigen B7. *Journal of Experimental Medicine*, **1743**, 561–9.

Linsley P.S., Clark E.A., Ledbetter J.A. (1990) T cell antigen CD28 mediates adhesion with B cells by interacting with activation antigen B7-BB1 *Proceedings of the National Academy of Sciences USA*, **87**13, 5031–5.

Linsley P. & Ledbetter J. (1993) The role of the CD28 receptor during T-cell responses to antigen. *Annual Review of Immunology*, **11**, 191–212.

Linsley P.S., Greene J.L., Tan P., Bradshaw J., Ledbetter J.A., Anasetti C., Damle N.K. (1992a) Co-expression and functional co-operation of CTLA-4 and CD28 on activated T lymphocytes. *Journal of Experimental Medicine*, **176**, 1595–604.

Linsley, P.S., Wallace P.M., Johnson J. et al. (1992b) Immunosuppression in vivo by a soluble form of the CTLA-4 T-cell activation molecule. *Science*, **257**, 792–5.

Murphy E.E., Terres G., Macatonia S.E. et al. (1994) B7 and Interleukin 12 co-operate for proliferation and interferon γ production by mouse T helper clones that are unresponsive to B7 co-stimulation. *Journal of Experimental Medicine*, **180**, 223–31.

Nickoloff B., Mitra R., Lee K., Turka L., Green J., Thompson G., & Shimizu Y. Discordant expression of CD28 ligands, BB1 and B7 on keratinocytes in vitro and psoriatic cells in vivo. *American Journal of Pathology*, **142**, 1029–40.

Noelle R.J., Roy M., Shepherd D.M., Stanmenkovic I., Ledbetter J.A., & Aruffo A. (1992) A 39-kDa protein on activated helper T-cells binds CD40 and transduces the signal for cognate activation of B cells. *Proceedings of the National Academy of Sciences USA*, **89**, 6550–4.

Nunes, J., Klasen S., Franco M.D., Lipcey C., Mawas C., Bagnasco M., & Olive D. (1993) Signalling through CD28 T-cell activation pathway involves an inositol phospholipid-specific phospholipase C activity. *Biochemical Journal*, **293**, 835–42.

Ostrand-Rosenberg S., Roby C. & Clements, V. (1991) Abrogation of tumorigenicity of MHC Class II antigen expression requires the cytoplasmic domain of the Class II molecule. *Journal of Immunology*, **147**, 2419–22.

Razi-Wolf Z., Galvin F., Gray G. & Reiser H. (1993) Evidence for an additional ligand, distinct from B7, for the CTLA-4 receptor. *Proceedings of the National Academy of Sciences USA*, **90**, 11182–6.

Roy M., Waldschmidt T., Aruffo A., Ledbetter J.A. & Noelle R.J. (1993) The regulation of the expression of gp39, the CD40 ligand, on normal and cloned CD4+ T-cells. *Journal of Immunology*, **151**, 2497–510.

Rudd C.E., Janssen O., Cai Y., deSilva A.J., Raab M., & Prasad K.V.S. (1994) Two-step TCRz/CD3-CD4 and CD28 signalling in T-cells: SH2/SH3 domains, protein-tyrosine and lipid kinases. *Immunology Today*, **15**, 225–34.

Shahinian A., Pfeffer K., Lee K.P. et al. Differential T-cell co-stimulatory requirement in CD28-deficient mice. *Science*, **261**, 609–12.

Stein P., Fraser J. & Weiss A. (1994) The cytoplasmic domain of CD28 is both necessary and sufficient for co-stimulation of IL-2 scretion and association with phosphatidylinositol 3′-kinase. *Molecular and Cellular Biology*, **14**, 3392–402.

Swartz R.H. (1989) Acquisition of immunological self tolerance. *Cell*, **57**, 1037–81.

Truitt K.E., Hicks C.M. & Imboden J.B. (1994) Stimulation of CD28 triggers an association between CD28 and phosphatidylinositol 3-kinasee and jurkat T-cells. *Journal of Experimental Medicine*, **179**, 1071–6.

Van Gool S.W., de Boer M., & Ceuppens J.L. (1994) The combination of Anti-B7 monoclonal antibody and cyclosporin A induces alloantigen-specific anergy during a primary mixed lymphocyte reaction. *Journal of Experimental Medicine*, **179**, 75–20.

Ward S.G., Westwick J., Hall N.D. & Sansom D.M., (1993) Ligation of CD28 receptor by B7 induces formation of D-3 phosphoinositides in T lymphocytes independently of T-cell receptor/CD3 activation. *European Journal of Immunology*, **23**, 2572–7.

Young J.W., Koulova L., Soergel S.A., Clark E.A., Steinmann R.M., & Dupont B. (1992) The B7/BB1 antigen provides one of several co-stimulatory signals for the activation of CD4+ T lymphocytes by human blood dendritic dells in vitro. *Journal of Clinical Investigation*, **90**, 229–37.

# 9

# The Role of Cytokines in Tumour Rejection

## GUIDO FORNI AND ROBIN FOA

## ■ INTRODUCTION

Cytokines are proteins that act as soluble cell to cell messengers, distinguished by their high interactivity, and can act in both an autocrine and paracrine manner. The effect of a single cytokine, however, cannot be readily predicted, since its presence induces other cytokines, which can significantly affect the primary actions. The progressive characterization of cytokines and the identification of their activity, both in vitro and particularly in vivo, are enabling some of the naturally occurring inter-actions between a tumour and its host to be teased apart. The resulting picture is, however, so complex and changeable that the role of an indi-vidual cytokine is difficult to elucidate in detail (Nathan & Sporn, 1991; Colombo et al., 1992a).

A given cytokine can, indeed, both promote and inhibit tumour growth. Whether it acts in one way or the other will depend on its con-centration, the characteristics of the tumour cell, other cell types, for example, stroma, the type of host reaction and the temporal stage of the tumour–host relationship.

First, neoplastic cells themselves characteristically produce cytokines spontaneously (Pekarek et al., 1993), and use them as: (1) autocrine fac-tors; (2) to recruit and suppress reactive leukocytes; and (3) to modulate the activity of endothelial and stromal cells. In their turn, cytokines pro-duced by the host in reaction to a tumour modify the scenario created by tumour expansion (Colombo et al., 1992a).

The existence of so many contrasting variables means that the part played by a cytokine can only be interpreted within the compass of a clearly defined context (Nathan & Sporn, 1991). Moreover, the ability to release a cytokine in an autocrine manner, could be a key factor in the promotion of neoplastic transformation and in permitting tumour growth in vivo (Sporn & Todaro, 1980). This progression may itself be

**199**

greatly influenced by the types of cytokines in the environment, since their range of influence occurs during long periods of tumour dormancy, extensive necrosis, or rapid growth.

A closer understanding of the roles played by a cytokine in the tumour microenvironment would clarify many features of both immunosurveillance and immunoenhancement (Prehn, 1994). The many parts played by various cytokines in the natural progression of any specific tumour are not easily elucidated.

When pharmacological concentrations of a single cytokine are made locally available, however, its effects are unambiguous, although they may often be surprisingly different from what might have been predicted on the basis of in vitro data.

# ■ LOCAL CYTOKINES IN TUMOUR GROWTH

A tumour can be characterized in terms of the cytokines it produces and the cytokine receptors it expresses. The distinct cytokine production (Giovarelli et al., 1988; Colombo et al., 1992b; Pikarek et al., 1993), and receptor expression patterns are often displayed by both haematopoietic and solid tumours (Weidmann et al., 1992; Obiri et al., 1994). Even those of the same histotype may have important consequences, which may be direct, by promoting or inhibiting tumour growth, or indirect, by promoting such growth through interactions on the microenvironment.

## Direct Action

If a tumour cell can both produce a cytokine, and express its receptor, the resultant autocrine loop may influence its growth either positively or negatively. Both autocrine promotion of growth and loss of growth inhibition by autocrine factors can convert nontumorigenic cells into fully malignant cells (Sporn & Todaro, 1980; Lang & Burgess, 1990; Haddow et al., 1991). Indeed, this is evident when the transforming growth factor-$\beta$ (TGF-$\beta$), interleukin (IL)-3, IL-5, IL-6, IL-9, or granulocyte–macrophage colony-stimulating factor (GM-CSF) genes are transfected into certain cells (Blankenstein et al., 1991b). IL-6 is a good example as it is secreted by a variety of cell types, and its biological action includes the growth and stimulation of plasmacytomas and some Epstein–Barr virus (EBV)-positive lymphoblastoid cells. Transgenic mice carrying the IL-6 gene frequently develop plasmacytomas and plasmacytoma cells often use IL-6 as an autocrine growth factor (Kishimoto, 1989). Transfection of an EBV line with this gene also leads to secretion of substantial levels of IL-6 and hence an altered growth pattern, as shown by clonogenicity in soft agar cultures. As a the result, these essentially nontumorigenic cells are able to form progressively growing tumours in *nu/nu* mice (Scala et al., 1990). IL-8 is a member of a family of related cytokines with inflammatory and growth-stimulating activity. It is produced by many tumour cells and may act as an important autocrine growth factor for several human melanomas (Schadendorf et al., 1993). Acute and chronic leukaemia B cells as well as acute myeloid cells can produce IL-8 constitutively, suggesting that it plays an autocrine regulatory role in B lymphocyte proliferation (Francia di Celle et al., 1994; Francia di Celle et al., submitted). In this context, the ability of cyclosporin A to inhibit cytokine secretion by blocking auto-crine regulation of tumour growth appears of particular interest (Nair et al., 1994).

Establishment of autocrine or paracrine circuits facilitating neoplastic growth, however, is not a generalized event. For example, IL-2 is an important growth-stimulation factor for lymphocytes (Smith, 1990) and macrophages (Espinoza-Delgado et al., 1990), and myeloid, B and T cell leukaemia cells may both express the IL-2 receptor and actively absorb paracrinally released IL-2, suggesting that IL-2 can induce a stimulatory signal on leukeamic cells (Giovarelli et al., 1988). By contrast, clonogenic proliferation assays and heterotransplantation in heavily immunosuppressed *nu/nu* mice have shown that IL-2 only occasionally induces a small stimulatory effect on acute leukaemia cells in vitro, whereas in vivo its presence hampers their expansion by eliciting a local, non T cell-dependent reactivity (Foa et al., 1990). Moreover, following IL-2 gene transduction into human acute leukaemia cells, no variation in cell phenotype, proliferation and IL-2 receptor expression is observed. However, the tumorigenicity of IL-2-transduced leukaemia cells was reduced or abrogated in immunosuppressed *nu/nu* mice in direct proportion to the amounts of IL-2 released. Histology shows that the rejection of IL-2-releasing leukaemia cells depends on macrophage killing activity (Cignetti et al., 1994).

By contrast, regression of some tumours following the local or systemic administration of a cytokine may be due to its interaction with its receptors on their cell membrane. Direct inhibition of this kind has been demonstrated in a few cases for exogenous IL-2 (Li et al., 1993) and IL-4 (Obiri et al., 1994; Topp et al., 1994), and is more readily shown with tumour necrosis factor (TNF) (Vassalli, 1992).

## Indirect Action

The growth of some tumour cells may also closely depend on their ability to induce local (and systemic) immunosuppression through the secretion of cytokines. However, tumour growth may also be the outcome of much more complex cytokine circuits. TGF-$\beta$ provides an exemplary illustration of this:

■ TGF-$\beta$ synthesis by tumour cells is often much greater than that of their normal counterparts.
■ TGF-$\beta$ usually inhibits tumour growth, although it may cause stimulation of tumour growth in some cases.
■ Loss of TGF-$\beta$ sensitivity is often a necessary step in the progression to malignancy.
■ By bringing about local inhibition of tumour growth and increasing the formation of the extracellular matrix, TGF-$\beta$ could provide a more favourable environment for the initial establishment of tumour cells.

The advantage conferred on a tumour by the paracrine action of TGF-$\beta$ often outweighs the disadvantage imposed by its inhibition of cell proliferation (Chang et al., 1993).

## ■ LOCAL CYTOKINES IN TUMOUR REJECTION

When pharmacological cytokine thresholds are reached at the site of a tumour, a strong immune reaction may lead to the establishment of an immune memory (Forni et al., 1994). Since most tumour cells do not express receptors for a given cytokine their rejection does not necessarily involve a cytokine-dependent inhibition of proliferation. Similar reactions are activated by repeated local injections of cytokines, by those released by cytokine gene-engineered (thereafter, referred to as engineered) tumour cells, and those released by other engineered cells, even those not antigenically related to the tumour itself. The efficacy of the reaction, however, varies significantly as a function of the amount of cytokine administered and the route chosen (Colombo & Forni, 1994) (Table 9.1).

It was originally supposed that a cytokine-triggered reaction depended on the direct activation of tumour-infiltrating lymphocytes (Bubenik et al., 1983), whereas in fact it requires a succession of four distinct, though interlinked, stages that can be better understood by examining what happens when live engineered cells are used (Forni et al., 1994).

### Initial Growth

Undisturbed growth on the part of engineered murine tumour cells occurs during the first 8–72 hours after a challenge (Figure 9.1). Histological examination shows that they retain their oncogenicity,

Table 9.1. Cytokine Gene Transfer into Murine Tumors: Range of Cytokines and Effect on Host Immunity

| Gene transferred | Targeted tumour | Cytokine production | Tumour inhibition in syngeneic mice | Host immune cells involved | References |
|---|---|---|---|---|---|
| mIL-1α (Tr) | Transformed NIH-3T3, met1 | 1 U[e] | Yes | n.d. | Douvdevani et al. (1992) |
| mIL-2 (Tr) | Colon carcinoma, CT-26 | 800 U[d] | Yes | CD8[+] | Fearon et al. (1990) |
| mIL-2 (Tr) | Melanoma, B16 | n.d. | Yes | n.d. | Fearon et al. (1990) |
| hIL-2 (I) | Fibrosarcoma, CMS- 5 | 2.5–15 U[c] | Yes | CTL | Gansbacher et al. (1990b) |
| mIL-2 (I) | Mastocytoma, P815 | 1500–7500 U[c] | Yes | CTL | Ley et al. (1991) |
| hIL-2 (I) | Rat sarcoma, HSNLV | 250–5000 U[c] | Yes | Most CD8[+] | Russell et al. (1991) |
| mIL-2 (Tr) | Mammary adenocarcinoma, T'SA | 300 U[c] | Weak | n.d. | Cavallo et al. (1992) |
| mIL-2 (Tr) | Mammary adenocarcinoma, T'SA | 60 000 U[c] | Yes | CD8[+], N | Cavallo et al. (1992) |
| hIL-2 (I) | Fibrosarcoma, MCA-102 | 60 000 pg | Yes | CD8[+], NK | Karp et al. (1993) |
| hIL-2 (I) | Bladder carcinoma, MBT-2 | 10 U[c] | Yes | CTL | Connor et al. (1993) |
| hIL-2(I) | Lung carcinoma, 3LL | 14 U[d] | Yes | CTL | Porgador et al. (1993a) |
| mIL-4 (Tr) | Plasmacytoma, J558L | 233 U[c] | Yes | E, M | Tepper et al. (1989) |
| mIL-4 (Tr) | Mammary adenocarcinoma, K485 | 56 U[c] | Yes | n.d. | Tepper et al. (1989) |
| mIL-4 (Tr) | Renal cell carcinoma, RENCA | 15 000 U[b] | Yes | T, E | Golumbeck et al. (1991) |
| mIL-4 (Tr) | Hamster ovary, CHO | 5000 U[c] | Yes (nude mice) | M | Platzer et al. (1992) |
| mIL-5 (Tr) | Plasmacytoma, J558L | 500 U[c] | No | E | Kruger-Krasagakes et al. (1993) |
| hIL-6 (Tr) | Melanoma, B16 | n.d. | Yes | M, N | Sun et al. (1992) |
| hIL-6 (Tr) | Lung carcinoma, 3LL | 0.6–3.9 U[d] | Yes | CTL | Porgador et al. (1992) |
| mIL-6 (I) | Sarcoma, MCA-207 | 200–250 U[b] | Yes | T | Mullen et al. (1992) |
| mIL-7 (Tr) | Plasmacytoma, J558L | 4–65 U[e] | Yes | CD4[+], M | Hock et al. (1991) |
| mIL-7 (Tr) | Mammary adenocarcinoma, T'SA | 50 U[e] | Yes | CD4[+] | Hock et al. (1991) |
| mIL-7 (I) | Fibrosarcoma, FSA | 20 ng[c] | Yes | T, E | McBride et al. (1992) |
| mIFN-α (Tr) | Friend leukaemia, 3C18 | 256–512 U[e] | Yes | n.d. | Ferrantini et al. (1993) |
| mIFN-γ (Tr) | Neuroblastoma, C1300 | 5–50 U[e] | Yes | CD8[+] | Watanabe et al. (1989) |

*(continued)*

Table 9.1. (contd.)

| Gene transferred | Targeted tumour | Cytokine production | Tumour inhibition in syngeneic mice | Host immune cells involved | References |
|---|---|---|---|---|---|
| mIFN-γ (I) | Fibrosarcoma, CMS-5 | 1.25 U$^c$ | Yes | CTL | Gansbacher et al. (1990a) |
| mIFN-γ (Tr) | Adenocarcinoma, SP1 | 256 U$^e$ | Yes | CTL | Esumi et al. (1991) |
| mIFN-γ (Tr) | Colon carcinoma, CT-26 | 8 U$^e$ | Yes | CTL | Esumi et al. (1991) |
| mIFN-γ (I) | Lung carcinoma, 3LL | 360–512 U$^d$ | Yes | CTL | Porgador et al. (1993b) |
| mIFN-γ (I) | Bladder carcinoma, MBT-2 | 75 U$^c$ | Yes | CTL | Connor et al. (1993) |
| mIFN-γ (Tr) | Mammary adenocarcinoma, T'SA | 20–60 000 U$^d$ | Weak | M | Lollini et al. (1993) |
| hTNF-α (Tr) | Skin tumor, 1591-RE | 50 000 pg$^a$ | Yes (nude mice) | NoT | Teng et al. (1991) |
| mTNF-α (I) | Plasmacytoma, J558L | 40 pg$^e$ | Yes | M | Blakenstein et al. (1991a) |
| hTNF-α (Tr) | Sarcoma, MCA-205 | 1200 pg$^b$ | Yes | CD4$^+$, CD8$^+$ | Asher et al. (1991) |
| hTNF-α (I) | Sarcoma, MCA-102 | 11000 pg$^b$ | No | n.d. | Karp et al. (1993) |
| hG-CSF (I) | Colon adenocarcinoma, C-26 | 20–90 pg$^c$ | Yes | N | Colombo et al. (1991) |
| hM-CSF (Tr) | Plasmacytoma, J558L | 10–100 U$^e$ | No | Mac-1$^+$ | Dorsh et al. (1993) |
| mGM-CSF (I) | Melanoma, B16 | 300 ng$^c$ | No | ND | Dranoff et al. (1993) |
| hMCP (Tr) | Melanoma, B16 | n.d. | Weak | M | Bottazzi et al. (1992) |
| hMCP (Tr) | Hamster ovary, CHO | n.d. | Yes (nude mice) | M | Rollins & Sunday (1991) |

m, mouse; h, human; IL, interleukin; IFN, interferon; TNF, tumour necrosis factor; G-CSF, granulocyte colony-stimulating factor; M-CSF, macrophage colony-stimulating factor; GM-CSF, granulocyte–macrophage colony-stimulating factor; MCP, monocyte chemoattractant protein; Tr, transfection; I, infection via retroviral vector; n.d., not determined or information not provided; CTL, cytotoxic T lymphocytes; N, neutrophils; NK, natural killer cells; E, eosinophils; M, macrophages; T, T cells

Cytokine production is reported as U ml$^{-1}$ 10$^{-6}$ cells when determined by bioassay and referred to a titration curve obtained with recombinant cytokines or to 1 U as the equivalent of the half maximal proliferation. Cytokine production is reported as pg or ng 10$^{-6}$ cells when determined by ELISA assay.

$^a$ Measured at 16 h; $^b$ measured at 24 h; $^c$ measured at 48 h; $^d$ measured at 72 h; $^e$ number of cells and time not reported.

Reproduced with permission from Colombo & Forni (1994).

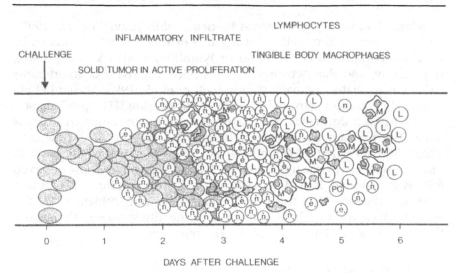

**Figure 9.1** Schematic representation of the kinetics of growth and rejection of T/SA adenocarcinoma cells releasing small amounts of IL-2 following IL-2-gene transduction. e, eosinophils; L, lymphocytes; M, macrophages; n, neutrophils; PC, plasma cells.

since they usually grow at the same rate as the parental cells. The importance of this initial growth lies in its supply of a sufficient antigen load to the immune system.

## Inflammatory Debulking Phase

The proliferation of engineered cells increases the cytokine release so that it increases in amount in the environment as the tumour expands until a pharmacological threshold is reached, and the biological activity of the cytokine begins. The most immediate effect produced by the majority of cytokines is an inflammatory reaction (days 1–5). Leukocytes are recruited in large numbers, and infiltrate the tumour mass and kill the engineered cells by damaging their membrane and cytoplasm (Forni et al., 1987; Cavallo et al., 1992; Modesti et al., 1993; Musiani et al., 1994). The debulking efficacy of this reaction depends on the kind, amount, and activity of the cytokine, the tumour histotype, and the extracellular matrix (Colombo et al., 1992a; Modesti et al., 1994). To study the influence of the distinct cytokines, we have used as a model a spontaneous mammary adenocarcinoma of Balb/c mice (TS/A). The mechanism whereby the TS/A adenocarcinoma is rejected varies according to the type of gene transduced. Rejection activated by cells engineered to release IL-2 is mainly sustained by neutrophils (Cavallo et al., 1992), while that activated by cells releasing IL-4 or IL-7 is largely mediated by eosinophils (Musiani et al., 1994) or lymphocytes (Hock et al., 1993), respectively, and that activated by cells releasing TNF-$\alpha$ or interferon-$\gamma$ (IFN-$\gamma$), is mediated by macrophages (Lollini et al., 1993; Musiani et al., 1994). Macrophages activated by TS/A cells releasing IFN-$\gamma$ produce prolonged tumour dormancy, but 'takes' are eventually observed in most mice. The reaction elicited by cells releasing IL-5 (Kruger-Krasagakes, 1993), IL-6 and GM-CSF (Allione, et al., 1994) is not strong enough to inhibit their growth. Each of these mechanisms resembles those observed following repeated local injection of the corresponding recombinant cytokine, showing that the reaction pattern is not influenced by the way in which the threshold is reached. Generally speaking, the greater the amount of cytokine, the quicker the rejection.

## The Arrival of T Cells

The mounting of a specific immune response requires 3–5 days, which means that a specific T cell-mediated reactivity is unlikely to make a significant contribution to tumour debulking. Later, however, the killer activity of the inflammatory cells is apparently sustained through their intense cross talk with T cells, since the dominant and recurrent ultrastructural hallmark of this stage is represented by the membrane contacts between granulocytes, macrophages, fibroblasts, and lymphocytes (days 3–7). T cells are too few to cause any significant tumour cell destruction on their own. Their continuous contact with the inflammatory cells, on the other hand, suggests that they act as guides, probably through the intense release of secondary cytokines revealed by in situ hybridization experiments (Stoppacciaro et al., 1994). The importance of this guidance is confirmed by the fact that, in mice selectively deprived of T cells, the antitumour reaction of inflammatory cells elicited by small amounts of IL-2, IL-4, and G-CSF becomes marginal (Forni et al., 1987; Bosco et al., 1990; Stoppacciaro et al., 1993). The effectiveness of the reaction elicited by several cytokines is thus significantly improved by T cell guidance, even if it is not mediated by T cells.

The fact that only the inflammatory cells kill neoplastic cells may be another result of this late guidance. The morphological evidence shows that local tumour cell destruction is not associated with damage to adjacent normal tissues. This selectivity is apparent both when engineered mouse cells and when recombinant cytokines are used. It could also stem from the fact that the T cells are guided by the concentration gradient of the secreted cytokine, or preferentially recognize certain aspects of the neoplastic cell membrane.

## The End of the Reaction

Progressive killing of the engineered cells and replacement of the tumour itself by granulation tissue represent the final stage of the reaction (days 5–10). In many cases, the engineered cells are totally destroyed, whereas in others a few remain intermingled in the granulation tissue, and may eventually form a new tumour after a period of dormancy. The transduced gene coding for the cytokine is occasionally lost by these survivors, although they may also continue to secrete cytokines. The granulation tissue is full of macrophages that have ingested the cell debris. Tumour-draining nodes often enlarge progressively during the rejection process, and display expanded cortical and paracortical areas, as well as numerous macrophages and granulocytes.

# ■ CLINICAL PERSPECTIVES OF LOCAL UTILIZATION OF CYTOKINES

Several, mostly anecdotal, studies (Pericle, Di Pierro & Forni, 1992) have shown that repeated local injections of a variety of cytokines are followed by impressive nonspecific reactions in human tumours that are as effective as surgery, and could perhaps be exploited for the management of in situ tumours, or of those located in only a few body cavities. However, the fact that their effects are often no more than temporary and confined to the lesions actually treated (Cortesina et al., 1994) means that their clinical significance may be small. Cancer is usually a chronic systemic disease, and local successes, however striking, are often devoid of long-term therapeutic consequences (Forni et al., 1993). In addition, these temporary effects have frequently been obtained in advanced tumours that seemed unlikely to respond owing to marked immunodepression preventing the establishment of any systemic reactivity (Cortesina et al., 1994).

The experimental data, therefore, suggest that tumour rejection induced by the local administration of cytokines could serve as the starting point for the creation of a new kind of antitumour vaccines.

# ■ THE RATIONALE OF GENE-ENGINEERED ANTITUMOUR VACCINES

Tumour rejection induced by cytokines in mice is often followed by protection against a subsequent challenge with nonengineered parental cells, and a systemic immune memory may also be established even after the rejection of apparently nonimmunogenic forms. In addition, a significant number of mice bearing established tumours have actually been cured by repeated injections of engineered cells.

Vaccination with engineered cells is thus an attractive prospect. Its exploitation, however, requires a deeper understanding of the mechanisms whereby the local presence of cytokines confers immunogenicity on a tumour.

The complexity of the reaction that results in the rejection of engineered cells means that direct activation of tumour-infiltrating lymphocytes by a cytokine cannot be the source of such immunogenicity. As we have seen, T cells guide the effector leukocytes during rejection. Afterwards, however, the dialogue between them flows in the opposite direction. The inflammatory setting and the presence of nonspecific leukocytes are instrumental for the indirect presentation of tumour antigens to CD4$^+$ and CD8$^+$ memory cells whose reactivity against poorly or nonimmunogenic tumours was unexpected. It is an outcome of the unique situation occurring during rejection. It would seem that establishment of an immune memory is dependent on the fulfilment of four conditions:

- Loading of the immune system with sufficient tumour antigen.
- Intervention of the host antigen-presenting cells (APC).
- Appropriate antigen presentation by APC.
- Presence of the appropriate cytokines.

These four features cannot be dissociated when engineered cells are used, since the cytokine is involved in rejection, APC recruitment, and activation of particular memory mechanisms.

Transfection of TS/A cells with the metabolic suicide gene cytosine deaminase (CD) is another engineering approach that enables the nontoxic prodrug 5-fluorocytosine (5-FC) to destroy these cells after their establishment and hence confer protection against a subsequent lethal challenge with the parental cells. This combination of CD engineering and 5-FC leads, indeed, to an elegant and repeatable equivalent of the early twentieth-century practice of ligating a tumour's blood vessel to provoke its necrosis. Regression, in fact, is itself a good immunogenic stimulus, even when it occurs slowly due to the presence of small quantities of a cytokine. A slow reaction, in fact, allows cells to grow before they are rejected, whereas the rapid disappearance of an incipient tumour as a result of a very intense and effective reaction does not load APC with enough antigen to elicit the establishment of an immune memory. Creation of a sound memory against a nonimmunogenic tumour on the part of a cytokine, therefore, requires induction of the slow regression of a tumour that has already grown to a certain degree (Consalvo et al., 1995). When regression takes place in the presence of a given cytokine, the selective promotion of particular memory mechanisms can be exploited by the promotion (or inhibition) of certain types of mechanisms to obtain a more effective response. A vigorous cytotoxic T lymphocyte (CTL)-mediated memory, for example, is acquired in the presence of the T helper 1 ($T_{H1}$) cytokines IL-2, IL-7, and IFN-$\gamma$ whereas the development of CTL is strongly inhibited, and the memory is mediated by antibodies, in the presence of the $T_{H2}$ cytokine, IL-4.

Inhibition of a subsequent challenge is conferred by both $T_{H1}$ and $T_{H2}$ reactivity. The regression of already established tumours, on the other hand, requires the reactivity induced by $T_{H1}$ cytokines. In addition to providing guidance towards the elaboration of an antitumour vaccine for human use, these experimental data suggest that such strategies should incorporate adequate presentation of tumour antigen, which is persistent and occurs in the presence of $T_{H1}$ cytokines (Cavallo et al., 1994).

## ■ SYSTEMIC UTILIZATION OF CYTOKINES

IFN-$\alpha$ and IL-2 are the two cytokines that have been extensively employed in the management of cancer patients and that have shown a variable degree of antitumour activity. IFN-$\alpha$ has shown activity, alone or in combination with chemotherapy and/or IL-2, in a proportion (10–20%) of patients with solid tumours, in particular those with renal cell carcinoma and malignant melanoma. Its efficacy has, however, been much more evident in haematological malignancies, including hairy cell leukaemia (HCL), chronic myeloid leukaemia (CML), multiple myeloma, non-Hodgkin's lymphoma, essential thrombocythaemia, and Waldestrom's macroglobulinaemia. In particular, IFN-$\alpha$ has a primary role in the management of HCL and CML. For many years, it has been the first line approach for patients with HCL, where the prolonged intramuscular or subcutaneous administration for 6–12 months induces partial, or less frequently, complete clinical and haematological remissions in the great majority of patients (Quesada, Reuben & Manning, 1984; Ratain, Golomb & Vardimann, 1985). Based on the experience accumulated over more than 10 years of clinical use, it is fair to say that IFN-$\alpha$ has had a major impact in the management of HLC because it has modified the natural prognostic course of the disease. It also represents the first demonstration that complete remissions can be induced in human cancer using only a cytokine. A higher rate of complete responses has recently been obtained following a single one-week course of the purine analogue 2-chlorodeoxyadenosine (Piro, Carrera & Carson, 1990) suggesting that this compound, which at present is not widely available, will most likely become the first therapeutic choice for the treatment of HCL. A combination of the two approaches may prove even more effective.

Similarly, IFN-α has had a major impact in CML. In addition to exert-
ing a marked effect on the white blood cell count, prolonged IFN-α
administration can also induce a decrease in the number of
Philadelphia⁺ cells and a complete cytogenetic conversion has been documented in some patients (Talpaz et al., 1986). This is an important result
because it shows for the first time that a complete cytogenetic eradication
can be achieved following the administration of a biological modifier,
especially as such responses have not been observed with conventional
chemotherapy. A recent update of an Italian multicentre study has con-
clusively shown that the administration of IFN-α has a clinical impact in
the course of CML because it can delay the time of blastic transformation
and prolong the overall survival (Italian Cooperative Study Group, 1994).

Following extensive preclinical studies in vitro (Grimm et al., 1982)
and in vivo in distinct experimental models (Mulé et al., 1984), IL-2 has
been widely utilized in the management of cancer patients. The first
encouraging report on the potential antitumour activity of the systemic
administration of high doses of IL-2, with or without lymphokine activated killer (LAK) cells activated ex vivo, was reported ten years ago
(Rosenberg et al., 1985). Based on the experience accumulated over this
decade, it can be stated that IL-2, alone or in combination with LAK cells,
may induce objective clinical responses in a proportion of patients with
advanced renal cell carcinoma and metastatic melanoma (Rosenberg et
al., 1989; Foa, Guarini & Gansbacher, 1992). Although responses have
been limited to a small proportion of patients (about 15%), it should be
noted that these have been obtained in patients with advanced and
refractory disease, and some have been long-lived. Responses have also
been documented in acute myeloid leukaemia (AML) (Foa et al., 1991). It
should be noted that the complete remissions induced by IL-2 alone have
so far been achieved only in AML patients with a small proportion of
residual bone marrow blasts, and that the effectiveness of IL-2 remains
limited (if any at all) in patients with advanced disease. We have recently
reported that, in five out of fourteen patients with limited disease, the
remission induced by IL-2 has been the longest in the natural history of
each patient (Meloni et al., 1994).

These encouraging results, however, have been achieved with high
doses of IL-2, an approach which has major limitations, including severe
systemic toxicity, an inability to predict the few clinical responses, and
the absence of any demonstration that IL-2 administration induces the
generation of specific antitumour cytotoxic lymphocytes. Moreover, it is
still not clear if the direct killing of tumour cells by specific or nonspecific
effector lymphocytes is the exact mechanism by which IL-2 achieves its
therapeutic effect. The IL-2 pleiotropic activity, as detected in vitro,
becomes even more evident in vivo because of the highly interactive

nature of the immune system. The efficacy of IL-2 in vivo may rest on the induction of a cascade of interconnected effector functions, each affecting neoplastic growth with distinct mechanisms and selectivity. LAK and tumour infiltrating lymphocytes (TIL) cells, either adoptively transferred or generated in vivo, may have an important debulking role, but, by releasing several cytokines, they may activate multiple host reaction mechanisms that play an even more substantial part in tumour inhibition.

These biological observations, coupled with the ability to transduce human tumour cells stably with cytokine genes (see section on engineered human tumor cells and the activation of vaccine protocols), have inevitably led to the expectation that clinical protocols with tumour cells engineered to release the wanted cytokine can be designed.

# ◾ ENGINEERED HUMAN TUMOUR CELLS AND THE ACTIVATION OF VACCINE PROTOCOLS

Following extensive experimental studies, it has recently been shown that human tumour cell lines can be successfully transduced with cytokine genes by using retroviral vectors. Because of the encouraging clinical results obtained with exogenous IL-2 in a proprotion of cancer patients and because transfer of the IL-2 gene into experimental tumour cells could induce the generation of a specific antitumour response and immunological memory, interest has been mainly focused on the possibility of transducing the IL-2 gene into human tumour cell lines. Productive transfer has been shown for melanoma, renal cell carcinoma, neuroblastoma, and acute leukaemia cell lines, etc. (Gansbacher et al., 1992; Gastl et al., 1992; Belldegrun et al., 1993; Cignetti et al., 1994; Forni et al., 1994). This approach results in a reduced or abrogated tumourigenic potential of the engineered neoplastic cells when injected into immunosuppressed nude mice. In view of a possible clinical utilization of the IL-2 engineered human tumour cells, attention has been centered on assessing the kinetics of IL-2 production after exposure of doses of gamma radiation sufficient to block cell growth.

Following the results obtained in experimental tumours and with human neoplastic cells over the last three years, several protocols based on the clinical use of engineered tumour cells or effector cells have been activated or approved (see Clinical Protocol List, 1994). Most investigators contemplate subcutaneous vaccination with allogenic and irradiated neoplastic cell lines transduced with retroviral vectors carrying cytokine genes, usually IL-2. Preliminary results in advanced and resistant metastatic melanoma and renal cell carcinoma indicate that this approach is feasible on an outpatient basis, and that the small quantities of IL-2 released by the engineered cells are devoid of systemic toxicity (Foa et al., 1994a, 1994b). It has not yet been established whether, through this strategy, specific antitumour cytotoxic effectors can commonly be generated. With regard to possible antitumour effects, it is likely that protocols enrolling patients with less advanced disease and, hence, with less compromised immune system will need to be activated.

Although several years will probably be required to establish the true impact of the gene-transfer modalities hereby discussed, technological advances have opened prospects for the management of cancer patients that, until recently, would have been regarded as no more than imaginary.

## ■ ACKNOWLEDGEMENTS

Work supported by Associazione Italiana per la Ricerca sul Cancro (AIRC), Milano, Special Project 'Gene Therapy', and by Consiglio Nazionale delle Ricerche (CNR), Roma, Special Project 'Applicazioni Cliniche della Ricerca Oncologica'.

### REFERENCES

Allione A., Consalvo M., Nanni P. et al. (1994) Immunizing and curative potential of replicating and nonreplicating murine mammary adenocarcinoma cells engineered with IL2, IL4, IL6, IL7, IL10, TNFα, GM-CSF, and IFNγ gene or admixed with conventional adjuvants. *Cancer Research*, **54**, 6022–6.

Asher A.I., Mule J.J., Kasid A. et al. (1991) Murine tumor cells transduced with the gene for tumor necrosis factor. *Journal of Immunology*, **146**, 3227–34.

Belldegrun A., Tso C.-L., Sakata T. et al. (1993) Human renal carcinoma line transfected with interleukin-2 and/or interferon α gene(s): implications for live cancer vaccines. *Journal of the National Cancer Institute*, **85**, 207–16.

Blankenstein T., Qin Z., Uberla K., Muller W., Rosen H., Volk H.D., Diamanstein T. (1991a) Tumor suppression after tumor cell targeted tumor necrosis factor alpha gene transfer. *Journal of Experimental Medicine*, **173**, 1047–52.

Blankenstein T., Rowley D.A. & Schreiber H. (1991b) Cytokines and cancer: experimental systems. *Current Opinion in Immunology*, **3**, 694–8.

Bosco M.C., Giovarelli M., Forni M., Modesti A., Scarpa S., Masuelli L. & Forni G. (1990) Low doses of interleukin-4 injected perilymphatically in tumour bearing mice inhibit the growth of poorly and apparently non-immunogenic tumours and induce a tumour specific immune memory. *Journal of Immunology*, **145**, 3136–43.

Bottazzi B., Walter S., Govoni D., Colotta F. & Mantovani A. (1992) Monocyte chemotactic cytokine gene transfer modulates macrophage infiltrations, growth and susceptibility to IL-2 therapy of a murine melanoma. *Journal of Immunology*, **148**, 1280–5.

Bubenik J., Perlmann P., Indrova M., Simova J., Jandlova T. & Neuwirt J. (1983) Growth inhibition of an MC-induced mouse sarcoma by TCGF (IL 2)-containing preparations. *Cancer Immunology and Immunotherapy*, **14**, 205–6.

Cavallo F., Colombo M.P., Allione A. et al. (1994) Antitumour responses elicited by mouse adenocarcinoma cells engineered to release IL-2 and IL-4. In G. Forni, R. Foa, A. Santoni & L. Frati (eds) *Cytokine-induced tumour immunogenicity. From exogenous molecules to gene therapy*, pp. 196–208. London, Academic Press.

Cavallo F., Giovarelli M., Gulino A. et al. (1992) Role of neutrophils and CD4+ T lymphocytes in the primary and memory response to nonimmunogenic murine mammary adenocarcinoma made immunogenic by IL-2 gene transfection. *Journal of Immunology*, 149, 3627–35.

Chang H.L., Gillet N., Figureari I., Lopez A.R., Palladino M.A. & Derynck R. (1993) Increased transforming growth factor β expression inhibits cell proliferation in vitro, yet increases tumourigenicity and tumour growth of Met A sarcoma cells. *Cancer Research*, 53, 4391–8.

Cignetti A., Guarini A., Carbone A. et al. (1994) Transduction of the IL2 gene into human acute leukemia cells induces tumor rejection without modifying cell proliferation and IL2 receptor expression. *Journal of the National Cancer Institute*, 86, 785–90.

Clinical Protocols List (1994) *Cancer Gene Therapy*, 1, 73–8.

Colombo M.P., Ferrari G., Stoppacciaro A. et al. (1991) Granulocyte colony-stimulating factor gene transfer suppresses tumorigenicity of a murine adenocarcinoma in vivo. *Journal of Experimental Medicine*, 173, 889–97.

Colombo M.P. & Forni G. (1994) Cytokine gene transfer in tumour inhibition and tentative tumour therapy: Where are we now? *Immunology Today*, 15, 48–51.

Colombo M.P., Modesti A., Parmiani G. & Forni G. (1992a) Local cytokine availability elicits tumour rejection and systemic immunity through granulocyte-T-lymphocyte cross-talk. *Cancer Research*, 52, 4853–7.

Colombo M.P., Maccalli C., Mattei S., Melani C., Radrizzani M. & Parmiani G. (1992b) Expression of cytoline genes, including IL-6, in human malignant melanoma cell lines. *Melanoma Research*, 2, 181–9.

Connor J., Bannerji R., Saito S., Heston W., Fair W. & Gilboa E. (1993) Regression of bladder tumors in mice treated with interleukin 2 gene-modified tumor cells. *Journal of Experimental Medicine*, 177, 1127–34.

Consalvo M., Mullen C., Modesti A. et al. (1995) Fluorocytosine induced eradication of murine adenocarcinomas engineered to express the cytosine deaminase suicide gene requires host immune competence and leaves an efficient memory. *Journal of Immunology*, 154, 5302–12.

Cortesina G., De Stefani A., Galeazzi E. et al. (1994) Temporary regression of recurrent squamous cell carcinoma of the head and neck achieved with low but not with high dose of recombinant interleukin-2 injected perilymphatically. *British Journal of Cancer*, 69, 572–6.

Dorsh M., Hock H., Kunzendorf U., Diamanstein T. & Blankenstein T. (1993) Macrophage colony-stimulating factor gene transfer into tumor cells induces macrophage infiltration but not tumor suppression. *European Journal of Immunology*, 23, 186–90.

Douvdevani A., Huleihel M., Zoller M., Setal S. & Apte R.N. (1992) Reduced tumorigenicity of fibrosarcomas which constitutively generate IL-1α either spontaneously or following IL-1α gene transfer. *International Journal of Cancer*, 51, 822–30.

Dranoff G., Jaffee E., Lazenby A. et al. (1993) Vaccination with irradiated tumor cells engineered to secrete murine granulocyte macrophage colony-stimulating factor stimulates potent, specific, and long-lasting antitumor immunity. *Proceedings of the National Academy of Sciences USA*, 90, 3539–43.

Espinoza-Delgado I., Ortaldo J.R., Winkler-Pickett R., Sugamura K., Varesio L. & Longo D.L. (1990) Expression and role of p75 interleukin-2 receptor on human monocytes. *Journal of Experimental Medicine*, 171, 1821–6.

Esumi N., Hunt B., Itaya T. & Frost P. (1991) Reduced tumorigenicity of murine tumor cells secreting γ-interferon is due to non specific host responses and is unrelated to Class I major histocompatibility complex expression. *Cancer Research*, 51, 1185–9.

Fearon E.R., Pardoll D.M., Itaya T. et al. (1990) Interleukin 2 production by tumor cells by passes T helper function in the generation of an antitumour response. *Cell*, 60, 397–403.

Ferrantini M., Proietti E., Santodonato L. et al. (1993) α1-Interferon gene transfer into metastatic Friend leukemia cells abrogated tumorigenicity in immunocompetent mice: Antitumor therapy by means of interferon-producing cells. *Cancer Research*, 53, 1107–12.

Foa R., Caretto P., Fierro M.T. et al. (1990) Interleukin 2 does not promote the in vitro and in vivo proliferation and growth of human acute leukaemia cells of myeloid and lymphoid origin. *British Journal of Haematology*, 75, 34–40.

Foa R., Guarini A. & Gansbacher B. (1992) IL2 treatment for cancer: from biology to gene therapy. *British Journal of Cancer*, 66, 992–8.

Foa R., Guarini A., Cignetti A., Cronin K., Rosenthal F. & Gansbacher B. (1994a) Cytokine gene therapy: a new strategy for the management of cancer patients. *Natural Immunity*, 13, 65–75.

Foa R., Guarini A., Gillio-Tos A., Riera L. & Cignetti A. (1994b) Immunorecognition of human leukemic cells elicited by IL-2. In G. Forni, R. Foa, A. Santoni & L. Frati (eds) *Cytokine-induced tumour immunogenicity. From exogenous molecules to gene therapy*, pp. 385–402. London, Academic Press.

Foa R., Meloni G., Tosti S. et al. (1991) Treatment of acute myeloid leukaemia patients with recombinant interleukin 2: A pilot study. *British Journal of Haematology*, 77, 491–7.

Forni G., Foa R., Santoni A. & Frati L. (eds) (1994) *Cytokine-induced tumour immunogenicity. From exogenous molecules to gene therapy*. London, Academic Press.

Forni G., Giovarelli M., Cavallo F. et al. (1993) Cytokine induced tumour immunogenicity: from exogenous cytokines to gene therapy. *Journal of Immunotherapy*, 14, 253–7.

Forni G., Giovarelli M., Santoni A., Modesti A. & Forni M. (1987) Interleukin-2 activated tumour inhibition in vivo depends on the systemic involvement of host immunoreactivity. *Journal of Immunology*, 138, 4033–41.

Francia di Celle P., Carbone A., Marchis D. et al. (1994) Cytokine gene expression in B-cell chronic lymphocytic leukemia: evidence of constitutive interleukin-8 (IL-8) mRNA expression and secretion of biologically active IL-8 protein. *Blood*, 84, 220–8.

Gansbacher B., Bannerji R., Daniels B., Zier K., Cronin K. & Gilboa E. (1990a) Retroviral vector-mediated gamma-interferon gene transfer into tumor cells generates potent and long lasting antitumor immunity. *Cancer Research*, 50, 7820–5.

Gansbacher B., Zier K., Cronin K. et al. (1992) Retroviral gene transfer induced constitutive expression of interleukin-2 or interferon-γ in irradiated human melanoma cells. *Blood*, 80, 2817–25.

Gansbacher B., Zier K., Daniels B., Cronin K., Bannerji R. & Gilboa E. (1990b) Interleukin 2 gene transfer into tumor cells abrogates tumorigenicity and induces protective immunity. *Journal of Experimental Medicine*, 172, 1217–24.

Gastl G., Finstad C.L., Guarini A. et al. (1992) Retroviral vector-mediated lymphokine gene transfer into human renal cancer cells. *Cancer Research*, 52, 6229–36.

Giovarelli M., Foa R., Benetton G., Lusso P., Fierro M.T. & Forni G. (1988) Release of interleukin-2-like material by B-chronic lymphocytic leukemia cells. A Paracrine model of production and utilization. *Leukemia Research*, 12, 201–9.

Golumbek P.T., Lazenby A.J., Levitsky H.J. et al. (1991) Treatment of established renal cancer by tumor cells engineered to secrete interleukin-4. *Science*, 245, 713–6.

Grimm E.A., Mazumder A., Zhang H.Z. & Rosenberg S.A. (1982) Lymphokine-activated killer cell phenomenon. Lysis of natural killer-resistant fresh solid tumour cells by interleukin 2-activated autologous human peripheral blood lymphocytes. *Journal of Experimental Medicine*, 155, 1823–41.

Haddow S., Fowlis D.J., Parkinson K., Akhurst R.J. & Balmain A. (1991) Loss of growth control by TGF-$\beta$ occurs at a late stage of mouse skin carcinogenesis and is independent of ras gene inactivation. *Oncogene*, 6, 1465–70.

Hock H., Dorsch M., Diamanstein T. & Blankenstein T. (1991) Interleukin 7 induces CD4$^+$ T cell-dependent tumour rejection. *Journal of Experimental Medicine*, 174, 1291–8.

Hock H., Dorsch M., Kunzendorf U., Qin Z., Diamantstein T. & Blankenstein T. (1993) Mechanisms of rejection induced by tumour cell-targeted gene transfer of interleukin 2, interleukin 4, interleukin 7, tumour necrosis factor, or interferon gamma. *Proceedings of the National Academy of Sciences USA*, 90, 2774–8.

Italian Cooperative Study Group on Chronic Myeloid Leukemia (1994) Interferon alfa-2a as compared with conventional chemotherapy for the treatment of chronic myeloid leukemia. *New England Journal of Medicine*, 330, 820–5.

Karp S.E., Farber A., Salo J.C. et al. (1993) Cytokine secretion by genetically modified nonimmunogenic murine fibrosarcoma. Tumor inhibition by IL-2 but not tumor necrosis factor. *Journal of Immunology*, 150, 896–908.

Kishimoto T. (1989) The biology of interleukin-6. *Blood*, 74, 1–6.

Kruger-Krasagakes S., Li W., Richter G., Diamanstein T. & Blankenstein T. (1993) Eosinophils infiltrating interleukin-5 gene-transfected tumours do not suppress tumour growth. *European Journal of Immunology*, 23, 992–5.

Lang R.A. & Burgess A.W. (1990) Autocrine growth factors and tumourigenic transformation. *Immunology Today*, 11, 244–9.

Ley V., Langlade-Demoyen P., Kourilsky P. & Larsson-Sciard E.L. (1991) Interleukin 2 dependent activation of tumor-specific cytotoxic T lymphocytes in vivo. *European Journal of Immunology*, 21, 851–4.

Li W.C., Yasumura S. & Whiteside T.L. (1993) Transfer of interleukin 2 receptor genes into squamous cell carcinoma. Modification of tumour cell growth. *Archives of Otolaryngology and Head Neck Surgery*, 119, 1229–35.

Lollini P. L., Bosco M.C., Cavallo F. et al. (1993) Inhibition of tumour growth and enhancement of metastasis after transfection of the $\gamma$-interferon gene. *International Journal of Cancer*, 55, 320–9.

McBride W.H., Thacker J.D., Comora S. et al. (1992) Genetic modification of a murine fibrosarcoma to produce interleukin 7 stimulates host cell infiltration and tumor immunity. *Cancer Research*, 52, 3931–7.

Meloni G., Foa R., Vignetti M. et al. (1994) Interleukin-2 may induce prolonged remissions in advanced acute myelogenous leukemia. *Blood*, 84, 2158–73.

Modesti A., Masuelli L., Modica A. et al. (1993) Ultrastructural evidence of the mechanisms responsible for interleukin-4 activated rejection of a spontaneous murine carcinoma. *International Journal of Cancer*, 53, 988–93.

Modesti A., Musiani P., Cortesina G. & Forni G. (1994) Cytokine dependent tumour recognition. In G. Fornia, R. Foa, A. Santoni and L. Frati (eds) *Cytokine-induced tumour immunogenicity. From exogenous molecules to gene therapy.* pp. 385–402. London, Academic Press.

Mulé J.J., Shu S., Schwarz R. & Rosenberg S.A. (1984) Successful adoptive immunotherapy of established pulmonary metastases with LAK cells and recombinant IL-2. *Science*, **255**, 1487–9.

Mullen C.A., Coale M.M., Levy A.T. et al. (1992) Fibrosarcoma cells transduced with the IL-6 gene exhibited reduced tumorigenicity, increased immunogenicity and decreased metastatic potential. *Cancer Research*, **52**, 6020–4.

Musiani P., Modesti A., Brunetti M. et al. (1994) The nature and potential of the reactive response to mouse mammary adenocarcinoma cells engineered with IL-2, IL-4 or IFN-γ gene. *Natural Immunity*, **13**, 93–101.

Nair A.P., Hahn K., Banholzer S., Hirsh R. & Moroni C. (1994) Cyclosporin A inhibits growth of autocrine tumour cell lines by destabilizing interleukin-3 mRNA. *Nature (London)*, **369**, 239–42.

Nathan C. & Sporn M. (1991) Cytokines in context. *Journal of Cell Biology*, **113**, 981–6.

Obiri N.I., Siegel J.P., Varricchio F. &. Puri R.K. (1994) Expression of high-affinity IL-4 receptors on human melanoma, ovarian and breast carcinoma cells. *Clinical and Experimental Immunology*, **95**, 148–55.

Pekarek L.A., Weichselbaum R.R., Beckett M.A., Nachman J. & Schreiber H. (1993) Footprinting of individual tumours and their variants by constitutive cytokine expression patterns. *Cancer Research*, **53**, 1978–81.

Pericle F., Di Pierro F. & Forni G. (1992) Clinical trials with local administration of lymphopoietic growth factors. In R. Mertelsmann (ed.) *Lympho-hematopoietic growth factors in cancer therapy II*, pp. 87–96. Berlin, Springer-Verlag.

Piro L.D., Carrera C.J. & Carson D.A. (1990) Lasting remissions in hairy-cell leukemia induced by a single infusion of 2-chlorodeoxy-adenosine. *New England Journal of Medicine*, **322**, 1117–20.

Platzer C., Richter G., Uberla K., Hock H., Diamantstein T. & Blankenstein T. (1992) Interleukin 4 mediated tumor suppression in nude mice involves interferon-gamma. *European Journal of Immunology*, **22**, 1729–33.

Porgador A., Bannerji R., Watanabe Y., Feldman M., Gilboa E. & Eisenbach L. (1993b) Antimetastatic vaccination of tumor-bearing mice with two types of IFN-gamma gene-inserted tumor cells. *Journal of Immunology*, **150**, 1458–70.

Porgador A., Gansbacher B., Bannerji R. et al. (1993a) Anti-metastatic vaccination of tumor-bearing mice with IL-2-gene-inserted tumor cells. *International Journal of Cancer*, **53**, 471–7.

Porgador A., Tzehoval E., Katz A. et al. (1992) Interleukin 6 gene transfection into Lewis lung carcinoma tumor cells suppresses the malignant phenotype and confers immunotherapeutic competence against parental metastatic cells. *Cancer Research*, **52**, 3679–86.

Prehn R.T. (1994) Stimulatory effects of immune reactions upon the growth of untransplanted tumours. *Cancer Research*, **54**, 908–14.

Quesada J.R., Reuben J.R. & Manning J.T. (1984) Alpha interferon for induction of remission in hairy cell leukemia. *New England Journal of Medicine*, **310**, 15–8.

Ratain M.J., Golomb H.M. & Vardimann J.W. (1985) Treatment of hairy cell leukemia with recombinant alpha2 interferon. *Blood*, **65**, 644–9.

Rollins B.J. & Sunday M.E. (1991) Suppression of tumor formation in vivo by expression of the JE gene in malignant cells. *Molecular and Cellular Biology*, **11**, 3125–31.

Russell S.J., Eccles S.A., Flemming C.L., Johnson C.A. & Collins, M.K.L. (1991) Decreased tumorigenicity of a transplantable rate sarcoma following transfer and expression of an IL-2 cDNA. *International Journal of Cancer*, **47**, 244–51.

Rosenberg S.A., Lotze M.T., Muul L.M. et al. (1985) Observations on the systemic administration of autologous lymphokine-activated killer cells and recombinant interleukin-2 to patients with metastatic cancer. *New England Journal of Medicine*, **313**, 1485–92.

Rosenberg S.A., Lotze M.T., Yang J.C. et al. (1989) Experience with the use of high-dose interleukin-2 in the treatment of 652 cancer patients. *Annals of Surgery*, 210, 474–84.

Scala G., Quinto E., Ruoco M.R. et al. (1990) Expression of an exogenous IL6 gene in human EBV B cells confers growth advantage and in vitro tumourigenicity. *Journal of Experimental Medicine*, **172**, 61–8.

Schadendorf D., Moller A., Algermissen B., Worm M., Sticherling M. & Czarnetzki B.M. (1993) IL-8 produced by human malignant melanoma cells in vitro is an essential autocrine growth factor. *Journal of Immunology*, **151**, 2667–75.

Smith K.A. (1990) Cytokines in the nineties. *European Cytokine Network*, 1, 7–12.

Sporn M.B. & Todaro T. (1980) Autocrine secretion and malignant transformation of cells. *New England Journal of Medicine*, **303**, 878–81.

Stoppacciaro A., Forni G. & Colombo M.P. (1994) Different tumours transduced with different cytokine genes as G-CSF and IL-2 show inhibition of tumour take through neutrophil activation but differ in T cell functions. *Folia Biologica*, **40**, 89–99.

Stoppacciaro A., Melani C., Parenza M. et al. (1993) Regression of an established tumour genetically modified to release granulocyte colony-stimulating factor requires granulocyte-T cell cooperation and T cell-produced interferon gamma. *Journal of Experimental Medicine*, **178**, 151–61.

Sun W.K., Kreisle R.A., Philips A.W. & Ershler W.B. (1992) In vivo and in vitro characteristics of interleukin-6 transduced B16 melanoma cells. *Cancer Research*, **52**, 5412–5.

Talpaz M., Kantarjiian H.M., McCredie K., Trujillo J.M., Keating M.J. & Gutterman J.U. (1986) Hematologic remission and cytogenetic improvement induced by recombinant human interferon alpha in chronic myelogeneous leukemia. *New England Journal of Medicine*, **314**, 1065–9.

Teng M.N., Park B.H., Koeppen H.K., Tracey K.J., Fendly B.M. & Schreiber H. (1991) Long-term inhibition of tumor growth by tumor necrosis factor in the absence of cachexia or T-cell immunity. *Proceedings of the National Academy of Sciences USA*, **88**, 3535–9.

Tepper R.L., Pattengale K., Leder P. (1989) Muring interleukin 4 displays a potent anti-tumor activity in vivo. *Cell*, **57**, 503–12.

Topp M.S., Koenigsmann M., Mire Sluis A. et al. (1994) Recombinant human interleukin-4 inhibits growth of some human lung tumour cell lines in vitro and in vivo. *Blood*, **82**, 2837–44.

Vassalli P. (1992) The pathophysiology of tumour necrosis factor. *Annual Review of Immunology*, **10**, 411–52.

Watanabe Y., Kuribayashi K., Miyatake S. et al. (1989) Exogenous expression of mouse interferon gamma cDNA in mouse neuroblastoma Cl300 cells results in reduced tumorigenicity by augmented anti-tumor immunity. *Proceedings of the National Academy of Sciences USA*, **86**, 9456–60.

Weidmann E., Sacchi M., Plaisance S. et al. (1992) Receptors for interleukin 2 on human squamous cell carcinoma cell lines and tumour in situ. *Cancer Research*, 52, 5963–70.

# —10

## Inhibition of Nonhemopoietic Cancer Cell Growth by Interleukin-4 and Related Cytokines

DAVE S.B. HOON, TAKASHI MORISAKI AND RICHARD ESSNER

## ■ INTRODUCTION

Cytokines, particularly those produced from immune cells, have been studied with regard to tumor immunology in terms of their effect on activating immune cells towards recognizing and inhibiting growth of tumors. However, recent studies indicate that immune cytokines can have a significant direct effect on cancer cells. These observations have come from hypotheses, experiments, and serendipitous findings. It has become increasingly clear now that the immune cells can release a number of soluble factors to regulate normal nonhemopoietic cell growth as well. Most of the studies on these factors show that they can potentially regulate cancer cell function and growth as well. The majority of the studies on these factors have focused on cytokine autocrine and paracrine growth regulation. As we unravel the functions of the immune system, it becomes obvious that cytokines play an important role in regulating functions of nonimmune cell systems in our body. In the last two decades, the tumor growth inhibitory effect by the cytokines tumor necrosis factor (TNF) and interferons (INFs) have been well studied (Baron et al., 1992; Tracey & Cerami, 1994). A large number of reviews have focused on these two cytokines and therefore they will not be discussed in any further detail.

The review will focus on immune cytokines that have a direct effect on the growth or function of tumor cells that leads to cell death, growth inhibition, and/or modulation of overall tumor progression. The focus will be on several of the cytokines using the class I hemopoietin receptor superfamily that includes interleukin (IL)-2,3,4,5,6,9,11,13,15, ciliary neurotrophic factor (CNTF), oncostatin M (OSM), leukemia inhibitory factor (LIF), erythropoietin (EPO), prolactin (PRL), growth hormone (GH), and granulocyte–macrophage colony-stimulating factor (GM-CSF). IL-1, which is often grouped with these cytokines because of its many similar activities, uses the immunoglobulin (Ig) superfamily receptors. Most of these cytokines are primarily released from immune cells, and have been well defined in regulating growth and function of immune cells (Cosman, 1993). These same cytokines have also now been shown to regulate nonimmune cell functions in normal and disease states (Phillips et al., 1990; Dinarello and Wolff, 1993; Lewis et al., 1993). The majority of these cytokines have positive growth effects on hemopoietic cells or non-hemopoietic cells. The interesting findings that we are now becoming more aware of are the growth inhibitory effects on cancer cells by these cytokines. The review will highlight on the cancer cell growth cytokines IL-4 and several family members, which include IL-2, IL-6, and OSM. Also included will be IL-1, which has been demonstrated to have significant direct antitumor cell activity. Other cytokines of the hemopoietin receptor family are not discussed because there are few available reports on their direct effect on nonhemopoietic cancers.

There is increasing evidence that human tumor cells of different histologic origin can express receptors for various immune cytokines. Many of these receptors expressed on the tumor cells are functional (Braunschweiger et al., 1988; Chen, Shulman & Revel, 1991; Tungekar et al., 1991; Morisaki et al., 1922; Weidmann et al., 1992; Obiri et al., 1993). These cytokine receptors are also expressed on normal cells, but only in low quantities and are difficult to detect (Idzerda et al., 1990). Receptor amplification on tumor cells, and the ready availability of tumor cell lines has allowed us to evaluate their function in more detail on tumor cells than normal cells. The role of immune cytokine receptors on tumor cells still remains a mystery. In many in situ analyses of normal tissue and disease states, tumor immune cell infiltrates have been well documented (Barnes et al., 1989; Belldegrun et al., 1989; Fisher et al., 1989; Balch et al., 1990). These immune cell infiltrates, when activated, release various cytokines. Therefore, cells in their nearby environment such as other immune cells, normal nonhemopoietic cells, or tumor cells with specific receptors will be influenced by the cytokines. This describes a microenvironment where nonimmune cells and the immune system interact quite extensively. Active cytokine release in this micro-environment will modulate cell to cell interaction and functions. It is now known that an activated receptor can deliver signal(s) that are interpreted in a different manner depending on the type of host cell histology and physiological state. In addition, it is now becoming known that activated receptors on cancer cells can induce different signal pathways compared to their normal counterpart cells.

Tissue destruction is often associated with the presence of T cell infiltrates, particularly in tumors (Belldegrun et al., 1989; Balch et al., 1990). However, there are many situations in which no significant tissue destruction is present but the T cells are very active in releasing cytokines. These immune cytokines can also be neutralized by antagonistic factors released by various types of cells (Tilg et al., 1994).

In recent years, there has been an intensive effort by many laboratories to develop reagents to block these immune cytokines, particularly if they augment the pathological condition. Immune cytokines, which are primarily associated with regulation of normal cell growth and differentiation, are of particular interest in their direct role on tumor cells. In many different cancers, they have been shown to have positive autocrine and/or paracrine effects. Although there are many descriptions of expression of cytokine receptors on various solid tumors, the reports on their functional activity is very limited. The level of expression of these receptors usually play a significant role in the cells responsiveness to the respective cytokine.

## ■ INTERLEUKIN-4

### Characterization

IL-4, a member of the immune cytokine family, is derived primarily from CD4+ T cells, mast cells, and basophils (Paul & Ohara, 1987; Bradding et al., 1992). The CD4+ T helper 2($T_{H2}$) has been defined as the major T cell type releasing IL-4 (Mosmann & Coffman, 1989). However, CD8+ T cells can also release IL-4 (Seder et al., 1992; Morisaki et al., 1994b). IL-4 is encoded by a gene consisting of four exons located on chromosome 5 (Sorg et al., 1993). Human IL-4 is composed of about 153 amino acids with a molecular weight of 15–20 kDa, depending on glycosylation (Paul & Ohara, 1987). IL-4 responses are induced through the IL-4 receptor (IL-4R) encoded by a gene on chromosome 16 (Pritchard et al., 1991). The IL-4R is a member of the class I hematopoietin receptor superfamily and to date has been defined only as a single class of high-affinity binding receptor ranging from 100 to 5,000 sites per cell (Idzerda et al., 1990). The receptor has characteristic cysteine residues and the WSXWS motif also found on other members of the receptor family (Boulay & Paul, 1992; Cosman, 1993). Recently, the IL-2 receptor (IL-2R) gamma chain has been identified to be associated with IL-4R and contributes to its binding affinity (Russell et al., 1993)

## Antiproliferative Activity

Human IL-4 has been shown to possess a broad spectrum of biological activities on normal immune and nonimmune cells (Defrance et al., 1987; Spits et al., 1987; Essner et al., 1989; Phillips et al., 1990; Toi, Harris & Bicknell, 1991; Hoon et al., 1993a; Lewis et al., 1993). This cytokine is most recognized for its function as a growth regulator and differentiation factor of B cells. T cells, granulocytes, and macrophages (Te Velde et al., 1988; Tepper, Coffman & Leder, 1992). IL-4 has significant inhibitory effects on both human hemopoietic and nonhemopoietic malignancies. Significant growth inhibition of human lymphomas and leukemias have been demonstrated (Akashi et al., 1991; Pandreau et al., 1992; Defrance et al., 1992; Okabe et al., 1991). Cell growth inhibition of hemopoietic cancers by IL-4 is understandable in that IL-4 plays a major role in the regulation of normal cell proliferation of T and B cells. The cytokine has been shown to inhibit cell proliferation of melanoma (Hoon et al., 1991a, 1993a), renal carcinomas (Hoon et al., 1991b; Obiri et al., 1993), gastric carcinomas (Morisaki et al., 1992; 1994a), lung carcinomas (Tungekar et al., 1991; Topp et al., 1993), gliomas (Iwasaki et al., 1993), breast carcinomas (Totpal and Aggarawal 1991; Toi, Bicknell & Harris, 1992) and colon carcinomas (Toi et al., 1992). IL-4 has been shown to inhibit and stimulate nonhemopoeitic cell proliferation as well (Dechanet et al., 1993; Monroe et al., 1988). The tumor cell proliferation inhibition has been demonstrated to be IL-4 dose-dependent and not the result of a direct toxic effect (Hoon et al., 1991a; Morisaki et al., 1992; Topp et al., 1993). Studies have been primarily performed on cell lines and verified to some extent on primary cultures (Obiri et al., 1993). There can be considerable variability between different cell lines of similar histological origins. It has been demonstrated that the effect of IL-4 on tumor cells is related to the level of IL-4R expression (Morisaki et al., 1992). Cells with a very low level of or no IL-4R do not respond. IL-4R has been demonstrated on a wide variety of tumor cells with labelled IL-4, specific mRNA detection, and monoclonal antibodies (Jabaari et al., 1989; Mat et al., 1990; Morisaki et al., 1992; Obiri et al., 1993). IL-4 effect on tumor cells can be neutralized with anti-IL-4 antibodies (Morisaki et al., 1992; Topp et al., 1993). Experiments have shown that the IL-4 antiproliferative effect is not due to production of other possible secondary cytokines such as IFN, TNF, IL-1, and IL-6 (Topp et al., 1993).

IL-4R-positive lung carcinomas and gastric carcinomas appear to be more sensitive to IL-4 than other types of carcinoma. IL-4R has been demonstrated on non small-cell carcinomas but not on small-cell carcinomas (Tungekar et al., 1991). Recent studies have shown human IL-4 treatment can inhibit growth of xenografts of human nonsmall-cell lung carcinomas transplanted in Balb *nu/nu* mice (Topp et al., 1993). Although IL-4 can activate effector T cells and eosinophils (Teppler et al., 1992; Hoon et al., 1993), the studies demonstrate it has a direct antiproliferative effect on tumors in vivo. These studies are supported by the demonstration of a direct antiproliferative effect of IL-4 on primary tumor cultures. The experiments provide important evidence for the use of IL-4 on primary tumor cultures. The experiments provide important evidence for the use of IL-4 as a therapeutic agent towards IL-4R-positive carcinomas. Currently, IL-4 clinical trials are in progress.

Analysis of gastric carcinomas have shown the presence of IL-4 mRNA expression (Morisaki et al., 1992). The expression level was low and infrequently expressed amongst the cell lines studied. Interestingly, the cell lines with higher expression of IL-4R also expressed IL-4. This suggests that there may be a negative autocrine growth regulatory effect by IL-4. Human IL-4 transfected into various tumor lines has demonstrated similar effects to those of exogenous added IL-4 (Hoon et al., 1994). IL-4-transfected melanoma cells showed modulation of cell surface antigens, morphology changes, and growth inhibition.

## Synergistic Effects

Several of the cytokines when combined have shown additive or synergistic effects. The latter results are the most interesting. Our studies demonstrated that IL-4 combined with TNF-$\alpha$ or IFN-$\gamma$ significantly enhanced inhibition of cell proliferation (Hoon et al., 1991a, 1991b). The effect was most significant with IL-4 plus TNF. This effect has been confirmed by other investigators (Totpal & Aggarawal, 1991). Interestingly, this synergism was only prevalent when the cancer cells that were studied were sensitive to IFN or TNF alone. For example, gastric carcinomas that were highly sensitive to IL-4, but weakly responsive to IFN or TNF had no additional growth inhibition when the cytokines were combined. In melanoma, renal cell carcinomas, and lung carcinomas, the combination of IL-4 plus TNF at low concentrations was shown to be highly significant in inhibiting cancer cell growth. The studies demonstrate that low concentrations of the individual cytokines used together can have more potent effects than higher concentrations of the cytokines used individually. Immune cell infiltrates of tumors often release IL-4, and TNF. Therefore the synergistic effect of these cytokines may be a natural host defense mechanism against tumor progression. The mechanism of the synergistic effects of IL-4 with IFN-$\gamma$ or TNF is not known. One possible explanation is that they all block $G_0/G_1$ cell cycle progression and, although the receptors belong to different receptor families, their pathway of signal transduction may coincide at some point.

IL-4 has also been shown to block growth-factor-induced stimulation of carcinoma cell growth. Studies have shown that IL-4 can inhibit hormones such as insulin- and estrogen-induced proliferation of carcinoma cells (Toi et al., 1992; Morisaki et al., 1994a). The mechanism of this inhibitory effect is unknown. IL-4 had no effect on the expression on estrogen and insulin receptor expression or their binding affinity. These studies suggest that IL-4 antiproliferative effect may be related to blockage of a specific nuclear signal-transduction pathway activating cell cycle progression. Interestingly, the human insulin and estrogen receptors to date have shown limited common elements with IL-4 in their signal transduction pathways. IL-4 inhibition of breast carcinomas is most effective during $17\beta$-estradiol-induced cell proliferation (Toi et al., 1992). Similarly, insulin-induced gastric and lung carcinoma cell proliferation was significantly inhibited by IL-4 (Morisaki et al., 1994a; Essner & Hoon, submitted). Both insulin and estrogen play a significant role in carcinoma cell proliferation and normal cell growth. Epithelial cells of the digestive tract lining have a very high proliferation and turnover rate. IL-4 may be an important host mechanism to control abnormal epithelial cell growth.

## Cell-cycle Blocking

To further understand the mechanism of the inhibitory effect of cell proliferation by IL-4, postreceptor genetic factors that potentially could transduce the signals of this effect were examined. The initial focus of the study was on cell cycle-controlling nuclear factors. IL-4 treatment of carcinomas could lock cells in the $G_0/G_1$ phase of the cell cycle and significantly reduce cells in the S-phase (Morisaki et al., 1994a). This observation was correlated to the cell growth inhibition on IL-treatment. The effect was observed within 24 hours of IL-4 treatment and would peak after 72 hours (Morisaki et al., 1994a). To further evaluate the IL-4 blocking effect on $G_0/G_1$ phase cell cycle progression, we examined several regulatory factors known to regulate $G_1$ phase transition to S-phase. Retinoblastoma protein (Rbp) has been identified as a key nuclear factor regulating $G_0/G_1$ phase transition that leads to cell proliferation (Goodrich et al., 1991; Dowdy et al., 1993). The phosphorylation state of Rbp controls cell cycle progression (Lin et al., 1991; Meek & Street, 1992). Rbp, when hyperphosphorylated, produces an 112–116 kDa band and, when hypo(un)phosphorylated, it produces an 110 kDa band; the former induces cells to enter into the S-phase (Morisaki et al., 1994a) (Figure 10.1). On examining carcinoma cells treated with IL-4, it was demonstrated that, after 24 hours, an Rbp 110 kDa band begins to appear and the Rbp 112–116 kDa band disappears. After 48–72 hours, the Rbp 112–116 kDa band disappears and the 110 kDa band becomes prominent.

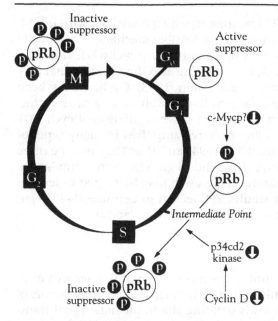

**Figure 10.1**  The effect of IL-4 on the cell cycle of carcinomas. A description of the possible cell nuclear events occurring post IL-4 receptor activation is shown schematically. Cell-cycle progression blockage occurs as the $G_1$ phase and IL-4 events inhibit hyperphosphorylation of retinoblastoma protein (Rpb). Possible events leading to this include down-regulation of p34cdc2 activity, cyclin D1 activity, and c-Myc protein expression.

The experiments suggest that IL-4 blocks proliferation by locking cells in the $G_{1/0}$ phase through preventing Rbp phosphorylation. This evidence provides important clues as to the mechanism of IL-4 inhibition on cell-cycle progression leading to inhibition of proliferation.

The phosphorylation of Rbp has been strongly suggested to be regulated by p34cdc2 kinase (Lin et al., 1991; Meek & Street, 1992). There are several consensus sequence recognition sites for this kinase on Rbp. In our studies p34cdc2 was shown to be markedly down-regulated after IL-4 treatment (Morisaki et al., 1994a). Cyclin D1 has recently been implicated as an important regulator of $G_1$/S-phase transition (Hunter & Pines, 1991; Sherr, 1993). In actively proliferating cells, cyclin D1 is amplified. Cyclin D1 has been suggested to be an oncogene (Hinds et al., 1994) and indicated to regulate p34cdc2 kinase activity and Rbp function (Dowdy et al., 1993; Sherr, 1993). However, the interacting roles of these three key molecules in regulating cell-cycle progression is still not clear. We demonstrated that the level of cyclin D1 decreased at 24 and 48 hours

(Morisaki et al., 1994a) after IL-4 treatment, which coincided with inhibition of cell proliferation. This suggested a possible mechanism of how IL-4 may regulate cell proliferation by down-regulating cyclin D1. However, there are other cyclins such as A, B, and E, and also the D family that play important roles in cell cycle progression (Sherr, 1993). Cyclin D1 has been suggested as a sensor for growth factors. IL-4 inhibition of growth-factor-induced cell proliferation may be through down-regulation of cyclin D1 and interacting molecules. Cyclin D1 is overamplified in many types of carcinomas (Sherr, 1993; Hinds et al., 1994) and thus they may be more sensitive to activation at a lower threshold of growth factor stimulation. IL-4 down-regulation of carcinoma cell growth may be related to level of cyclin D1 expression. Further studies are needed in defining IL-4's regulatory role on these $G_1$–S-phase cell-cycle-regulating factors.

## Signal Transduction

Our initial approach in defining the mechanism of IL-4 growth inhibitory effect has been on defining changes in nuclear regulatory factors of the cell cycle. Another approach is defining the immediate signal transduction pathway(s) after IL-4 activation. A common feature of the hemopoietin receptor family is that they do not have cytoplasmic tyrosine kinase domains; however, their activation triggers phosphorylation of proteins. The IL-4R to date is defined as a homodimer with a large cytoplasmic domain of approximately 500 amino acids (Boulay & Paul, 1992). The cytoplasmic domain has no consensus sequences for serine/threonine or tyrosine kinases. IL-4 has been shown to induce tyrosine phosphorylation of cellular substrates in murine hemopoietic cells (Wang et al., 1993; Keegan et al., 1994a; Schindler et al., 1994). The mechanism(s) of this event(s) have not been unraveled yet. Many studies have been performed in examining potential IL-4-induced cytoplasmic signal-transducing factors of murine hemopoietic cells. There are no major studies on human tumors. IL-4R on murine hemopoeitic cells has been demonstrated to be phosphorylated on IL-4 binding. In these studies, IL-4 has a mitogenic effect on hemopoietic cells (Harada et al., 1992). Corresponding studies in human cell hemopoietic and nonhemopoietic cells have not been well defined.

Recent studies in our laboratory suggest that IL-4 significantly induces phosphorylation of multiple cellular substrates in the range of 50–200 kDa (Essner & Hoon, submitted). Studies are underway in defining specific substrates that have been phosphorylated and their linkage to regulating the cell cycle. Mechanisms need to be determined why IL-4 induces a signal(s) to inhibit proliferation carcinoma cells, whereas in hemopoietic cells the signal(s) often induces proliferation. In studying this problem, we have assessed insulin, which is a well-known $G_1$–S-phase progression factor that can stimulate carcinoma cells of different organs to proliferate. IL-4 was demonstrated to inhibit insulin-induced cell proliferation (Morisaki et al., 1994a). However, both insulin and IL-4 separately and together induced tyrosine phosphorylation of many similar cellular substrates. This may suggest that both factors activate similar pathways and the message to the nuclear factors regulating cell cycle is interpreted differently.

The search is still on for identification of specific cytoplasmic signal-transducting factors that are activated by tyrosine phosphorylation and regulate cell growth. Molecules identified to be phosphorylated on activation of IL-4R include the 170 kDa (4PS) protein and insulin receptor substrate 1 (IRS-1), which have been found in murine lymphoid cells (Wang et al., 1993; Keegan et al., 1994a). These two molecules are functionally similar. The studies suggest that IL-4R and the insulin receptor may have overlapping signal-transduction pathways in the lymphoid system whereby activation of both induces cell proliferation (Keegan et al., 1994b). However, in the human tumor system, the functional effects of the individual factors are quite opposite. Studies of IL-4-induced protein phosphorylation of T cell lines have shown that 4PS phosphorylation is not observed. These data suggest that there may be multiple signal pathways induced by IL-4. Many of the hemopoietic receptor cytokines have growth-promoting activity and activate $p21^{ras}$–GTP complexes, however, IL-4 does not (Keegan et al., 1994b).

The growth inhibitory effect of IL-4 is quite remarkable as it has been duplicated in cancer cells of different histological origins by many laboratories. It is the only member of the interleukin family that uses the hemopoietin receptor superfamily and has shown significant consistent inhibitory effects on solid cancers. Overall, it appears that the carcinomas are the most sensitive to IL-4. Interestingly, IL-4 in general promotes T cell and B cell growth. This suggests that activation of IL-4R on tumor cells induces different signal transductions or the tumor cells respond in a different manner compared to the normal cells. IL-4R is found on many types of normal cells but in very low levels (Idzerda, 1990). One can interpret this as IL-4 has regulatory function(s) on normal cells. IL-4R may be up-regulated during certain physiologic states therefore more susceptible to exogenous factors. Some elegant studies have demonstrated that IL-4 can activate ion flow and trancytosis of antigen–antibody complexes in epithelial cells particularly of the gut. IL-4 has been shown to up-regulate the expression of polymeric Ig receptor, which facilitates transcytosis of IgA–antigen complexes (Phillips et al., 1990).

## Antigen Modulation

IL-4 has other effects on tumor cells than growth inhibition. Studies on tumor cells have shown that IL-4 can enhance human leukocyte antigen (HLA) class I and II antigens as well as tumor-associated antigens (Hoon et al., 1991, 1991b). Studies on melanoma and renal cell carcinomas showed that IL-4 could up-regulate HLA antigens similar to immune cells particularly when they are expressed in low levels. Gangliosides on the cell surface of melanoma and other tumors play important roles in cell–cell interaction and antigenicity (Hoon et al., 1993b). Several antigenic tumor-associated antigens, particularly the cell-surface ganglioside antigen $GD_2$, was significantly elevated on melanoma and renal cell carcinomas when treated with IL-4. Expression of other gangliosides such as $GM_3$, $GM_2$, and $GD_3$ were modulated depending on their level of expression (Hoon et al., 1991a, 1991b). These studies demonstrate that carbohydrate antigen expression can be modulated similar to histocompatibility antigens by IL-4. Modulation of gangliosides could be due to direct modulation of specific carbohydrate synthesis enzymes such as transferases or through an indirect effect due to modulation of the physiologic state of the cells. In related studies, we demonstrated that this up-regulation of cell surface antigens can potentially make the tumor cells more antigenic and be better targets for cytotoxic T cells (Hoon et al., 1993a). Also the adhesion molecule ICAM (intracellular adhesion molecule) on melanoma cells was shown to be up-regulated after IL-4 treatment. ICAM serves as a very important adhesion molecule for T cell docking to tumor cells. These effects by IL-4 may represent host T helper cell mechanisms in preparing the tumor cell to be a better target for attack. Modulation of cell-surface antigen expression by IL-4 may also represent changes in physiologic activity of the cells in preparation for death.

## Antimetastatic Effect

In recent studies we have demonstrated that IL-4 may have an important role in controlling metastasis particularly cell migration. Hepatocyte growth factor (HGF) also referred to as scatter factor has been shown to induce cell migration and invasion of tumor cells that express HGF receptor (c-MET) (Furlong et al., 1991). c-met expression has been demonstrated on carcinomas, other tumors, and normal epithelial cells (Prat et al., 1991). We have demonstrated that IL-4 can significantly inhibit colon carcinoma cell migration induced by HGF on established cell lines and primary cultures (Uchiyama & Hoon, submitted). IL-4 was able to inhibit HGF-induced proliferation only for certain c-MET expressing colon carcinomas. In Boyden chamber migration and collagen matrix invasion assays IL-4 was able to inhibit HGF-induced migration and invasion in a dose-dependent manner. The role of HGF on normal and cancer cells is still not fully understood. IL-4 antagonistic effect on HGF functions may represent a normal host mechanism in regulating epithelial cell growth, invasion, and migration. These studies and others on the down-regulation by IL-4 of the effects of growth factors on carcinomas indicate how significant a role it plays in controlling IL-4R-positive carcinoma progression.

## Summary

IL-4 direct inhibitory effect on tumor cells still remains a mystery. The cytokine is a strong regulator of IL-4R-positive immune cell growth and has now been shown to have similar effects on carcinoma cells. The mechanism of IL-4 effect on tumors may be understood better if we knew of its physiologic role on normal epithelial cells. Current clinical trials are underway in the treatment of various types of human tumors. However, these trials are complicated to interpret in that IL-4 also activates many immune effector cells and directly effects tumor cells. Overall, it seems this dual function may be very advantageous. Understanding the mechanism of the IL-4 direct growth inhibitory effect on carcinomas should provide further insight into carcinoma cell growth regulation. IL-4 regulation of other factors which promote tumor progression is an important host defense mechanism as well.

## ■ INTERLEUKIN-2

### Characteristics

IL-2 was originally described in 1976 as a T cell growth factor from mitogen-activated human lymphocyte culture supernatants that supported the growth and proliferation of T lymphocytes (Morgan, Ruscetti & Gallo 1976). This approximately 15 kDa glycoprotein is secreted primarily by T helper and cytotoxic T cells in response to antigen and/or other cytokine stimulation (Smith, 1988). IL-2 exerts a variety of biological effects on hemopoietic cells that include activation of cytotoxic T cells, helper T cells, macrophages, natural killer cells, and B cells. In vitro studies and in vivo adoptive immunotherapy studies have shown that IL-2 can activate antigen-specific and nonspecific T cell responses against tumors (Schwartzentruber et al., 1994; Oppenheimer

& Lotze 1994). IL-2 is one of the most extensive clinically studied cytokines of the hemopoietin receptor family. IL-2R is expressed as a single a chain (p55), single $\beta$-chain (p70) or as a heterodimer of $\alpha\beta$ chains (Minami et al., 1993). Recently, the gamma chain has been shown to play an important role in IL-2R signal transduction (Takeshita et al., 1992; Russell et al., 1993).

### Antiproliferative Activity

Recent investigations have demonstrated a direct cytotoxic effect of IL-2 on human carcinomas. Studies have shown IL-2R$\alpha$ chain on pancreas by mRNA analysis and by flow cytometric analysis with anti-IL-2R$\alpha$ monoclonal antibody (Kawami et al., 1993). IL-2R have been demonstrated on squamous cell carcinoma of the head and neck (SCCHN) (Cortesina et al., 1992; Weidmann et al., 1992), normal keratinocytes (Weidmann et al., 1992) and sarcomas (Carloni et al., 1989). IL-2 inhibition of SCCHN did not affect cell viability. The effect was almost completely blocked by anti-IL-2 p70 monoclonal antibody and partially by anti-IL-2 p55. This suggests the effect may be largely due to IL-2R p70. The receptors have been shown to be functional in vivo in that low doses of IL-2 were able to inhibit growth of carcinomas in vivo. IL-2 has been also shown to inhibit growth of breast cancer cell lines in vitro and cell lines transplanted on fresh biopsy tissues such as SCCHN. As more studies are conducted, we will probably observe that other cell types have functional IL-2R. The physiological role of these IL-2R on cells of nonhemopoietic origin remains a mystery similar to IL-4. IL-2 therapy to IL-2R positive tumors has an advantage in that it has direct effect on the tumor cells and indirect effect through activating many types of immune effector cells against the tumor.

## ■ INTERLEUKIN-6

### Characteristics

IL-6 was initially reported as a fibroblast-derived glycoprotein, although it is now known to be secreted by T and B lymphocytes, endothelial cells, and macrophages (Van Snick, 1990). The human IL-6 protein is about 21 kDa. IL-6 has multifunctional activity on a variety of cell types and function. In general IL-6 is related to IL-1 and TNF in that they are released from monocytes and can regulate induction of one another. It is also well recognized as a positive growth factor of many cell types. The IL-6 low-affinity receptor on cells is 80 kDa and referred to as IL-6Rα (Yamaski et al., 1988). A 130 kDa glycoprotein (gp130) associated with IL-6Rα enhances the binding affinity of the IL-6R and is an essential component for signal transduction (Murakami et al., 1991). The gp130 protein is shared with OSM and LIF also thus allowing for cross competition amongst these cytokines in receptor binding (Gearing et al., 1992; Cosman, 1993).

IL-6 has been shown to be a positive growth factor for hemopoietic and nonhemopoietic tumors. The cytokine is produced as an autocrine factor in Kaposi's sarcomas, renal cell carcinomas, glioblastomas, osteosarcomas, bladder carcinoma, cervical carcinomas, and myelomas (Miki et al., 1989; Watson et al., 1990; Takizawa et al., 1992; Stephanou et al., 1992). IL-6 is most well known for its autocrine growth factor effect on myelomas (Kawano et al., 1988). IL-6 has been shown to have antiproliferative effects on lung carcinomas (Takizawa et al., 1993) and breast carcinomas (Chen et al., 1991). Although exogenously added IL-6 can not completely suppress growth of lung cancer cell lines (Takizawa et al., 1992). Other studies on similar cell lines with IL-6 have shown no significant effect (Serve et al., 1991). This discrepancy may be due to culture conditions or assay systems. Studies have shown that anti-IL-6 antibodies can accelerate IL-6-producing lung carcinoma cell lines (Takizawa et al., 1992). The affinity and number of IL-6R varies from cell types, however, there was no correlation to IL-6 inhibitory activity. IL-6 has been shown to up-regulate IL-6R on cells.

Studies on breast carcinoma cells show that IL-6 can inhibit growth in a cell-density-dependent manner and is not due to a cytotoxic effect (Chen et al., 1991). IL-6 was found to induce morphological changes of epithelial characteristics and loss of cell–cell adhesion. Studies have shown that IL-6 combined with TNF-α has a synergistic action and blocks cells in the S-phase of the cell cycle of MCF7 (human or breast cancer) cells (Bajaj et al., 1993). Neither of these agents alone had any significant effect on MCF7 cells. IL-6 behaves in a similar manner to TGF-β in that it can stimulate and inhibit cell growth depending on the cell type and physiological state of the cell. IL-6 inhibition of lung carcinomas was not through the induction of TGF-β (Takizawa et al., 1992). Understanding of the signal transduction pathways on activation of IL-6R on nonhemopoietic normal and neoplastic cells will help unravel why, in some cells, IL-6 has a positive effect and, in others, a negative effect on proliferation. The effect of this cytokine on different types of tumors is unique compared to other cytokines in that it can enhance or inhibit growth.

# ■ INTERLEUKIN-1

## Characteristics

IL-1 at approximately 17.5 kDa occurs as two forms, IL-1α and IL-1β with only about 25% homology between the two. IL-α exists primarily as a membrane-bound glycoprotein and IL-β is secreted, although the mechanism for secretion has not been elucidated (Dinerallo & Wolff, 1993). The cytokine has been demonstrated to exert a wide variety of biologic functions, including participation in inflammatory responses, septic shock, T helper cell responses, B cell activation, and the induction of other cytokines and modulation of adhesion molecule expression (Lipsky et al., 1983; Bani et al., 1991; Dinerallo & Wolff 1993). IL-1 activity on cells is mediated through IL-1 type I receptor (IL-1RI) or type II receptors (IL-RII). Both receptors are members of the Ig superfamily (Rosiff, 1990; Dinarello & Wolff, 1993). IL-1 receptors are found on a variety of hemopoietic cells and nonhemopoietic cells (Dower & Urdal, 1987; Gaffney et al., 1988; Rosoff, 1990). IL-1 is known to be produced by a wide variety of cell types.

## Antiproliferative Activity

IL-1 has been shown to have direct cytotoxic effects on certain tumors. Tsai & Gaffney (1986) demonstrated that IL-1 coeluted with a growth inhibitory factor of the mammary cell line MCF7 and a number of other malignant lines tested. In these experiments the effects of IL-1 were not mediated by prostaglandin synthesis. IL-1 was shown to inhibit growth of breast carcinoma and osteosarcoma cells (Sgagious, Kasid & Danforth, 1991; Jia & Kleinerman, 1991). One mechanism by which IL-1 has been shown to inhibit breast carcinoma cell proliferation is by antagonizing oestradiol stimulation of proliferation and reducing oestrogen receptor levels (Danforth & Sgagias, 1991). Several groups have demonstrated that IL-1 has inhibitory activity on melanoma (Lachman et al., 1986; Onozaki et al., 1985; Usui, Mimnaugh & Sinhe, 1991). Onozaki and associated (1985) demonstrated the effects of IL-1 on the human A375 melanoma cell line were not immediate but, over time, the tumor cells eventually lysed. Growth inhibition of colorectal carcinoma and NIH:OVCAR-3 ovarian carcinoma by IL-1 has also been demonstrated (Killian et al., 1991; Raitano & Korc, 1993).

The mechanism in which IL-1 exerts its effect on tumor cell growth is unknown. The IL-1R and release of IL-1 has been demonstrated on a number of tumor cell lines (Kock et al., 1989; Stenphanos et al., 1992). The presence of IL-1R is necessary for growth inhibition, although the density of IL-1R did not correlate with IL-1 inhibitory activity. IL-1 has been shown to block cells in $G_0/G_1$ phase, however, together they have no combinatory effect (Sgagious et al., 1991). As individual agents, IFN-$\alpha$ and IL-1 have been shown to inhibit NIH:OVCAR-3 cells and, when combined together, they have synergistic activity. Similarly TNF and IL-1 have been shown to have synergistic anti-proliferative activity (Ruggiero & Baglioni, 1987).

# ONCOSTATIN M

## Characteristics

OSM is a glycoprotein that is approximately 28 kDa is produced by activated T cells (Miles et al., 1992). Cells responding to OSM have been shown to express high- and low-affinity receptors of approximately 150–160 kDa. OSM has been shown to act as a differentiation factor of myeloid leukemia cells (Bruce et al., 1992). The OSM receptor belongs to the hemopoietic receptor superfamily, and has been suggested to include the gp130 subunit of the IL-6R and the $\alpha$ chain of LIF (leukemia inhibitory factor) receptor (Cosman, 1993).

## Antiproliferative Activity

OSM has been shown to have functional activity on normal and neoplastic human cells (Horn et al., 1990). Inhibition of proliferation of melanoma and other cancers by OSM treatment has been demonstrated (Lu et al., 1993; McDonald et al., 1993; Lu & Kerbel, 1994). Most studies on growth inhibitory effects by OSM have been on melanoma. Differential effects of OSM on melanoma have been observed depending on the stage of tumor progression from which the cells were derived. Primary melanomas of early stage were more sensitive than metastatic melanomas (Lu et al., 1993). OSM has recently been found to have a growth stimulatory effect on Kaposi's sarcoma and is suggested to be an autocrine growth factor (Miles et al., 1992; Cai et al., 1994). Signal transduction studies have shown that OSM, IL-6, LIF, and CNTF induce similar protein tyrosine phosphorylations regardless of the cell type. Gp130 is shared by IL-6, OSM, and LIF, and was a competitor for receptor binding with these cytokines (Gearing et al., 1992). This suggests that both IL-6 and OSM receptors on melanoma and Kaposi's sarcoma may be responsible for the effect of individual cytokines. Interestingly, OSM has been shown to regulate IL-6 expression (Brown et al., 1991). The divergent growth effects of OSM on cancers suggest that differential signal transduction pathways are activated on treatment with OSM. IL-6 and OSM both have positive and negative growth regulatory activities depending on the cell type. Melanoma and Kaposi's sarcoma are a good example of the divergent effects of OSM and IL-6.

# ■ CONCLUSION

We have reviewed some of the major findings on immune cytokines that have direct antiproliferative effects on human nonhemopoietic tumors. These studies suggest that immune cell cytokines with direct antiproliferative effects on cancer cells have a very important role in controlling tumor progression. In time we will be likely to see many more cytokines that have similar antitumor activity. Many of these cytokines activities are autocrine and/or paracrine. These studies indicate that soluble mediators released by immune cells in the nearby environment of tumors may have just as an important role as cytolytic immune cells and antibodies in controlling tumor progression.

The more we assess and learn about the expression and function of cytokine receptors on tumors and their normal cell counterparts, the better we will understand their physiologic roles. Activation of these cytokine receptor genes in tumor cells may represent abnormal gene activation related to the cancer cell genetic instability. Curiously, many of these receptors diminish when the cancer cell becomes poorly differentiated and are no longer responsive to the cytokines. Cancers, as they progress, become more autonomous from host regulatory factors. There appears to be a narrow window in the cancer cell's stage of progression when the receptors are maximally expressed. In general, the normal cell counterparts of the cancer cells express receptors at a far lower level. Although the cytokine receptors on tumor cells are much lower in expression compared to hemopoietic cells. The signal-transduction pathways of direct immune cytokine regulation of normal hemopoietic cell growth and differentiation may be present for all cell types. Cancer cells may activate genes and signal-transduction pathways that were present during embryonic or fetal stages when growth factors played a more significant role in cell growth and differentiation. It is well known that cancer cells, as they progress, revert back to fetal and embryonic characteristics. However, further understanding the role of these functional cytokine receptors on tumor cells will eventually lead to developing better antitumor therapeutic strategies.

## REFERENCES

Akashi K., Shibuya T., Harada M. et al., (1991) Interleukin 4 suppresses the spontaneous growth of chronic myelomonocytic leukemia cells. *Journal of Clinical Investigation*, **88**, 223–30.

Bajaj P., Lawry J., Shenton G. & Rees R.C. (1993) Interleukin-6 and tumor necrosis factor alpha synergistically block S-phase cell cycle and upregulate intercellular adhesion molecule-1 expression on MCF7 breast carcinoma cells. *Cancer Letters*, **71**, 143–9.

Balch C.M., Riley L.B., Bae Y.U. et al. (1990) Pattern of human tumor-infiltrating *lymphocytes* in 120 human cancers. *Archives of Surgey*, **125**, 200–9.

Bani M.R., Garofalo A., Scanziani E. & Givazzi R. (1991) Effect of interleukin-1-beta or metastasis formation in different tumor systems. *Journal of the National Cancer Institute*, **83**, 119–23.

Barnes P.F., Mistry S.D., Cooper S.L., Pirmez C. & Rea T.H. (1989) Compartmentalization of a CD4+ T lymphocyte subpopulation in tuberculosis pleuritis. *Journal of Immunology*, **142**, 1114–9.

Baron S., Coppenhaver D.H., Dianzani F. et al. (eds) (1992) Introduction to the interferon system. In *Interferon Principles and Medical Applications*, pp. 1–15. Galveston, University of Texas Medical Branch Press.

Belldegrun A., Kasid A., Uppenkamp M., Topalian S.L. & Rosenberg S.A. (1989) Human tumor infiltrating lymphocytes: analysis of lymphocytes mRNA expression and relevance to cancer immunotherapy. *Journal of Immunology*, **142**, 4520–5.

Boulay J.-L. & Paul W.P. (1992) The interleukin-4 related lymphokines and their binding to hematopoietic receptors. *Journal of Biological Chemistry*, **267**, 20525–8.

Bradding P., Feather I.H., Howarth P.H. et al. (1992) Interleukin 4 is localized to and released by human mast cells. *Journal of Experimental Medicine*, **176**, 1381–6.

Braunschweiger P.G., Johnson C.S., Kumar N., Ord V. & Furmanski P. (1988) Antitimour effects of recombinant human interleukin 1 alpha in RIF-1 and PANcO$_2$ solid tumors. *Cancer Research*, **48**, 6011–6.

Brown T.J., Rowe J.M., Liu J.W. & Shoyab M. (1991) Regulation of IL-expression by oncostatin M. *Journal of Immunology*, **147**, 2175–80.

Bruce G.A., Hoggatt H.I. & Rose T.M. (1992) Oncostatin M is a differentiation factor for myeloid leukemia cells. *Journal of Immunology*, **149**, 1271–5.

Cai J., Gill P.S., Masvel R. et al. (1994) Oncostatin-M is an autocrine growth factor in Kaposi's sarcomas. *American Journal of Pathology*, **145**: 74–79.

Carloni G., Paterson H., Mareel M., et al. (1989) N-ras dependent revertant phenotype in human HT 1980 fibrosarcoma cells is associated with loss of proliferation within normal tissues and expression of an adult membrane antigenic phenotype. *Oncogene*, **4**, 873–80.

Chen L., Shulman L.M., & Revel M. (1991) IL-6 receptors and sensitivity to growth inhibition by IL-6 in clones of human breast carcinoma cells. *Journal of Biological Regulators and Homeostatic Agents*, **5**, 125–36.

Cortesina G., Sacchi M., Galeazzi E., Johnson J.T., & Whiteside T.L. (1992) Interleukin 2 receptors on squamous cell carcinomas on the head and neck. Characterization and functional role. *Acta Oto-Laryngologica*, **112**, 370–5.

Cosman D. (1993) The hematopoietin receptor superfamily. *Cytokine*, **5**, 95–106.

Danforth D.N. & Sgagias M.K. (1991) Interleukin-1α blocks estradiol-stimulated growth and down-regulates the estrogen receptor in MCF-7 breast cancer cells in vitro. *Cancer Research*, **51**, 488–93.

Dechanet J., Briolay J., Rissoan M.-C. et al. (1993) IL-4 inhibits growth factor-stimulated rheumatoid synoviocyte proliferation by blocking the early phases of the cell cycle. *Journal of Immunology*, **151**, 4908–917.

Defrance T., Fluckiger A.C., Rosi J.F., Magaud J.P., Sotto J.J., & Banchereau J. (1992) Antiproliferative effects of interleukin-4 on freshly isolated non-Hodgkin malignant B-lymphoma cells. *Blood*, **79**, 990–6.

Defrance T., Vanbervliet B., Aubry J.P. et al. (1987) B cell growth-promoting activity of recombinant human interleukin 4. *Journal of Immunology*, **139**, 1135–41.

Dinarello C.A. & Wolff S.M. (1993) The role of interleukin-1 in disease. *New England Journal of Medicine*, **328**, 106–13.

Dowdy S.F., Hinds P.W., Louie K., Reed S.L., Arnold A. & Weinberg R.A. (1993) Physical interaction of the retinoblastoma protein with human D cyclins. *Cell*, 73, 499–511.

Dower S.K. & Urdal D.L. (1987) The interleukin-1 receptor. *Immunology Today*, **8**, 46–51.

Essner R., Rhodes K., McBride W.H., Morton D.L. & Economou J.S. (1989) IL-4 down-regulates IL-1 and TNF gene expression in human monocytes. *Journal of Immunology*, **142**, 3857–61.

Fisher E.R., Paik S.M., Rockette H. et al. (1989) Prognostic significance of eosinophils and mast cells in rectal cancer: Findings from the National Surgical Adjuvant Breast and Bowel Project (Protocol R-01) *Human Pathology*, **20**, 159–63.

Furlong R.A., Takehara T., Taylor W.G., Nakamura T. & Rabin S. (1991) Comparison of biological and immunochemical properties indicates that scatter factor and hepatocyte are indistinguishable. *Journal of Cell Science*, **88**, 7001–5.

Gaffney E.V., Kuch G., Tsai S.C., Loucks T., Lingenfelter S.E. (1988) Correlation between human cell growth response to interleukin 1 and receptor binding. *Cancer Research*, **48**, 5455–5.

Gearing D.P., Comeau M.R., Friend D.J. et al. (1992) The IL-6 signal transducer gp130: an oncostatin M receptor and affinity converter for the LIF receptor. *Science*, **255**, 143–7.

Goodrich D.W., Wang N.P., Quin Y-W., Lee E.P., & Lee W.-H. (1991) The retinoblastoma gene product regulates progression through the G1 phase of the cell cycle. *Cell*, **67**, 293–302.

Harada N., Yang G., Miyajima A. & Howard M. (1992) Identification of an essential region for growth signal transduction in the cytoplasmic domain of human interleukin-4 receptor. *Journal of Biological Chemistry*, **267**, 22752–8.

Hinds P.W., Dowdy S.F., Eaton E.N., Arnold A. & Weinberg R.A. (1994) Function of a human cyclin D gene as an oncogene. *Proceedings of the National Academy of Sciences USA*, **91**, 709–13.

Hoon, D.S.B., Banez M., Okun E., Morton D.L. & Irie R.F. (1991a) Modulation of human melanoma cells by interleukin-4 and in combination with gamma-interferon or alpha-tumor necrosis factor. *Cancer Research*, **51**, 2002–8.

Hoon D.S.B., Hayashi Y., Morisaki T., Foshag L.J. & Morton D.L. (1993a) Interleukin-4 plus tumor necrosis factor alpha augments the antigenicity of melanoma cells. *Cancer Immunology and Immunotherapy*, **37**, 378–84.

Hoon, D.S.B., Okun, E., Banez M., Irie R.F. & Morton D.L. (1991b) Interleukin 4 alone and with gamma-interferon or alpha-tumor necrosis factor inhibits cell growth and modulates cell surface antigens on human renal cell carcinoma. *Cancer Research*, **51**, 5687–93.

Hoon D.S.B., Uchiyama A. & Morton D.L. (1994) IL-4 can augment melanoma cell immunogenicity. *Biological Therapy of Cancer IX* (Meeting Abs., et al.) p.35.

Hoon D.S.B., Wang Y., Sze L. et al. (1993b) Molecular cloning of a human monoclonal antibody reaction to ganglioside GM3 antigen on human cancer. *Cancer Research*, **53**, 5244–50.

Horn D., Fitzpatrick W.C., Gompper P.T. et al. (1990) Regulation of cell growth by recombinant oncostatin M. *Growth Factor*, **2**, 157–65.

Hunter T. & Pines J. (1991) Cyclins and cancer. *Cell*, 66, 1059–65.

Idzerda R.L., March C.J., Mosley B. et al. (1990) Human interleukin 4 receptor confers biological responsiveness and defines a novel receptor superfamily. *Journal of Experimental Medicine*, 171, 861–73.

Iwaski K., Rogers L.R., Estes M.L. & Barnes B.P. (1993) Modulation of proliferation and antigen expression of a cloned human glioblastoma by interleukin-4 alone and in combination with tumor necrosis factor-alpha and/or interferon gamma. *Neurosurgery*, 33, 489–93.

Jabaari B.A., Ladyman H.M., Larche M., Sivolapenko G.B., Epenetos A.A. & Ritter M.A. (1989) Elevated expression of the interleukin 4 receptor in carcinoma: a target for immunotherapy? *British Journal of Cancer*, 59, 910–4.

Jia S.F. & Kleinerman E.S. (1991) Antitumor activity of TNF-alpha, IL-1, and OFN-gamma against three human osteosarcoma cell lines. *Lymphokine and Cytokine Research*, 10, 281–4.

Kawami H., Yoshida K., Yamaguchi Y., Saeki T. & Toge T. (1993) The expression and biological activity of IL-2 receptor on a human pancreas cancer cell line. *Biotherapy*, 6, 33–9.

Kawano M., Hirano T., Matsuda T. et al. (1988) Autocrine regulation and essential requirement of BSF-2/IL-6 for human multiple myelomas. *Nature (London)*, 332, 83–5.

Keegan A.D., Nelms K., Wang L.M., Pierce J.H. & Paul W.E. (1994b) Interleukin 4 receptor signaling mechanisms. *Immunology Today*, 15, 432–32.

Keegan A.D., Nelms K., White M., Wang L-M, Pierce J.H. & Paul W.E. (1994a) An IL-4/receptor region containing an insulin receptor motif is important for IL-4-mediated IRS-1 phosphorylation and cell growth. *Cell*, 76, 811–20.

Killian P.I., Kaaffka K.C., Biondi D.A. et al. (1991) Anti-proliferative effect of interleukin-1 on human ovarian carcinoma cell lines (NIH: OVCAR3). *Cancer Research*, 51, 823–8.

Kock A., Schwartz T., Urbanski A. et al. (1989) Expression and release of interleukin-1 by different human melanoma cell lines. *Journal of the National Cancer Institute*, 81, 39–41.

Lachman L.B., Dinarello C.A., Llansa N.D. & Fidler I.J. (1986) Natural and recombinant human interleukin 1-B is cytotoxic for human melanoma cells. *Journal of Immunology*, 136, 3098–102.

Lewis D.B., Liggitt H.D., Effmann E.L. et al. (1993) Osteoporosis induced in mice by overproduction of interleukin 4. *Proceedings of the National Academy of Sciences USA*, 90, 11618–22.

Lin B., Grunenwald S., Morla A.O., Lee W.-H. & Wang J.Y. (1991) Retinoblastoma cancer suppressor gene product is a substrate of the cell regulator cdc2 kinase. *EMBO Journal*, 10, 857–64.

Lipsky P.E., Thompson P.A., Rosenwasser L.J. & Dinarello C.A. (1983) The role of interleukin 1 in human B-cell activation: inhibition of B-cell proliferation and the generation of immunoglobulin-secreting cells by an antibody against human leukocytic pyrogen. *Journal of Immunology*, 30, 2708–16.

Lu C. & Kerbel R.S. (1994) Cytokines, growth factors and the loss of negative growth controls in the progression of human cutaneous malignant melanomas. *Current Opinion in Oncology*, 6, 212–20.

Lu C., Rak J.W., Kobayashi H. & Kerbel R.S. (1993) Increased resistance to oncostatin M-induced growth inhibition of human melanoma cell lines derived from advanced-stage lesions. *Cancer Research*, 53, 2708–11.

Mat I., Larche M., Melcher D. & Ritter M.A. (1990) Tumor-associated upregulation of the IL-4 receptor complex. *British Journal of Cancer Research*, **62**, 96–8.

McDonald V.L., Dick K.O., Malik N. & Shoyab M. (1993) Selection and characterization of a variant of human melanoma cell line A375 resistant to growth inhibitory effects of oncostatin M (OM). *Growth Factors*, **9**, 176–75.

Meek D.W. & Street A.J. (1992) Nuclear protein phosphorylation and growth control. *Biochemical Journal*, **287**, 1–15.

Miki S., Iwano M., Miki Y. et al. (1989) Interleukin-6 (IL-6) functions as an in vitro autocrine growth factor in renal cell carcinomas. *FEBS Letters*, **250**, 607–10.

Miles S.A., Martinez-Maza O., Rezai A. et al. (1992) Oncostatin M as a potent mitogen for AIDS-Kaposi's sarcoma derived cells. *Science*, **255**, 1432–4.

Minami Y., Kono T., Miyazaki T. & Taniguichi T. (1993) The IL-2 receptor complex: its structure, function and target genes. *Annual Review of Immunology*, **11**, 245–68.

Monroe J.G., Halder S., Prystowsky M.B. & Lammie P. (1988) Lymphokine regulation of inflammatory processes: interleukin-4 stimulates fibroblasts proliferation. *Clinical Immunology and Immunopathology*, **49**, 292–5.

Morgan D.A., Ruscetti F.W. & Gallo R.C. (1976) Selective in vitro growth of T lymphocytes from normal human bone marrows. *Science*, **193**, 1007–10.

Morisaki T., Morton D.L., Uchiyama A., Yazuki D., Barth A. & Hoon D.B. (1994b) Characterization and augmentation of CD4+ cytotoxic T cell lines against melanoma. *Cancer Immunology and Immunotherapy*, **39**, 172–8.

Morisaki T., Uchiyama A., Yazuki D., Essner R., Morton D.L. & Hoon S.B. (1994a) Interleukin 4 regulates G1 cell cycle progression in gastric carcinoma cells. *Cancer Research*, **54**, 1113–1118.

Morisaki T., Yazuki D.H., Lin R.T., Foshag L.J., Morton D.L. & Hoon D.S.B. (1992) Interleukin 4 receptor expression and growth inhibition of gastric carcinoma cells by interleukin 4. *Cancer Research*, **52**, 6059–65.

Mosmann T.R. & Coffman R.L. (1989) TH1 and TH2 cells: different patterns of lymphokine secretion lead to different functional properties. *Annual Review of Immunology*, **7**, 145–74.

Murakami M., Nazarek M., Hibi M. et al. (1991) Critical cytoplasmic region of the interleukin 6 signal transducer gp130 is conserved in the cytokine receptor family. *Proceedings of the National Academy of Sciences USA*, **88**, 11349–53.

Obiri N.I., Hillman G.G., Haas G.P., Sud S. & Puri R.K. (1993) Expression of high affinity interleukin-4 receptors on human renal cell carcinoma cells and inhibition of tumor cell growth in vitro by interleukin-4. *Journal of Clinical Investigation*, **91**, 88–93.

Okabe M., Kunieda Y., Sugiwura T. et al. (1991) Inhibitory effect of interleukin-4 on the in vitro growth of Ph-positive acute lymphoblastic leukemia cells. *Blood*, **6**, 1574–80.

Onozaki K., Matsushima K., Aggarwal B.B. & Oppenheim J.J. (1985) Role of interleukin 1 is a cytocidal factor for several tumor cell lines. *Journal of Immunology*, **135**, 3926–8.

Oppenheimer M.H. & Lotze M. (1994) Interleukin-2: solid tumor therapy. *Oncology*, **51**, 154–69.

Paciotti G.F. & Tamarkin L. (1988) Interleukin-2 differentially affects the proliferation of a hormone-dependent and a hormone-independent human breast cancer cell line in vitro and in vivo. *Anticancer Research*, **8**, 1233–9.

Pandrau Q., Saeland S., Duront I. et al. (1992) Interleukin 4 inhibits in vitro proliferation of leukemic and normal human B cell precursors. *Journal of Clinical Investigation*, **90**, 1697–706.

Paul W.E. & Ohara J. (1987) B-Cell stimulatory factor interleukin 4. *Annual Review of Immunology*, 5, 429–59.

Phillips J.O., Everson M.P., Moldoveanu Z., Lue C. & Mestecky J. (1990) Synergistic effect of IL-4 and IFN-gamma on the expression of polymeric Ig receptor (secretory component) and IgA binding by human epithelial cells. *Journal of Immunology*, 145, 1740–4.

Prat M., Narsimhan R. P., Crepaldi T., Nicotra R., Natali P.G. & Comoglio P.M. (1991) The receptor encoded by the human c-Met oncogene is expressed in hepatocyte epithelial cells and solid tumors. *International Journal of Cancer*, 49, 323–8.

Pritchard M.A., Baker E., Whitmore S.A. et al. (1991) The interleukin-4 receptor gene (IL4R) maps to 16p112-16p12.1 in human and to the distal region of mouse chromosome. *Genomics*, 10, 801–6.

Raitano A.B. & Korc M. (1993) Growth inhibition of a human colorectal carcinoma cell line by interleukin 1 is associated with enhanced expression of t-interferon receptors. *Cancer Research*, 53, 636–40.

Rosoff P.M. (1990) IL-1 receptors: structure and signals. *Seminars in Immunology*, 2, 129–37.

Ruggiero V. & Baglioni C. (1987) Synergistic anti-proliferative activity of interleukin 1 and tumor necrosis factor. *Journal of Immunology*, 138, 661–3.

Russell S.M., Keegan A.D., Harada N. et al. (1993) The interleukin-2 receptor gamma chain is a functional component of the interleukin-4 receptor. *Science*, 262, 1880–3.

Schindler C., Kashleva H., Pernis A., Pine R. & Rothman P. (1994) STF:IL-4: a novel IL-4 induced signal transducing factor. *EMBO Journal*, 13, 1350–6.

Schwartzentruber D.J., Hom S.S., Dadmarz R. et al. (1994) In vitro predictors of therapeutic response in melanoma patients receiving tumor-infiltrating lymphocytes and interleukin-2. *Journal of Clinical Oncology*, 12, 1475–83.

Seder R.A., Boulay J.-L., Finkelman F. et al. (1992) CD8+ T cells can be primed in vitro to produce IL-4. *Journal of Immunology*, 148, 1652–5.

Serve H., Steinhauser G., Oberberg D. et al. (1991) Studies on the interaction between interleukin-6 and human malignant non-hematopoietic cell lines. *Cancer Research*, 51, 3856–66.

Sherr C.J. (1993) Mammalian G1 cyclins. *Cell*, 73, 1059–65.

Sgagius M.K., Kasid A. & Danforth D.N. Jr. (1991) Interleukin-1 alpha and tumor necrosis factor-alpha (TNF-alpha) inhibit growth and induce TNF messenger RNA in MCF human breast cancer cells. *Molecular Endocrinology*, 5, 1740–7.

Smith K.A. (1988) Interleukin-2: receptor, impact, and amplification. *Science*, 240, 1169–73.

Sorg R.V., Enczmann J., Sorg U.R., Schneider E.M. & Wernet P. (1993) Identification of an alternatively spliced transcript of human interleukin-4 lacking the sequence encoded by exon 2. *Experimental Hematology*, 21, 560–3.

Spits H., Yssel H., Takebe Y. et al. (1987) Recombinant interleukin 4 promotes the growth of human T cells. *Journal of Immunology*, 139, 1142–7.

Stephanou A., Knight R.A., Annichiariro-Petruzelli M., Finazzi-Agro A., Lightmann S.L. & Melino G. (1992) Interleukin:1 beta and interleukin-6 mRNA are expressed in human glioblastoma and neuroblastoma cells respectively. *Functional Neurology*, 129, 33.

Takeshita T., Asao H., Ohtani K. et al. (1992) Cloning of the gamma chain of the human IL-2 receptor. *Science*, 257, 379–83.

Takizawa H., Ohtoshi T., Ohta K. et al. (1992) Interleukin 6/beta cell stimulatory factor-II is expressed and released by normal and transformed human bronchial epithelial cells. *Biochemical and Biophysical Research Communications*, **187**, 596–602.

Takizawa H., Ohtoshi T., Ohta K. et al. (1993) Growth inhibition of human lung cancer cell lines by interleukin 6 in vitro: a possible role in tumor growth via an autocrine mechanism. *Cancer Research*, **53**, 4175–81.

Tepper R.I., Coffman R.L. & Leder P. (1992) An eosinophil-dependent mechanism for the antitumor effect of interleukin-4. *Science*, **247**, 548–51.

Te Velde A.A., Klomp J.P.G., Yard B.A., DeVries J.E. & Figdor C.G. (1988) Modulation of phenotypic and functional properties of human peripheral blood monocytes by IL-4. *Journal of Immunology*, **140**, 1548–54.

Tilg H., Shapiro L., Vannier E. et al. (1994) Induction and their effects on IL-2 induced cytokine production in vitro. *Journal of Immunology*, **153**, 3189–98.

Toi M., Bicknell R. & Harris A.L. (1992) Inhibition of colon and breast carcinoma cell growth by interleukin-4. *Cancer Research*, **52**, 275–9.

Toi M., Harris A.L. & Bichnell R. (1991) Interleukin-4 is a potent mitogen for capillary endothelium. *Biochemical and Biophysical Research Communications*, **174**, 1287–93.

Topp M.S., Koenigsmann M., Mire-Sluis A. et al. (1993) Recombinant human interleukin-4 inhibits growth of some human lung tumor cell lines in vitro and in vivo. *Blood*, **82**, 2837–44.

Totpal K. & Aggarawal B.B. (1991) Interleukin 4 potentiates the anti-proliferative effects of tumor necrosis factor on various tumor cell lines. *Cancer Research*, **51**, 4266–70.

Tracey K.J. & Cerami A. (1994) Tumor necrosis factor: a pleiotropic cytokine and therapeutic target. *Annual Review of Medicine*, **45**, 491–503.

Tsai S.-.C. & Gaffney E.V. (1986) Inhibition of cell proliferation by interleukin-1 derived from monocytic leukemia cells. *Cancer Research*, **46**, 1471–7.

Tungekar M.F., Turkey H., Dunhill M.S., Gatter K.C., Ritter M.A. & Harris A.L. (1991) Interleukin-4 receptor expression on human lung tumors and normal lung. *Cancer Research*, **51**, 261–4.

Usui N., Mimnaugh E.G. & Sinha B.K. (1991) A role for the interleukin 1 receptor in the synergistic antitumor effects of human interleukin 1 alpha and etoposide against human melanoma cells. *Cancer Research*, **51**, 769–74.

Van Snick J. (1990) Interleukin-6: an overview. *Annual Review of Immunology*, **81**, 253–78.

Yamaski K., Taga T., Hirata Y. et al. (1988) Cloning and expression of the human interleukin-6 (BSF-2/IFNβ2) receptor. *Science*, **241**, 825–8.

Wang L.-M., Keegan A.D., Li W. et al. (1993) Common elements in interleukin 4 and insulin signaling pathways in factor-dependent hematopoietic cells. *Proceedings of the National Academy of Sciences USA*, **90**, 4032–6.

Watson J.M., Sensintaffar J.L., Berek J.S. & Martinez-Maza O. (1990) Constitutive production of interleukin 6 by ovarian cancer cell lines and primary ovarian tumor cultures. *Cancer Research*, **50**, 6959–65.

Weidmann E., Sacchi M., Plaisance S. et al. (1992) Receptors for interleukin 2 on human squamous cell carcinoma cell lines and tumor in situ. *Cancer Research*, **52**, 5963–70.

# 11

## Current Concepts Concerning Melanoma Vaccines

DONALD L. MORTON AND
MEPUR H. RAVINDRANATH

## ■ THE ORIGIN AND EVOLUTION OF A THERAPEUTIC VACCINE CONCEPT

Active specific immunotherapy with tumor cell vaccines has received considerable attention in the past two decades and provides hope for an efficient treatment of cancer. In general, cancer vaccines are not used to induce prophylactic immunity, but rather to enhance the appropriate immune response (cell-mediated or humoral) to relevant tumor antigens, which retards or arrests tumor growth after the advent of neoplasia. Cancer vaccines may reduce tumor-induced immunosuppression and selectively augment long-lasting humoral and cellular antitumor immunity.

The early literature on cancer vaccines has been reviewed elsewhere (Morton & Ravindranath, 1993). Briefly, the clinical use of cancer vaccines was initiated in 1902 by von Leyden and Blumenthal, and the clinical benefit of cancer vaccines was first documented by Coca and co-workers (Coca & Gilman, 1909; Coca, Dorrance & Lebredo, 1912), who observed several instances of tumor regression after repeated administration of viable autologous and allogeneic tumor cells in large numbers at 14-day intervals. Administering soluble proteins from cancer cells, Vaughan (1914) observed a better response in patients with a small tumor burden. Graham & Graham (1962) injected irradiated tumor cells in patients after surgical reduction of tumor burden and noted that the vaccine 'radiosensitized the residual disease.' Although these early studies do not meet today's standards for clinical trials, the data suggest that occasional clinical responses were clearly observed.

Since 1970, several kinds of tumor vaccines have been developed. Thus far, the most promising cancer vaccines are those developed against

**241**

melanoma. Melanoma vaccines are administered to patients with high-risk recurrent and regional disease, after surgical removal of the tumor, and to patients who have measurable metastatic melanoma poorly responsive to other currently available therapies.


# ■ MELANOMA VACCINE PREPARATIONS

The design of a melanoma vaccine must consider intra-individual and inter-individual tumor heterogeneity, factors augmenting immuno-genicity of melanoma-associated antigens (MAAs), unfavorable immuno-logical responses, tumor-derived or host-derived circulating immunosuppressive factors causing general immunosuppression (as well as specific immunosuppression caused by tumor antigens), tumor infiltration of immune effector cells, such as lymphocytes and macro-phages, and in vivo fixation of antibodies to tumor cells. In addition to being therapeutically effective, the ideal melanoma vaccine should be easy and inexpensive to manufacture, safe to administer, and stable to store. Most melanoma vaccines are based on whole autologous or allogeneic tumor cells, or cell extracts/lysates, with or without an immunostimulant such as bacille Calmette–Guerin (BCG) (Mehigan, Gray & Morton, 1971; Morton et al., 1971, 1972, 1973; Morton, 1972; Laucius et al., 1977; Hadley et al., 1978; Fisher et al., 1981; Leong 1983), Freund's complete adjuvant (Hollinshead et al., 1982), Newcastle disease virus (Cassel, Murray & Phillips, 1983; Cassel et al., 1984), vaccinia virus (Wallack et al., 1983; Hersey et al., 1987), vesicular stomatitis virus (Livingston et al., 1985a), alum (Bystryn et al., 1988), purified protein derivative from *Mycobacterium tuberculosis* (Tallberg et al., 1986), or DETOX (a combination of mycobacterial cell wall with trehalose dimycolate and monophosphoryl lipid A, derived from *Salmonella*) (Mitchell et al., 1988, 1993). Their usual route of administration is intradermal, although subcutaneous administration is not uncommon (Cassell et al., 1983; Slingluff, Vollmer & Seigler, 1988), and some investigators have observed a clinical response after intralymphatic administration (Weisenburger et al., 1982). Several trials have admin-istered cyclophosphamide, an immunosuppressive drug, prior to the vaccine to induce cell-mediated immunity, since a subset of T lym-phocytes can specifically suppress immunological responses to the tumor antigens (Morton et al., 1987; Mitchell et al., 1988, 1993; Bystryn et al., 1988; Berd, Maguire & Mastrangelo, 1986).

# ■ CURRENT TYPES OF MELANOMA VACCINES

## Soluble and Purified Vaccines

Melanoma vaccines may be prepared from tumor cells in fully or partially purified form. The purified HLA-depleted vaccines include ganglioside vaccines, recombinant protein vaccines, antiidiotypic antibody vaccines, and polyvalent shed antigen vaccines. The major advantage of purified vaccines is that they can be characterized easily and reproduced accurately; in addition, they do not induce anti-human leukocyte antigen (HLA) class I and II antibodies, which may confound measurement of cellular immune functions involved in vaccine responses.

**Univalent and Polyvalent Ganglioside Vaccines**    The concept that purified vaccines are superior to whole cell vaccines was first proposed by Livingston and co-workers (Livingston, Calves & Natoli, 1987a; Livingston et al., 1987b; Livingston, 1989). These investigators immunized early-stage metastatic melanoma patients intradermally or subcutaneously with a series of ten different cell vaccines consisting of irradiated autologous (Livingston et al., 1982) or allogeneic (Livingston et al., 1983, 1985a) melanoma cell lines mixed with adjuvants, such as BCG or *Corynebacterium parvum* or vesicular stomatitis virus (Livingston et al., 1985a), or treated with neuraminidase or trypsin or glutaraldehyde (Livingston et al., 1985b). Extensive analysis of preimmune and postimmune sera of vaccine recipients revealed very high antibody titers against HLA, viral antigens, bovine proteins used in culture of melanoma cells, and several nonspecific antigens, but only 'occasional' responses to MAAs, specifically gangliosides $GM_2$ and $GD_2$. Based on this study, Livingston (1991, 1993) concluded that $GM_2$ and $GD_2$ were immunogenic, and initiated a clinical trial with purified $GM_2$. In this trial, 122 patients with resected regional melanoma [American Joint Committee on Cancer (AJCC) stage III disease] were treated with low-dose cyclophosphamide followed by BCG with or without $GM_2$. After median follow-up of 63 months, the increases in disease-free survival (DFS) and overall survival were insignificant (18% and 11% respectively). However, exclusion of patients with elevated prestudy anti-$GM_2$ antibody levels significantly increased DFS ($P = 0.02$). These investigators are currently testing the immunogenicity of gangliosides coupled to keyhole limpet hemocyanin (KLH) and administered with QS-21 adjuvant in melanoma patients (Helling et al., 1993, 1994).

Immune responses to univalent ganglioside vaccines may have severe limitations as documented in the works of Houghton and co-workers

(Vadhan-Raj et al., 1986). Although all tumor cells expressing the targeted ganglioside can be eliminated, residual tumor cells with no or low levels of the ganglioside antigen may proliferate and create a tumor that is resistant to therapy. The heterogeneity of melanoma-associated gangliosides can be the major impediment to success of therapies with univalent ganglioside antigens.

Portoukalian and co-workers (1991) therefore developed a polyvalent purified ganglioside vaccine that can elicit immunoglobulin M (IgM) and particularly immunoglobulin G (IgG) responses against all the melanoma gangliosides. Patients responding to the ganglioside vaccine seemed to have significantly fewer recurrences (eleven out of seventeen) than those who did not have elevated IgG antibody titers (thirteen out of fifteen) ($P < 0.001$). The median disease-free interval was 71 weeks for responders versus 26 weeks for nonresponders. A major concern in the preparation of this vaccine is the possible phase transition, denaturing, and even rancification of gangliosides during the autoclaving that is necessary to ensure sterility.

**Recombinant Protein Antigens**   Van der Bruggen and co-workers (1991) found that many human melanoma tumors express antigens that are recognized in vitro by a panel of cytotoxic T lymphocyte (CTL) clones derived from the human melanoma cells. They identified a gene called MAGE-1 that directs expression of an MAA recognized by CTLs derived from patients with melanoma. The MAGE-1 protein, a nine amino-acid epitope sequence restricted by HLA-A1, has been identified in fresh tumor tissues from some patients with melanoma, small-cell lung cancer and breast cancer, but not in normal tissue (except testis) from patients without malignancy. Therefore, immunization with MAGE-1 protein is a potential approach to developing an antigen-specific vaccine for melanoma and other malignancies. Recent data (Oaks, Hanson & O'Malley, 1994) show that MAGE family genes are located at X chromosome (Xq27-qter). Because of lyonization in females and monosomy X in males, each sex is considered hemizygous for the MAGE genes and, as a result, one would expect more frequent spontaneous or 'iatrogenic' antigen-loss variants for the MAGE system than for antigens encoded by genes on autosomes. Efforts are being made to identify autosomal gene families expressed in human melanomas to explore the possibility of developing purified univalent protein vaccines. We have recently observed that patients immunized with a whole cell vaccine expressing the MAGE-1 gene form antibodies to recombinant MAGE-1 protein antigen (Hoon et al., 1995).

**Antiidiotypic Antibody Vaccines** Antiidiotypic antibodies (anti-ids) are used to mimic MAAs, or to stimulate or suppress regulation of the host's immune response to tumors (Kennedy, 1991). In a phase I clinical trial, Ferrone & Kageshita (1988) administered intradermally (0.5– 4 mg) a monoclonal anti-id mimicking the epitope of a high-molecular-weight (HMW) MAA (HMW-MAA) to 24 patients with AJCC stage IV melanoma. The monoclonal anti-id was specific for a monoclonal antibody that recognized HMW-MAA (Kusuma et al., 1987). Of the 24 patients, one demonstrated a partial response and eight others had minor responses or stabilization of disease. However, disease progression was observed in ten of the twenty-four anti-id vaccine recipients. It is noteworthy that anti-id monoclonal antibody bearing the internal image of HMW-MAA induced anti-HMW-MAA antibodies in hosts that expressed HMW-MAA in their normal tissues, whereas HMW-MAA bearing melanoma cells did not (Chattopadhyay et al., 1991, 1992; Ferrone, 1993). These findings may account for the induction of anti-HMW-MAA antibodies by anti-id monoclonal antibodies in patients with malignant melanoma, despite the lack of a detectable immune response to HMW-MAA expressed in melanoma lesions (Hamby et al., 1987). Ferrone (1993) hypothesizes that 'anti-id antibodies mimic the corresponding antigenic determinants in an imperfect way and therefore may stimulate B cell clones that have not been deleted during the establishment of self-tolerance because of their low affinity for the corresponding antigen. By contrast, TAA [tumor-associated antigens], which are auto antigens, are not immunogenic, because the responsive B cell clones have been deleted during the establishment of self-tolerance'.

A polyclonal anti-id was generated in rabbits against a murine monoclonal antibody specific for one of the epitopes on p97 (Nepom et al., 1984), a transferrin-like glycoprotein expressed on most melanoma cells. The polyclonal anti-id not only induced an antibody response against p97 but also induced a p97-specific cell-mediated response in BALB/c mice. Further animal studies examined different epitopes on p97 and the generation of monoclonal anti-ids (Kahn et al., 1989). Interestingly, the anti-p97 antibodies elicited by monoclonal anti-ids could not protect mice against transplanted p97 mouse melanoma cells. This suggests that polyclonal anti-ids mimicking p97 epitopes are superior to monoclonal anti-ids. However, Ferrone (1993) does not consider them to be practical therapeutic agents because they are difficult to mass produce and standardize.

**HLA-depleted Polyvalent Shed Antigen Vaccines** Within a period of 3 hours, melanoma cells release approximately half of the material expressed on their external surface but only a fraction of their internal molecules (Bystryn, Tedholm & Heaney-Kieras, 1981). The shed material primarily comprises highly enriched cell surface macromolecules and antigens in a fairly purified form. The polyvalent nature of the vaccine increases its chances of stimulating protective immunity. Bystryn harvested polyvalent shed antigens from four melanoma cell lines (three human and one hamster), purified these antigens to deplete their HLA component, and then tested the HLA-depleted antigens as a vaccine in a phase I clinical trial for patients with AJCC stage IV melanoma. The vaccine was nontoxic in all thirteen patients and caused complete regression of cutaneous metastases in one patient, who had no evidence of disease for more than 60 months (Bystryn et al., 1986). In a subsequent trial, the vaccine stimulated both humoral and cellular responses to melanoma in approximately 50% of ninety-four evaluable sequential patients with surgically resected regional (AJCC stage III) disease (Bystryn et al., 1991, 1992). There was a relation between antimelanoma cellular immune responses and favorable clinical outcome: median DFS was 4.7 years longer and overall survival was 3.7 years longer in patients with a strong vaccine-induced delayed-type hypersensitivity (DTH) response. Three years after the onset of treatment, 70% of patients with a strong DTH response but only 31% of nonresponders were still disease-free. A similar correlation was observed between vaccine-induced antimelanoma antibodies and improved survival. Overall median DFS was 30 months for vaccine recipients versus 18 months for historical controls; overall 5-year survival was 50% for vaccine recipients versus 33% for historical controls.

Although this shed-antigen vaccine is easy to prepare and reproduce, a major disadvantage is its xenogeneic antigens. The nature of any undesirable immunological responses to the xenogeneic proteins is unclear. Although the protein profile of the shed antigens has been characterized, the nature of allogeneic and xenogeneic carbohydrate residues and glycolipids deserves further analysis. Also, recent reports document that melanoma cells in culture down-regulate synthesis and expression of some protein MAAs (Savage et al., 1986; Bertheir-Vergnes et al., 1994); this suggests that the polyvalent shed antigens might not represent a true profile of melanoma antigens encountered in vivo.

### Cell Lysate Vaccines

The principle that attachment of a foreign component to tumor cells would augment immune recognition and antitumor response was first proposed by Kobayashi et al. (1969). The foreign component could be a virus or a bacterial derivative, or even a chemical capable of stimulating immune response. A number of investigators have used the principle of viral or bacterial xenogenization to augment the immunogenicity of melanoma vaccines. Some investigators have induced xenogenization with chemical haptens.

  **Viral Melanoma Oncolysate Vaccine**   Recently, it was documented that vaccinia virus-treated melanoma cells express some melanoma antigens that are lost in vitro (Savage et al., 1986; Bertheir-Vergnes et al., 1994) and, as a sequel, the viral melanoma lysate was found to elicit a better immune response. Reports on tumor-regressive effects of viral infections in cancer patients are not uncommon (Pasquinucci, 1971; Bluming & Ziegler, 1971; Sinkovics & Horvath, 1993). Roenigle and co-workers (1976) reported positive results for intralesional inoculation of vaccinia virus in patients with malignant melanoma. Significant tumor regression was observed in all eight patients with stage II disease; however, treatment of patients with stage III disease produced little or no regression. Austin & Boone (1979) reviewed virus augmentation of the antigenicity of tumor cell extracts.

  The tumor-regressive effects of viral infections prompted Wallack and co-workers (1977) to study the oncolytic actions of six nonpathogenic viruses on human cancer cell lines. Because of its efficient oncolytic activity and safety, they used the vaccinia virus to prepare a viral melanoma oncolysate (VMO) from cell lines established from four patients with primary and metastatic melanoma (Wallack et al., 1981, 1983). Each cell line was infected with vaccinia virus at a ratio of one cell to ten $TCID_{50}$ (50% tissue culture infectious dose). The four nucleus-free cell lysates were pooled at equal concentrations (in terms of total cell count) to obtain a polyvalent VMO vaccine.

  One of the major concerns about VMO vaccine is the presence of allogeneic major histocompatibility complex (MHC) antigens. The induction of antibodies to polymorphic MHC antigens was thoroughly analyzed in 25 vaccine recipients: only four patients showed evidence of anti-MHC antibodies. Wallack & Sivanandham (1993) envisage downregulation of MHC antigens consequent to vaccine virus infection. Most of the VMO recipients have developed DTH reactions. Evidence for induction of cytolytic cellular responses in VMO recipients is awaited.

  In a phase I trial, forty-eight patients with stage I and II melanoma were treated with the allogeneic VMO vaccine at different dose levels (0.05, 0.1, 0.5, 1.0, 1.5, and 2.0 mg protein). Since the sera of patients receiving 2 mg protein (weekly for 13 weeks and then every other week for 1 year or until recurrence) showed the highest antitumor activity, this dose and treatment was chosen for a phase II trial (Wallack et al., 1984, 1986). All pretreatment sera of the thirty-nine patients in the phase II trial were negative for antibodies to MAAs (Wallack & Michaelides, 1984); during or after treatment, the sera of twenty-four patients became positive for these antibodies. Statistical comparison of VMO recipients with thirty-nine matched controls (patients treated with BCG or *Corynebacterium parvum*) revealed a significant ($P = 0.04$) increase in the DFS of VMO recipients (Wallack et al., 1987). In a separate phase II study of VMO vaccine, Hersey and co-workers (1987) reported improved survival of VMO recipients. Interestingly, VMO recipients with the highest antimelanoma IgM and IgG antibody titers had a better survival than did patients with low titers. The results of this trial led to a phase III randomized, multiinstitutional prospective, double-blind trial of VMO versus vaccinia virus in 215 evaluable patients with high-risk stage II melanoma, which thus far has not shown a significant therapeutic benefit for VMO. A recent update by Wallack's group failed to show a significant difference in disease-free interval or overall survival between recipients of VMO and recipients of vaccinia virus only (Wallack et al., 1994, 1995). Median overall survival is not available because VMO recipients have not yet reached the 50% mark and the median overall survival is 45 months for the control group (Wallack et al., 1995).

Although VMO is polyvalent and allogeneic (which is an advantage with respect to melanoma's heterogeneity), and which reportedly can be produced without significant batch-to-batch variation, Wallack & Sivanandham (1993) concede that VMO 'could be more beneficial in patients with early stage disease, because patients with advanced melanoma may be somewhat more immunosuppressed.' Nevertheless, it is still possible that VMO vaccine may be useful in augmenting humoral and possibly cell-mediated antitumor immunity following surgical resection of all gross disease, even though it is not effective in established disease.

Another study documents a humoral immune response after immunizing melanoma patients with a vaccinia virus oncolysate (Dore et al., 1990). Thirty-two patients who were clinically disease-free following appropriate surgical treatment of high-risk melanoma (primary melanoma of the limbs or trunk, or recurrent melanoma) were immunized with a vaccinia virus oncolysate made from a pool of four human melanoma cell lines. Intradermal injections were given weekly for 3 months, and then bimonthly for 21 months or until relapse. Treated patients received a full 24-month treatment. Three relapsed and ten are alive (nine are disease-free) with a survival of 34–72 months. An analysis of DFS and overall survival to 5 years was made using the actuarial method: the DFS curve shows a 35% plateau reached after 40 months, and the overall survival curve shows a 60% plateau reached after 30 months, the significance of which cannot be evaluated in the absence of an adequate control group. Lymphocytes from vaccine recipients responded in vitro to the stimulation by oncolysate in the presence of low doses of interleukin-2 (IL-2), and this response was greater than that of normal individuals.

Dore's group (1990) found that IgG antibody production to gangliosides with N-glycolyl neuraminic acid (NeuGc) was of prognostic significance: the increase in antiganglioside IgG antibody after 3 and 6 months of treatment was linked to the absence of relapse. It is not clear whether the IgG antibodies were directed against melanoma-associated gangliosides or against gangliosides found in the fetal calf serum used to grow the melanoma cells. There is only one report documenting the presence of NeuGc gangliosides in human melanoma biopsies (Hirabayashi et al., 1987); subsequent investigators (Furukawa et al., 1988) have attributed the presence of NeuGc gangliosides to contamination from fetal calf serum. It remains to be documented whether human melanoma cell lines used for vaccine contain NeuGc gangliosides or synthesize these unique gangliosides after exposure to vaccinia virus, and whether human melanoma biopsies contain these gangliosides that disappear under culture conditions.

Bertheir-Vergenes and co-workers (1994) recently reported that sera of VMO vaccine recipients contain IgG antibodies not found in preimmune sera, which react to a 31-kDa melanoma antigen. Western blot immunostaining revealed that this protein is not found in the allogeneic melanoma cell lines used to prepare VMO vaccine or in the vaccinia virus preparation, or in the fetal calf serum used to culture the tumor cells, but it is found in tumor metastases of the patients. Interestingly, this antigen disappears within 5 days after culturing the tumor cells in vitro but is synthesized after exposure to vaccinia virus. Expression of this antigen in tumor metastases and induction of IgG antibodies against this protein antigen in patients immunized with VMO vaccine indicate the possible therapeutic benefit of VMO vaccine in human melanoma.

These findings are remarkably parallel to those of Savage et al. (1986), who reported antibody development in six melanoma patients following 6 weeks of immunization with allogeneic melanoma oncolysates prepared from three Newcastle virus-infected melanoma cell lines. Most of the elicited antibodies reacted with antigens found in extracts of virus-infected cells but not in extracts of noninfected tumor cells. Viral oncolysates may boost production of antigens which have been lost during culture of melanoma cells in vitro. The restoration of native tumor-associated antigens and the down-regulation of HLA antigens appear to be unique features of viral-induced melanoma oncolysates.

**Bacterial DETOX-coupled Lysate Vaccine**   It is often recognized that human MAAs are weakly immunogenic or a state of tolerance exists such that introducing purified MAAs alone, or tumor cells not admixed with viral or bacterial antigens may not be efficient for inducing active specific immunotherapy. Mitchell et al. (1988, 1993) suspect that treating tumor cells with chemicals or irradiation may alter their immunogenicity. They have prepared a vaccine containing bacterial cell-wall derivatives and tumor-cell membranes by mixing tumor-cell lysate with DETOX, which contains nontoxic lipid A (monophosphoryl lipid A from *Salmonella minnesota*) and cell-wall skeletons of *Mycobacterium phlei* in squalene oil and Tween-80. The mixed lysate is referred to as Melanoma Theracine, and a lyophilized preparation (Melacine) was made by Ribi Immunochemical Research, Inc. (Montana). The immunization dose contained about $2 \times 10^7$ tumor cell equivalents of allogeneic melanoma cell lysate with DETOX. The treatment is restricted to patients with measurable lesions of metastatic melanoma. Melanoma Theracine was administered on days 1, 8, 15, 22, and 36. In several patients cyclophosphamide was given 5–7 days before the first Theracine injection, in an effort to inhibit possible suppressor T cells. The reported response rate was approximately 20%, 20 of the 106 evaluable patients. Approximately 5% of the patients had complete remission and 15% had partial remission. The median duration of response was 17 months and the median duration of remission was 21 months. Median survival was approximately 6–12 months from the appearance of metastatic disease. Dramatic progress was reported in two patients who still survive without disease. The investigators strongly believe that Theracine significantly retarded tumor growth in patients whose disease was progressing before treatment. Data from phase II multicenter trials of Melacine conducted by Ribi Immunochem (Elliot et al., 1992) appeared to confirm Mitchell's results and also suggested that the DETOX melanoma lysate vaccine contributed to improved survival. However, a recent phase III randomized trial sponsored by Ribi has failed to confirm the earlier phase II results.

In the investigations of Mitchell et al. (1993), the strongest correlate of clinical response was an increase in CTL precursors. Before immunization, patients had one CTL in 10,000–50,000 lymphocytes. Three to six weeks after immunization, this ratio increased to one CTL in 2,500–5,000 lymphocytes. Interestingly, patients who failed to generate CTLs against at least one component of the vaccine uniformly failed to have a clinical response. CTL generation was documented in 58% of 111 patients. Of those who generated CTLs, 30% had objective remission or long-term stability. The effector lymphocytes were CD3$^+$. In cold target competition assay with various cell lines, different melanoma cell lines but not cell lines from other cancers blocked CTL reactivity against melanoma antigens on the vaccine, suggesting that cross reactivity of T cells against MAAs is unrestricted by self-MHC.

In a separate study, clones of T cells were derived from the tumor tissues of immunized patients (Harel et al., in press). Of the 117 clones produced, sixty-four were CD4$^+$CD8$^-$ phenotype and fifty-three were CD8$^+$. Intensive analysis of specificity and HLA-restricted studies utilizing matched lymphoblastoid cell lines proved that CTL reactivity is specific to melanoma. In one patient, seven of sixteen CD8$^+$ clones cytotoxic to autologous tumor cells were exclusively class I restricted, whereas five others were restricted by either class I or II, that is, they were blocked by pretreatment with monoclonal antibodies against class I or II antigens. One clone was not inhibited by either anti-class I or class II. Only two exclusively class II restricted CD4$^+$ T cells were recognized. In another analysis, lysis by eight of the eleven melanoma-reactive CD4$^+$ cells was exclusively HLA class I-restricted, as judged by blocking with monoclonal antibodies. Five of these HLA class I-restricted clones were reactive only with the autologous melanoma cells, whereas the other three clones were also reactive with allogeneic melanoma cells sharing HLA-A2/A28 (Kan-Mitchell et al., 1993).

The results of this study also revealed that the cytotoxicity of CD4$^+$ T cells was weaker than that of CD8$^+$ T cells, in that they required longer assays, a higher effector/target ratio, and most importantly pretreatment of the melanoma cells with gamma interferon, which mainly up-regulated tumor antigen expression. Furthermore, analysis of the first seventy-seven patients treated with Theracine revealed an association between three HLA class I alleles and clinical response to therapy: only patients whose lymphocytes shared one or more of these alleles with the vaccine had clinical remission. The three alleles were HLA-A2 (and HLA-A28, serologically cross reactive), HLA-B12 (including HLA-B44 and B45), and HLA-C3. HLA-A2/A28 and HLA-B12/44/45 are strong presenting molecules for melanoma-associated epitopes (Darrow, Slingluff & Seigler, 1989; Wolfel et al., 1989) and may permit CTLs from patients sharing these alleles to recognize and kill melanoma cells most efficiently after immunization with the allogeneic Theracine. It is not clear whether the similarity between alleles of the immunizing melanomas and those on the autologous tumors accounted for their improved effectiveness in eliciting a tumor response. However, autologous immunization (by definition fully 'matched') has thus far been less successful than allogeneic vaccine therapy. This study emphasizes the need to determine whether the HLA class I antigens of an allogeneic vaccine must match those of the cancer patient for efficient induction of CTLs.

Because Mitchell's investigations did not include a control group of patients receiving the vaccine without DETOX, his studies do not indicate to what extent this adjuvant augmented immunological activity or clinical efficacy. Recently, Schultz et al. (1995) examined the ability of

DETOX to potentiate the immunogenicity of a melanoma antigen vaccine and affect the clinical outcome of vaccine-treated patients. When compared with alum, DETOX augmented the antibody response to melanoma vaccine immunization but did not further increase cellular response. Interestingly, the antibody response was fourfold higher when DETOX was administered in low doses with shed melanoma antigens (see Bystryn's preparations for melanoma vaccine). Thus, this non-randomized study shows that DETOX did not improve the clinical outcome of patients treated with a melanoma vaccine.

## Whole Cell Vaccines

**Hapten-attached Cell Vaccines**   Recognition of the important role of T cells in antitumor activity led several investigators to develop strategies to induce better T cell responses to melanoma antigens. Based on an idea that the T cell response to a strongly immunogenic, hapten-modified tumor antigen might be followed by development of immunity to unmodified tumor antigens (Galili et al., 1976), analogous to the phenomenon of chemical-induced autoimmunity (Roth et al., 1975; Gilliland, 1991), Berd et al. (1990) attached the hapten dinitrophenol (DNP) to melanoma cells and administered this preparation to forty-six patients with surgically incurable metastatic melanoma. The patients were sensitized to DNP by topical application of 1% dinitrofluorobenzene (DNFB) in acetone–corn oil on 2 consecutive days. Cyclophosphamide was administered 3 days before the sensitization. Two weeks later, patients were again given cyclophosphamide, followed 3 days later by injection of DNP-conjugated melanoma vaccine. The vaccine included autologous, irradiated, cryopreserved cells ($10–25 \times 10^6$) mixed with BCG. Cyclophosphamide+DNP-conjugated vaccine was repeated every 28 days. The development of DTH was tested with DNP-conjugated autologous peripheral blood mononuclear cells: a DTH response was not present before treatment but was induced in all patients by DNFB sensitization.

Twenty of forty-six patients had clinically evident inflammatory responses in metastatic tumors 2–4 months after initiation of treatment. The tumors were infiltrated with $CD8^+$ T cells, in contrast to tumors derived from control subjects not treated with vaccine. In a panel of fourteen subcutaneous melanoma metastases from untreated patients, T cells ($CD3^+$) constituted $10.2 \pm 2.2\%$ of the total viable cells, compared with 40% in DNFB vaccine-treated patients. The CD8:CD4 ratio of T cells in treated patients was about 5:1.

T cell clones were generated from the tumor metastases of vaccine recipients. Of 140 clones generated, 70 killed cultured autologous melanoma cells but not natural killer (NK)-sensitive K562 cells. Further characterization of one clone revealed that it reproducibly killed autologous melanoma cells but failed to kill a panel of four allogeneic melanoma cell lines. The clinical impact of DNP-conjugated vaccine in patients with a lower tumor burden, that is, surgically curable regional metastases, was examined in a separate study. Forty-one patients with large (>3 cm), clinically palpable lymph nodes received the vaccine as adjuvant therapy following regional lymph node dissection. Eight injections of DNP-conjugated vaccine were administered at 4-week intervals. Cyclophosphamide was administered 3 days before the first two vaccine treatments. Of twenty-seven disease-free patients, twenty-two have survived more than 1 year after surgery and eleven have survived 2 years. This clinical outcome is reportedly better than that of a similar group of twenty-two patients previously treated with the nonhapten vaccine. However, the small number of patients and the use of selected historical controls prohibit any conclusions regarding therapeutic effectiveness. Although hapten conjugation appeared to augment infiltration of T lymphocytes into the residual metastases and destroy tumor, there is no information on the humoral antibodies elicited after immunization.

**Allogeneic Cell Vaccines: Polyvalent Antigen-adjusted Melanoma Cell Vaccine** While the results obtained with purified melanoma vaccines and xenogenized melanoma lysate are encouraging, no definitive conclusions on the efficacy of the vaccines for advanced-stage metastatic melanoma can be reached. Xenogenized melanoma lysate may be therapeutically beneficial for patients with early-stage melanoma, although randomized trials have thus far been negative. The proponents of viral oncolysates acknowledge that the efficacy of their vaccine may be affected by immunosuppression, a major problem encountered in the late stage of disease. It appears that vaccines would be most effective after minimizing immunosuppression due to tumor burden. As we have previously reported, immunosuppression is induced by the tumor-associated antigens shed from growing tumor (Ravindranath & Morton, 1991). A recent study (Kaucic et al., 1994) documents that tumor-driven gangliosides such as $GD_2$ can suppress the hematopoiesis (production of stem cells, undifferentiated lymphocytes and white blood cells) frequently associated with human malignancy. Antiganglioside antibodies elicited by a vaccine might minimize such ganglioside-induced immunosuppression before augmenting antitumor activity (Tai et al., 1985; Ravindranath et al., 1993; Morton, Ravindranath & Irie, 1994). In this regard, whole cell melanoma vaccine in combination with appropriate immunostimulants may reduce or eliminate tumor-induced immunosuppression, and also elicit antitumor immune responses against heterogeneous tumor-associated antigens.

The primary goal of our research during the past 25 years has been to develop a vaccine with high efficacy. The conceptual basis stems from our initial observation (Morton et al., 1970, 1974) that injecting BCG into the cutaneous metastases of melanoma patients produced a systemic enhancement of active immunity. Biopsy of uninjected melanoma lesions showed remarkable tumor infiltration and distinct clinical regression. Our early efforts at immunization with autologous irradiated tumor cells met with limited success (Morton et al., 1971, 1972, 1973; Morton, 1972) and produced results similar to those of Currie et al. (1971).

Efforts to reproduce these effects by intradermal or intralymphatic injection of randomly selected, irradiated allogeneic whole melanoma cells mixed with BCG was of limited success (Morton et al., 1978; Ahn et al., 1982; Morton, 1986). Only 35% of immunized patients responded by formation of antibodies to cell surface antigens. In 1984, a new improved polyvalent melanoma cell vaccine (MCV) was developed. MCV consists of three allogeneic melanoma cell lines containing high concentrations of the six MAA defined in our laboratory or demonstrated by us or others to be immunogenic in melanoma patients (Morton et al., 1989). These vaccine cell lines, selected from a large pool of melanoma cell lines, were chosen for their content of specific melanoma antigens including glycoproteins, lipoproteins, and gangliosides. Immunofluorescence studies showed that the antigens are on the cell surface. Cell-surface expression of MAA was considered a prerequisite for effective immune responses.

In late 1984, a phase II trial was initiated to evaluate MCV in melanoma patients with regional soft tissue metastases (AJCC stage IIIA disease) or distant metastases (AJCC stage IV disease). MCV was produced in large batches and analyzed for MAA expression to determine variance between lots. An outside laboratory screened MCV for viral, bacterial, and fungal infectious organisms. Before cryopreserving the vaccine, the cells were irradiated to 100–150 Gy. Vaccine was injected intradermally in axillary and inguinal regions on a schedule of every 2 weeks for 4 weeks, then monthly for 1 year. For the first two treatments, MCV was mixed with BCG (Glaxo, England) ($24 \times 10^6$ organisms/vial). After one year, the immunization interval was increased to every 3 months $\times$ 4, then every 6 months. One of the following biological response modifiers known to down-regulate suppressor cell activity was administered to some groups of patients receiving MCV: cimetidine, indomethacin, or cyclophosphamide.

Survival after MCV immunization correlated significantly with DTH ($P = 0.0066$) and antibody response to MCV ($P = 0.0117$). Of forty AJCC stage IV patients with evaluable disease, nine (23%) had regression (three complete). MCV patients experienced increased median and 5-year survival (stage IIIA twofold [$P = 0.00024$] and stage IV threefold [$P = 0.0001$]), compared with patients in our historical database receiving non-MCV immunotherapy and other treatments (Morton et al., 1992).

Our results show the following interesting findings not hitherto observed with other vaccines.

1. IgM antibodies to cell surface antigens correlated best with survival (Morton et al., 1992, 1993); there was no significant correlation between survival and IgG antibody to melanoma cell surface antigens. Patients developing high IgM titers (immunofluorescence index ≥ 50%) had almost a threefold increase in 5-year survival (9.6–26.8%) and a twofold increase in median survival (16–30 months). IgM antibodies were directed against a variety of melanoma-associated gangliosides (Ravindranath et al., 1989, 1991, 1993; Morton et al., 1994).
2. There was a highly significant ($P = 0.0066$) correlation between survival and DTH response (Morton et al., 1992, 1993). Median survival was 30 months for those whose DTH reaction exceeded 10 mm and only 17 months for those whose DTH was less than 10 mm. Respective 5-year survival rates were 27.7% and 10.0%. A significant association between survival and DTH was also noted after immunization with HLA-depleted polyvalent melanoma shed antigen (Bystryn et al., 1992) and autologous whole cell vaccine (Berd et al., 1990).
3. There was a significant ($P = 0.013$) positive correlation between in vivo DTH response and in vitro mixed lymphocyte tumor reaction (MLTR) (Morton et al., 1992, 1993). Of the forty patients for whom these data were available, 82% showed significantly ($P = 0.005$) enhanced stimulation to one or more MCV cell lines at either week 4 or 16 compared with week 0. Of these, 91% showed sensitization to at least two MCV lines.
4. Autologous MLTR studies revealed that immunization with allogeneic MCV enhanced the response to autologous melanoma cells, confirming the existence of cross-reacting antigens demonstrated by antibodies to membrane-associated antigens (Morton et al., 1992, 1993).
5. MLTR responses correlated with survival. Two-year DFS was 53% for patients responding to one or more MCV lines in the MLTR, compared with 20% for patients who showed no response ($P = 0.055$).
6. MCV immunization changed the profile of tumor-infiltrating lymphocytes: activated T and B cells (CD25) and NK cells (CD56) were

significantly enhanced, and the CD4/CD8 ratio was markedly elevated (Morton et al., 1992).

7.  In our recent study of 135 AJCC stage III melanoma patients, 83% responded by a positive DTH reaction ($\geqslant 6$ mm) during the first 4 months of MCV therapy (Barth et al., 1994a). Sixteen of thirty-three developed more than a 50% increase in CTL activity against one of MCV's cell lines during this period. Overall survival was significantly prolonged in patients with a positive DTH ($P = 0.0054$) and/or increased CTL activity ($P = 0.02$), suggesting that MCV induces specific T cell responses that are correlated with the clinical course.

8.  In a separate study of fifty-three melanoma patients immunized with MCV, we found that 57% had significantly elevated anti-MAGE-1 IgG serum levels after immunization with MCV (Hoon et al., 1995).

One of the crucial issues surrounding allogeneic vaccines is whether autologous melanoma cells have cross-reactive antigens. There are five lines of evidence indicating that an allogeneic whole cell vaccine (MCV) can induce an enhanced immune response against autologous melanoma cells:

1.  The strong correlation observed between humoral and cell-mediated immune responses to allogeneic melanoma cells and survival (Morton et al., 1992, 1993).

2.  The complete and partial regressions in patients with evaluable disease (Morton et al., 1992, 1993).

3.  The concomitant increase in CTL activity, MLTR, and humoral antibodies to allogeneic and autologous melanoma cells (Barth et al., 1994a; Morton et al., 1992, 1993).

4.  The changes in tumor-infiltrating lymphocytes in melanoma metastases (Morton et al., 1992).

5.  The ability of allogeneic melanoma cells to induce sensitization to autologous melanomas that share HLA class I antigens, and thereby render the autologous cells susceptible to in vitro killing by CTLs (Hayashi et al., 1993).

The question of MHC class I or II restriction has been raised as an argument against the use of allogeneic vaccines. We selected allogeneic melanoma cells that share MHC class I cross-reactive antigens with more than 90% of melanomas. We have noted that MCV augments T cell responses (Barth et al., 1994a). The enhanced T cell response to autologous melanoma cells may result from direct recognition of MAA presented by shared or cross reactive HLA molecules on MCV lines, as demonstrated in vitro (Hayashi et al., 1992a, 1992b). It is also possible that MAA recognition occurs through antigen processing and presentation of MCV's MAA by antigen-presenting cells. The allogeneic HLA antigens on the vaccine may stimulate alloreactive T cells that infiltrate the site of MCV injection, resulting in production of cytokines to attract nearby antigen-presenting cells. Recently, Nabel and co-workers (1993) have shown that in vivo transfection of the gene for an allogeneic HLA class I antigen into a patient's melanoma induced specific systemic T cell immunity.

In our study, approximately 20% of patients did not show a T cell response to MCV (Barth et al., 1994a), which could be due to T cell anergy or to T cell-specific immunosuppression.

**Genetically Altered Cell Vaccines: Cytokine-producing Cell Vaccines** To examine the molecular mechanisms underlying in situ cytokine regulation of immune responses, recent animal studies have incorporated the genes encoding various cytokines into tumor cells. Murine tumor cells expressing genes for IL-2 (Bubenik, Simova & Jandlova, 1990; Levitsky et al., 1990; Gansbacher et al., 1990a, 1990b), IL-4 (Tepper, Pattengale & Leder, 1989; Li et al., 1990), gamma interferon (Watanabe et al., 1989; Gansbacher et al., 1990b), or tumor necrosis factor-$\alpha$ (Blankenstein et al., 1991) retarded tumor growth; notably, mice that had eliminated the primary tumor frequently developed lasting tumor immunity. These findings strongly suggest that, by amplifying the immune response, cytokines can promote tumor rejection. This in turn indicates that cytokines can play a crucial role in vaccines for cancer treatment and provides hope for tumor cell vaccines that are genetically engineered to produce cytokines. There is no doubt that these agents can induce T cell responsiveness.

We recently developed a preclinical model to determine whether transfection of IL-2 gene into human melanoma cells would augment the response of autologous and allogeneic peripheral blood lymphocytes (PBLs) from melanoma patients (Uchiyama et al., 1993). IL-2 gene was transfected into three human melanoma cell lines, and the secretion of IL-2 from stable transfected cells was confirmed by ELISA. The PBL response to these melanoma cells was then examined in an MLTR using PBLs from eight melanoma patients. The PBL response was significantly higher to autologous ($P = 0.01$) or HLA-A cross reactive ($P = 0.05$) transfected melanoma cells than to nontransfected melanoma cells. These data suggest that IL-2 gene transfection may be an important strategy for enhancing specific immune responses induced by a polyvalent melanoma cell vaccine.

Cytokines are also used to enhance the expression of MAA in melanoma vaccines. We have observed that IL-4, gamma interferon, and tumor necrosis factor augment the expression of HLA class I and HLA-

DR antigens. IL-4 alone or in combination with interferon or tumor necrosis factor increased $GD_2$ expression (Hoon et al., 1991, 1993).

# ■ FUTURE DIRECTIONS: IN SEARCH OF A UNIVERSAL MELANOMA VACCINE

Formulation of a nontoxic, reproducible, universal melanoma vaccine requires recognition of its specific functions. The first and foremost function of a vaccine for patients with advanced-stage melanoma is to reduce or eliminate immunosuppression. Identification of tumor-induced direct and indirect immunosuppressive factors is necessary to outline the strategies to combat immunosuppression and allow the vaccine to induce an effective rejection response in the immunized host.

Vaccines cannot restore immunocompetence without eliminating or reducing immunosuppression. Our MCV trials document improved survival of patients who respond with high IgM antibody titers. The role of antimelanoma IgM antibody in direct killing of the tumor may be minimal, particularly considering the short half-life (5 days) of IgM and its poor ability to penetrate the tumor mass. Our preliminary studies document that IgM antibodies are directed against carbohydrate domains of glycoconjugates such as gangliosides. Gangliosides are known to be immunosuppressive. Recent studies show that gangliosides shed from melanoma cells can bind to IL-2 (Chu & Sharom, 1993) and inhibit hematopoiesis (Kaucic et al., 1994). Gangliosides elicit T cell-independent antibody responses (Freimer et al., 1993); the antibodies thus elicited are invariably IgM. Many of the IgM antibodies elicited by MCV may be directed against gangliosides (Tai et al., 1985; Ravindranath et al., 1989, 1993; Morton et al., 1994). Animal experiments show that augmentation of the antibodies may be useful in clearing the shed immunosuppressive gangliosides (Ravindranath, Brazeau & Morton, 1994a; Ravindranath, Morton & Irie, 1994b). Therefore, formulation of a universal vaccine should first attempt to eliminate immunosuppression, so that immunocompetence can be restored.

The second function of a universal vaccine is to stimulate CTLs. There is no doubt that vaccines augment infiltration of lymphocytes into residual tumors. The nature of infiltrating lymphocytes may differ with the immunostimulant administered with the vaccine. Mitchell and co-workers (1993) showed that DETOX stimulates infiltration of both $CD4^+$ and $CD8^+$ CTL phenotypes. BCG-MCV significantly stimulated infiltration of $CD4^+$, $CD25^+$ (activated T cells) and $CD56^+$ (NK cells) lymphocytes (Morton et al., 1992). A study linking different adjuvants to tumor infiltration of specific lymphocytes would be invaluable.

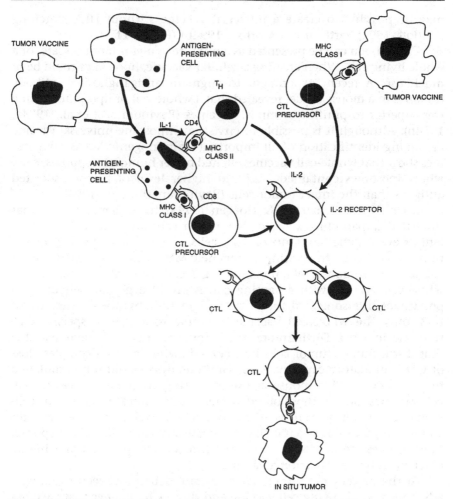

**Figure 11.1** Schematic diagram of possible mechanisms for T cell response to the MAAs of MCV. MCV cells may be degraded so that their MAAs can be presented to T cells by antigen-presenting cells (left); alternatively, T cells may recognize MAA peptides in shared HLA molecules on the surface of intact MCV cells, in which case the MCV cells act as antigen-presenting cells (right). Reprinted with permission from Barth et al. (1994b)

A universal vaccine must be designed with attention to MHC restriction elements. At the present time, it is unclear whether an HLA match between the cellular vaccine and the recipient is necessary to induce effective antitumor immune rejection responses. Since tumor-associated antigens can be presented in the context of host (self) HLA antigens, it may be possible to create a universal vaccine without HLA matching (Pardoll, 1991; Barth, Irie & Morton, 1994b) (Figure 11.1).

The antigen can be presented as a mixture, a membranous lysate, or a whole living cell. When creating a cellular vaccine, liposomes could be of much use. A recent experiment to augment antiganglioside antibody response in a mouse model revealed that a whole cell or liposome vaccine was superior to purified or mixed vaccines (Ravindranath et al., 1994a, 1994b). Although it is possible to envisage a liposome universal vaccine (assuming identification of all important immunogenic MAAs), our studies show that whole-cell vaccines elicited better humoral responses, even when liposomes contained a 27-fold higher level of tumor-associated antigens than the intact tumor cells (Ravindranath et al., 1994b).

Recently, Schirrmacher & Hoegen (1993) have demonstrated that irradiated trypan blue-excluding live tumor cells are superior to equivalent or even higher amounts of dead cells, or crude membrane preparations (oncolysates) in eliciting a syngeneic MHC class I-restricted tumor-specific CTL response. When comparing T cell stimulatory capacity of a whole-cell vaccine with a vaccine consisting of a glutaraldehyde-fixed polyvalent ultrasonicated tumor extract, in the absence or presence of IL-2, only the whole-cell vaccine was able to trigger a specific CTL response in vitro. Furthermore, these investigators have demonstrated that disruption of tumor cells by freeze–thawing led to a complete loss of CTL stimulatory capacity. Also, viral oncolysates did not stimulate a tumor-specific CTL response in tumor-bearing animals, whereas whole-cell vaccines did. All these observations clearly indicate that tumor cell-membrane integrity (as revealed by trypan blue exclusion) is required for stimulating a tumor-specific class I MHC-restricted CD8+ CTL response. More studies are needed to select the integral components of a highly efficient universal melanoma vaccine.

At the present time, there is an intense debate between those who advocate a whole living cell vaccine and those who believe that vaccines based on highly defined cellular components or highly defined, highly purified tumor antigens or peptides are better for cancer immunotherapy. Recent experimental studies in animal models clearly document that a whole cell vaccine is superior to soluble vaccines or oncolysates in eliciting CTL responses (Schirrmacher & Hoegen, 1993), or humoral responses leading to antitumor activity (Ravindranath et al., 1994a, 1994b). Review of melanoma vaccine clinical trials suggests that irradiated whole cell preparations administered with appropriate adjuvants are superior to other vaccine preparations. Living cell vaccines are generally the most effective formulation against infectious disease; the available evidence in tumor immunity and cancer immunotherapy appears to validate this concept. Furthermore, in syngeneic animal tumor-host models, irradiated tumor cells are invariably more effective immunogens than parts of cells, dead cells, cell lysates, or purified tumor-associated antigens or peptides. In addition, for effective gene therapy, highly immunogenic whole tumor cells could serve as suitable carriers for the transfected gene.

## ■ ACKNOWLEDGMENTS

From the Roy E. Coats Research Laboratories of the John Wayne Cancer Institute at Saint John's Hospital and Health Center. Supported by grants CA 12582 and CA 29605 from the National Cancer Institute and by funding from the Joyce and Ben Eisenberg Foundation and the Wrather Family Foundation, Los Angeles, California.

### REFERENCES

Ahn S.S., Irie R.F., Weisenburger T.H. et al. (1982) Humoral immune response to intra-lymphatic immunotherapy for disseminated melanoma: correlation with clinical response. *Surgery*, **92**, 362–7.

Austin F.C. & Boone W.B. (1979) Virus augmentation of the antigenicity of tumor cell extracts. *Advances in Cancer Research*, **30**, 301–45.

Barth A., Hoon D.S.B., Foshag L.J. et al. (1994a) Polyvalent melanoma cell vaccine induces delayed-type hypersensitivity and in vitro cellular immune response. *Cancer Research*, **54**, 3342–5.

Barth A.M., Irie R.F. & Morton D.L. (1994b) Update on immunotherapy for advanced melanoma. *Contemporary Oncology*, **4**, 52–60.

Berd D., Maguire H.C. Jr. & Mastrangelo M.J. (1986) Induction of cell-mediated immunity to autologous melanoma cells and regression of metastases after treatment with a melanoma cell vaccine preceded by cyclophosphamide. *Cancer Research*, **46**, 2572–7.

Berd D., Maguire H.C. Jr., McCue P. & Mastrangelo M.J. (1990) Treatment of metastatic melanoma with an autologous tumor-cell vaccine: Clinical and immunological results in 64 patients. *Journal of Clinical Oncology*, **8**, 1858–67.

Berthier-Vergnes O., Portoukalian J., Lefheriotis E. & Dore J.F. (1994) Induction of IgG antibodies directed to a $M_r$ 31,000 melanoma antigen in patients immunized with vaccinia virus melanoma oncolysates. *Cancer Research*, **54**, 2433–9.

Blankenstein T., Qin Z., Uberla K. et al. (1991) Tumor suppression after tumor cell-targeted tumor necrosis factor $\alpha$ gene transfer. *Journal of Experimental Medicine*, **173**, 1047–52.

Bluming A.Z. & Ziegler J.L. (1971) Regression of Burkitt's lymphoma in association with measles infection. *Lancet*, **ii**, 105–6.

Bubenick J., Simova J. & Jandlova T. (1990) Immunotherapy of cancer using local administration of lymphoid cells transformed by cDNA and constitutively producing IL2. *Immunology Letters*, **23**, 287–92.

Bystryn J.-C., Jacobsen S., Harris M., Roses D., Speyer J. & Levin M. (1986) Preparation and characterization of a polyvalent human melanoma antigen vaccine. *Journal of Biological Response Modifiers*, **5**, 211–23.

Bystryn J.-C., Oratz R., Harris M.N., Roses D.F., Golomb F.M. & Speyer J.C. (1988) Immunogenicity of a polyvalent melanoma antigen vaccine in humans. *Cancer*, **61**, 1065–72.

Bystryn J.C., Oratz R., Henn M., Adler A., Harris M.N. & Roses D.F. (1992) Relationship between immune response to melanoma vaccine and clinical outcome in stage II malignant melanoma. *Cancer*, **69**, 1157–64.

Bystryn J.C., Oratz R., Roses D.F., Harris M.N., Henn M. & Lew R. (1991) Improved survival of melanoma patients with delayed hypersensitivity response to melanoma vaccine immunization. *Clinical Research*, **39**, 503A.

Bystryn J.-C., Tedholm C.A. & Heaney-Kieras J. (1981) Release of surface macromolecules by human melanoma and normal cells. *Cancer Research*, **41**, 91–9.

Cassel W.A., Murray D.R. & Phillips H.S. (1983) A phase II study on the postsurgical management of stage II malignant melanoma with a Newcastle disease virus oncolysate. *Cancer*, **52**, 856–63.

Cassel W.A., Weidenheim K.M., Campbell W.G. & Murray D.R. (1984) Malignant melanoma: inflammatory mononuclear cell infiltrates in cerebral metastases during concurrent therapy with viral oncolysate. *Cancer*, **57**, 1302–9.

Chattopadhyay P., Kaveri S.V., Byars N., Starkey N.J., Ferrone S. & Raychaudhuri S. (1991) Human high molecular weight-melanoma associated antigen mimicry by an anti-idiotypic antibody: Characterization of the immunogenicity and the immune response to the mouse monoclonal antibody IMel-1. *Cancer Research*, **51**, 6045–51.

Chattopadhyay P., Starkey J., Morrow W.J.W. & Raychaudhuri S. (1992) Murine monoclonal anti-idiotope antibody breaks unresponsiveness and induces a specific antibody response to human melanoma-associated proteoglycan antigen in cynomolgus monkeys. *Proceedings of the National Academy of Sciences USA*, **89**, 2689–8.

Chu J.W.K. & Sharom F.J. (1993) Gangliosides inhibit T-lymphocyte proliferation by preventing the interaction of interleukin-2 with its cell surface receptors. *Immunology*, **79**, 10–17.

Coca A.F., Dorrance G.M. & Lebredo M.G. (1912) Vaccination in cancer: A report of the results of vaccination therapy as applied to seventy-nine cases of human cancer. *Journal of Immunology and Experimental Therapeutics*, **13**, 543–51.

Coca A.F. & Gilman G. (1909) The specific treatment of carcinoma. *Philosophical Journal of Science and Medicine*, **4**, 381–92.

Currie G.A. (1973) Effect of active immunization with irradiated tumor cells on specific serum inhibition of cell-mediated immunity in patients with disseminated cancer. *British Journal of Cancer*, **28**, 25–36.

Currie G.A., Lejeune F. & Fairley G.H. (1971) Immunization with irradiated tumor cells and specific lymphocyte cytotoxicity in malignant melanoma. *British Medical Journal*, **2**, 305–11.

Darrow T.L., Slingluff C.L. Jr. & Seigler H.F. (1989) The role of HLA class I antigens in recognition of melanoma cells by tumor-specific cytotoxic T lymphocytes. Evidence for shared tumor antigens. *Journal of Immunology*, **142**, 3329–35.

Dore J.F., Portoukalian J., Berthier-Vergnes O. et al. (1990) Responses de malades atteints de melanome a l'immunisation par onoclysats de melanomes au virus de la vaccine. *Bulletin de Cancer*, **77**, 881–91.

Elliott G.T., McLeod R.A., Perez J. & Von Eschen K.B. (1992) Results of phase II multicenter trial evaluating the activity of melacine melanoma theraccine in the treatment of disseminated melanoma. *Proceedings of the American Association of Cancer Research*, **33**, 332.

Ferrone S. (1993) Human tumor-associated antigen mimicry by anti-idiotypic antibodies. Immunogenicity and clinical trials in patients with solid tumors. *Annals of the New York Academy of Sciences*, **690**, 214–24.

Ferrone S. & Kagashita T. (1988) Human high molecular weight-melanoma associated antigen as a target for active specific immunotherapy: A phase I clinical trial with murine monoclonal antibodies. *Journal of Dermatology*, **15**, 457–65.

Fisher R.I., Terry W.D., Nodes R.J. et al. (1981) Adjuvant immunotherapy or chemotherapy for malignant melanoma. *Surgical Clinics of North America*, **61**, 1267–72.

Freimer M.L., McIntosh K., Adams R.A., Alving C.R. & Drachman D.B. (1993) Gangliosides elicit a T-cell independent antibody response. *Journal of Autoimmunity*, **6**, 281–9.

Furukawa K., Yamaguchi H., Oettgen H.F., Old L.J. & Lloyd K.D. (1988) Analysis of the expression of N-glycolylneuraminic acid-containing gangliosides in cells and tissues using two human monoclonal antibodies. *Journal of Biological Chemistry*, **263**, 8507–12.

Galili N., Naor D., Asjo B. & Klein G. (1976) Induction of immune responsiveness in a genetically low-responsive tumor-host combination by chemical modification of the immunogen. *European Journal of Immunology*, **6**, 473–6.

Gansbacher B., Zier K., Daniels B., Cronin K., Bannerji R. & Gilboa E. (1990a) Interleukin-2 gene transfer into tumor cells abrogates tumorigenicity and induces protective immunity. *Journal of Experimental Medicine*, **172**, 1271–24.

Gansbacher B., Bannerji R., Daniels B., Zier K., Cronin K. & Gilboa E. (1990b) Retroviral vector-mediated gamma-interferon gene transfer into tumor cells generates potent and long lasting antitumor immunity. *Cancer Research*, **50**, 7820–5.

Gilliland B.C. (1991) Drug-induced autoimmune and hematologic disorders. *Immunology and Allergy Clinics of North America*, **11**, 525–53.

Graham J.B. & Graham R.M. (1962) Autologous vaccine in cancer patients. *Surgery Gynecology and Obstetrics*, **109**, 121–9.

Hadley D.W., McElwain T.J. & Currie G.A. (1978) Specific active immunotherapy does not prolong survival in surgically treated patients with stage IIB malignant melanoma and may promote early recurrence. *British Journal of Cancer*, **37**, 491–8.

Hamby C.V., Liao S.K., Kanamaru T. & Ferrone S. (1987) Immunogenicity of human melanoma-associated antigens defined by murine monoclonal antibodies in allogeneic and xenogeneic hosts. *Cancer Research*, **47**, 5284–9.

Harel W., Goedegebuure P.S., LeMay L.G., Huang X.Q., Kan-Mitchell J. & Mitchell M.S. (in press) Melanoma-specific lysis by cloned CD4[+] and CD8[+] T cells from actively immunized melanoma patients. *Vaccine Research*.

Hayashi Y., Hoon D.S.B., Park M.S., Terasaki P.I., Foshag L.J. & Morton D.L. (1992a) Induction of CD4[+] cytotoxic T cells by sensitization with allogeneic melanomas bearing shared or cross-reactive HLA-A. *Cellular Immunology*, **139**, 411–25.

Hayashi Y., Hoon D.S.B., Park M.S., Terasaki P.I. & Morton D.L. (1992b) Cytotoxic T cell lines recognize autologous and allogeneic melanomas with shared or cross-reactive HLA-A. *International Archives of Allergy and Immunology*, **97**, 8–16.

Hayashi Y., Hoon D.S.B., Foshag L.J., Park M.S., Terasaki P.I. & Morton D.L. (1993) A preclinical model to assess the antigenicity of an HLA-A2 melanoma cell vaccine. *Cancer*, **72**, 750–9.

Helling F., Calves M., Shang Y., Oettgen H.F. & Livingston P.O. (1993) Construction of immunogenic GD3-conjugate vaccine. *Annals of the New York Academy of Sciences*, **690**, 396–7.

Helling F., Shang A., Calves M. et al. (1994) GD$_3$ vaccines for melanoma: superior immunogenicity of keyhole limpet hemocyanin conjugate vaccines. *Cancer Research*, **54**, 197–203.

Hersey P., Edwards A., Coates A., Shaw H., McCarthy W.H. & Milton G.W. (1987) Evidence that treatment with vaccinia melanoma cell lysates (VMCL) may improve survival of patients with stage II melanoma. *Cancer Immunology and Immunotherapy*, **25**, 257–63.

Hirabayashi Y., Higashi H., Kato S., Taniguchi M. & Matsumoto M. (1987) Occurrence of tumor associated ganglioside antigens with Hanganutziu–Deicher antigenic activity on human melanomas. *Japanese Journal of Cancer Research*, **78**, 614–20.

Hollinshead A., Arlen M., Yonemoto R. et al. (1982) Pilot studies using melanoma tumor-associated antigens (TAA) in specific active immunochemotherapy of malignant melanoma. *Cancer*, **49**, 1387–92.

Hoon D.S.B., Banez M., Okun E., Morton D.L. & Irie R.F. (1991) Modulation of human melanoma cells by interleukin-4 and in combination with gamma-interferon or α-tumor necrosis factor. *Cancer Research*, **51**, 2002–8.

Hoon D.S.B., Hayashi Y., Morisaki T., Foshag L.J. & Morton D.L. (1993) Interleukin-4 plus tumor necrosis factor α augments the antigenicity of melanoma cells. *Cancer Immunology and Immunotherapy*, **37**, 378–84.

Hoon D.S.B., Yuzuki D., Hayashida M. & Morton D.L. (1995) Melanoma patients immunized with melanoma cell vaccine induce antibody responses to recombinant MAGE-1 antigen. *Journal of Immunology*, **154**, 730–7.

Kan-Mitchell J., Huang X.Q., Steinman L. et al. (1993) Clonal analysis of in vivo-activated CD8$^+$ cytotoxic T lymphocytes from a melanoma patient responsive to active specific immunotherapy, *Cancer Immunology and Immunotherapy*, **37**, 15–25.

Kahn M., Hellstrom I., Estin C.D. et al. (1989) Monoclonal antiidiotypic antibodies related to p97 human melanoma antigen. *Cancer Research*, **49**, 3157–62.

Kaucic K., Grovas A., Li R., Quinones R. & Ladisch S. (1994) Modulation of human myelopoiesis by human gangliosides. *Experimental Hematology*, **22**, 52–9.

Kennedy R.C. (1991) The impact of idiotype-based strategies on cancer immunity. *Immunology and Allergy Clinics of North America*, **11**, 425–44.

Kobayashi H., Sendo F., Shirai T., Kaji H., Kodama T. & Saito H. (1969) Modification in growth in transplantable rat tumors exposed to Friend Virus. *Journal of the National Cancer Institute*, **42**, 3–8.

Kusuma M., Kageshita T., Tsugisaki M. & Ferrone S. (1987) Syngeneic anti-idiotypic antisera to murine anti-human high-molecular-weight-melanoma-associated antigen monoclonal antibodies. *Cancer Research*, **47**, 4312–7.

Laucius J.F., Bodurtha A.J., Mastrangelo M.J. & Bellet R.E. (1977) A phase II study of autologous irradiated tumor cells plus BCG in patients with metastatic malignant melanoma. *Cancer*, **40**, 2091–7.

Leong S.P.L. (1983) Detection of human malignant melanoma antigens by immuno-fluorescence and autologous postimmune antimelanoma sera. *Annals of the New York Academy of Sciences*, **420**, 237–40.

Levitsky J.W., Simmons H., Vogelstein B. & Frost P. (1990) Interleukin-2 production by tumor cell bypasses T helper function in the generation of an antitumor response. *Cell*, **60**, 397–403.

Li J., Henn M., Oratz R.F. & Bystryn J.C. (1990) The antibody response to immunization to a polyvalent melanoma antigen vaccine. *Journal of Clinical Research*, **38**, 660A.

Livingston P.O. (1989) The basis for ganglioside vaccines in melanoma. In *Human tumor antigens and specific tumor therapy*, pp. 287–96. New York, Alan Liss.

Livingston P. (1991) Active specific immunotherapy in the treatment of patients with cancer. *Immunology and Allergy Clinics of North America*, **11**, 401–23.

Livingston P.O. (1993) Approaches to augmenting the IgG antibody response to melanoma ganglioside vaccines. *Annals of the New York Academy of Sciences*, **690**, 204–13.

Livingston P.O., Albino A.P., Chung T.J.C. et al. (1985a) Serological response of melanoma patients to vaccines prepared from VSV lysates of autologous and allogeneic cultured melanoma cells. *Cancer*, **55**, 713–18.

Livingston P.O., Calves M.J. & Natoli E.J. (1987a) Approaches to augmenting the immunogenicity of the ganglioside GM2 in mice: purified GM2 is superior to whole cells. *Journal of Immunology*, **138**, 1524–31.

Livingston P.O., Kaelin K., Pinsky C.M., Oettgen H.R. & Old L.J. (1985b) The serological response of patients with stage II melanoma to allogeneic melanoma cell vaccines. *Cancer*, **56**, 2194–9.

Livingston P.O., Natoli E.J., Calves M.J., Stockert E., Oettgen H.F. & Old L.J. (1987b) Vaccines containing purified GM2 ganglioside elicit GM2 antibodies in melanoma patients. *Proceedings of the National Academy of Sciences USA*, **84**, 2911–19.

Livingston P.O., Takeyama H., Pollack M.S. et al. (1983) Serological responses of melanoma patients to vaccines derived from allogeneic cultured melanoma cells. *International Journal of Cancer*, **31**, 567–73.

Livingston P.O., Watanabe T., Shiku H. et al. (1982) Serological response of melanoma patients receiving melanoma cell vaccines. 1. Autologous cultured melanoma cells. *International Journal of Cancer*, **30**, 413–18.

Mehigan J.T., Gray B.K. & Morton D.L. (1971) Serum cytotoxic antibody in human sarcoma following autologous cellular immunotherapy. *Surgical Forum*, **22**, 108–9.

Mitchell M.S., Harel W., Kan-Mitchell J. et al. (1993) Active specific immunotherapy of melanoma with allogeneic cell lysates. Rationale, results and possible mechanisms of action. *Annals of the New York Academy of Sciences*, **690**, 153–66.

Mitchell M.S., Kan-Mitchell J., Kempf R.A., Harel W., Shau H. & Lind S. (1988) Active specific immunotherapy for melanoma: Phase I trial of allogeneic lysates and a novel adjuvant. *Cancer Research*, **48**, 5883–93.

Morton D.L. (1972) Immunotherapy of human melanomas and sarcomas. *Journal of the National Cancer Institute*, **35**, 375–8.

Morton D.L. (1986) Adjuvant immunotherapy of malignant melanoma: status of clinical trials at UCLA. *International Journal of Immunotherapy*, **II**(1), 31–6.

Morton D.L., Eilber F.R., Holmes E.C. et al. (1974) BCG immunotherapy of malignant melanoma: summary of a seven year experience. *Annals of Surgery*, **180**, 635–43.

Morton D.L., Eilber F.R., Holmes E.C. & Ramming K.P. (1978) Preliminary results of a randomized trial of adjuvant immunotherapy in patients with malignant melanoma who have lymph node metastases. *Australian and New Zealand Journal of Surgery*, **48**, 49–52.

Morton D.L., Eilber F.R., Malmgren R.A. & Wood W.C. (1970) Immunological factors which influence response to immunotherapy in malignant melanoma. *Surgery*, **68**, 158–64.

Morton D.L., Foshag L.J., Hoon D.S.B. et al. (1992) Prolongation of survival in metastatic melanoma after active specific immunotherapy with a new polyvalent melanoma vaccine. *Annals of Surgery*, **216**, 465–82.

Morton D.L., Haskell C.M., Pilch Y.H., Sparks F.C. & Winters W.D. (1972) Recent advances in oncology. *Annals of Internal Medicine*, **77**, 431–54.

Morton D.L., Holmes E.C., Eilber F.R. & Wood W.C. (1971) Immunological aspects of neoplasia: a rationale basis for immunotherapy. *Annals of Internal Medicine*, **74**, 587–604.

Morton D.L., Hoon D.S.B., Gupta R.G. et al. (1989) Treatment of malignant melanoma by active specific immunotherapy in combination with biological response modifiers. In M. Torisu & T. Yoshida (eds) *New horizons of tumor immunotherapy*, pp. 665–83. Amsterdam, Elsevier Science Publishers B.V.

Morton D.L., Hoon D.S.B., Nizze J. et al. (1993) Polyvalent melanoma vaccine improves survival of patients with metastatic melanoma. *Annals of the New York Academy of Sciences*, **690**, 120–34.

Morton D.L., Joseph W.L., Ketcham A.S., Geelhoed G.W. & Adkins P.C. (1973) Surgical resection and adjunctive immunotherapy for selected patients with multiple pulmonary metastases. *Annals of Surgery*, **178**, 360–6.

Morton D.L., Nizze J.A., Gupta R.K., Famatiga E., Hoon D.S.B. & Irie R.F. (1987) Active specific immunotherapy of malignant melanoma. In J.P. Kim, B.S. Kim & J.G. Park (eds), *Current status of cancer control and immunobiology*, pp. 152–61. Seoul.

Morton D.L. & Ravindranath M.H. (1993) Active specific immunotherapy with vaccines. In J.F. Holland, E. Frei, R.C. Bast, D.W. Kufe, D.L. Morton & R.R. Weichselbaum (eds) *Cancer medicine, 3rd edn, vol. 1*, pp. 913–26. Philadelphia, Lea & Febiger.

Morton D.L., Ravindranath M.H. & Irie R.F. (1994) Tumor gangliosides as targets for active specific immunotherapy of melanoma in man. *Progress in Brain Research*, **101**, 251–75.

Nabel G.J., Nabel E.G., Yang Z.Y. et al. (1993) Direct gene transfer with DNA–liposome complexes in melanoma: expression, biology activity, and lack of toxicity in humans. *Proceedings of the National Academy of Sciences USA*, **90**, 11307–11.

Nepom G.T., Nelson K.A., Holbeck S.L. et al. (1984) Induction of immunity to a human tumor marker in vivo by administration of anti-idiotypic antibodies in mice. *Proceedings of the National Academy of Sciences USA*, **81**, 2864–7.

Oaks M.K., Hanson J.P. Jr. & O'Malley D.P. (1994) Molecular cytogenetic mapping of the human melanoma antigen (MAGE) gene family to chromosome region Xq27-qter: implications for MAGE immunotherapy. *Cancer Research*, **54**, 1627–9.

Pardoll D. (1992) New strategies for active immunotherapy with genetically engineered tumor cells. *Current Opinion in Immunology*, **4**, 619–23.

Pasquinucci G. (1971) Possible effect of measles on leukemia. *Lancet*, i, 136.

Portoukalian J., Carrel S., Dore J.F. & Rumke P. (1991) Humoral immune response in disease-free advanced melanoma patients after vaccination with melanoma-associated gangliosides. *International Journal of Cancer*, **49**, 893–9.

Ravindranath M.H., Brazeau S.M. & Morton D.L. (1994a) Efficacy of tumor cell vaccine after incorporating monophosphoryl lipid A (MPL) in tumor cell membranes containing tumor-associated ganglioside. *Experientia*, **50**, 648–53.

Ravindranath M.H., Guenther M., Kunnath S., Nizze A., Famatiga E. & Morton D.L. (1993) Antiganglioside IgM responses to a new melanoma cell vaccine (MCV) in melanoma patients. *Proceedings of the American Association of Cancer Research*, **84**, 2915.

Ravindranath N.H. & Morton D.L. (1991) Role of gangliosides in active immunotherapy with melanoma vaccine. *International Reviews in Immunology*, **7**, 303–29.

Ravindranath M.H., Morton D.L. & Irie R.F. (1989) An epitope common to gangliosides O-acetyl-GD3 and GD3 recognized by antibodies in melanoma patients after active specific immunotherapy. *Cancer Research*, **49**, 3891–9.

Ravindranath M.H., Morton D.L. & Irie R.F. (1994b) Attachment of monophosphoryl lipid A (MPL) to cells and liposomes augments antibody response to membrane-bound gangliosides. *Journal of Autoimmunity*, **7**, 803–16.

Ravindranath M.H., Tsuchida T., Morton D.L. & Irie R.F. (1991) Gangliosides GM3: GD3 ratio as an index for the management of melanoma. *Cancer*, **67**, 3029–35.

Roenigle H.H. Jr., Deodhar S., St. Jacques R. et al. (1976) Immunotherapy of malignant melanoma with vaccinia virus. *Archives of Dermatology*, **109**, 668–73.

Roth J.A., Eilber F.R., Nizze J.A. & Morton D.L. (1975) Lack of correlation between skin reactivity to dinitrochlorobenzene and croton oil in patients with cancer. *New England Journal of Medicine*, **293**, 388–9.

Savage H.E., Rossen R.D., Hersh E.M. et al. (1986) Antibody development to viral and allogeneic tumor cell-associated antigens in patients with malignant melanoma and ovarian carcinoma treated with lysates of virus-infected cells. *Cancer Research*, **46**, 2127–33.

Schirrmacher V. & Hoegen P.L. (1993) Importance of tumor cell membrane integrity and viability for cytotoxic T lymphocyte activation by cancer vaccines. *Vaccine Research*, **2**, 183–95.

Schultz N., Oratz R., Chen D., Zeleniuch-Jacquotte A., Abeles G. & Bystryn J.-C. (1995) Effect of DETOX as an adjuvant for melanoma vaccine. *Vaccine*, **13**, 503–8.

Sinkovics J. & Horvath J. (1993) New developments in the virus therapy of cancer: a historic review. *Intervirology*, **36**, 193–214.

Slingluff C.L., Vollmer R. & Seigler H.F. (1988) Stage II malignant melanoma: presentation of a prognostic model and assessment of specific active immunotherapy in 1,273 patients. *Journal of Surgical Oncology*, **39**, 139–43.

Tai T., Cahan L.D., Tsuchida T., Morton D.L. & Irie R.F. (1985) Immunogenicity of melanoma-associated gangliosides in cancer patients. *International Journal of Cancer*, **35**, 607–12.

Tallberg T., Kalimo T., Halttunen P. et al. (1986) Postoperative active specific immunotherapy with supportive measures in patients suffering from recurrent metastasized melanoma: case reports of six patients. *Journal of Surgical Oncology*, **33**, 115–24.

Tepper R.I., Pattengale P.K. & Leder P. (1989) Murine interleukin-4 displays potent anti-tumor activity in vivo. *Cell*, **57**, 503–12.

Uchiyama A., Hoon, D.S.B., Morisaki T., Kaneda Y., Yuzuki D.H. & Morton D.I. (1993) Transfection of interleukin 2 gene into human melanoma cells augments cellular immune response. *Cancer Research*, **53**, 949–52.

Vadhan-Raj S., Cordon-Cardo C., Carswell E. et al. (1986) Phase I trial of a mouse monoclonal antibody against $GD_3$ ganglioside in patients with melanoma: induction of inflammatory responses at the tumor sites. *Journal of Clinical Oncology*, **6**, 1636–48.

Van der Bruggen P., Traversari C., Chomex P. et al. (1991) A gene encoding an antigen recognized by cytolytic T-lymphocytes on a human melanoma. *Science*, **254**, 1643–7.

Vaughan J.W. (1914) Cancer vaccine and anti-cancer globulin as an aid in the surgical treatment of malignancy. *JAMA*, **63**, 1258–62.

Von Leyden V.E. & Blumenthal F. (1902) Vorlautige Mitteilungen uber einige Ergebnisse der krebsforschung auf der medizinischen Klinic. *Dr. Med Wschr.* **28**, 637–41.

Wallack M.C. (1981) Specific immunotherapy with vaccinia oncolysates. *Cancer Immunology and Immunotherapy*, **12**, 1–6.

Wallack M.C., Bash J.A., Leftheriotis E. et al. (1987) Positive relationship of clinical and serologic responses to vaccinia melanoma oncolysate. *Archives of Surgery*, **122**, 1460–3.

Wallack M.K., McNally K.R., Leftheriotis E. et al. (1986) A Southeastern cancer study group phase I/II trial with vaccinia melanoma oncolysates. *Cancer*, **57**, 649–55.

Wallack M.K., Meyer M., Bourgoin A. et al. (1983) A preliminary trial of vaccinia oncolysates in the treatment of recurrent melanoma with serologic responses to the treatment. *Journal of Biological Response Modifiers*, **2**, 586–92.

Wallack M.K. & Michaelides M. (1984) Serologic response to human melanoma lines from patients with melanoma undergoing treatment with vaccinia melanoma oncolysates. *Surgery*, **96**, 791–9.

Wallack M.K. & Sivanandham M. (1993) Clinical trials with VMO for melanoma. *Annals of the New York Academy of Sciences*, **690**, 178–89.

Wallack M., Sivanandham M., Balch C. et al. (1994) A phase III randomized multi-institutional double blind adjuvant study of vaccinia melanoma oncolysate (VMO) vs vaccinia (V) alone in stage II melanoma. *Proceedings of the American Society of Clinical Oncology*, **13**, 1352.

Wallack M., Sivandham M., Blach C.M. et al. (1995) A phase III randomized, double-blind, multi-institutional trial of vaccinia melanoma oncolysate-active specific immunotherapy for patients with stage II melanoma. *Cancer*, **75**, 34–42.

Wallack M.K., Steplewski Z., Koprowski H. et al. (1977) A new approach in specific, active immunotherapy. *Cancer*, **39**, 560–4.

Watanabe Y., Kuribayashi K., Miyatake S. et al. (1989) Exogenous expression of mouse interferon-gamma cDNA in mouse neuroblastoma C1300 cells results in reduced tumorigenicity by augmented anti-tumor immunity. *Proceedings of the National Academy of Sciences USA*, **86**, 9456–60.

Weisenburger T.H., Jones P.C., Ahn S.C., Irie R.F. & Juillard G.J.F. (1982) Active specific intralymphatic immunotherapy in metastatic malignant melanoma: evidence of clinical response. *Journal of Biological Response Modifiers*, **1**, 57–63.

Wolfel T., Klehmann E., Muller C., Schutt K.H., Bucschenfelde M.Z. & Knuth A. (1989) Lysis of human melanoma cells by autologous cytolytic T cell clones. Identification of human histocompatibility leukocyte antigen A2 as a restriction element for three different antigens. *Journal of Experimental Medicine*, **170**, 787–810.

# -12-

# Immune Responses to Mucins

ROSALIND A. GRAHAM AND
JOYCE TAYLOR-PAPADIMITRIOU

## ■ INTRODUCTION

Mucins are complex, heavily glycosylated molecules of high molecular weight, produced by a variety of glandular epithelial cells such as the salivary gland, breast, ovary, endometrium, and the gastrointestinal tract, and by carcinomas that arise from them. The carbohydrate content is generally more than 50% and the oligosaccharide side chains are O-linked to serine and threonine residues in core protein via the linkage sugar N-acetylgalactosamine (GalNAc). Great variability is seen in the carbohydrate side chains of mucins, for example, the ovine submaxillary mucin (OSM) contains chains made up of one type of disaccharide unit, whereas, in contrast, many of the gastric mucins carry complex, branching side chains made up of more than one type of sugar. Much attention has recently been given to epithelial-associated mucins as numerous antibodies raised against normal epithelial cells or malignant epithelial cells have been shown to react with mucin molecules.

Physicochemical techniques were traditionally used to study mucin molecules but their complexity made them difficult to analyse. The development of recombinant DNA technology has, however, enabled the structure of mucin core proteins to be elucidated. To date, seven human mucin genes have been cloned, or partially cloned and sequenced, MUC1 being the first mucin gene to be cloned and partially sequenced (Gendler et al., 1987, 1988). The full cDNA sequence has subsequently been established (Gendler et al., 1990; Lan et al., 1990; Ligtenberg et al., 1990). A feature common to all the mucin molecules cloned so far is the presence of a tandem repeat domain that forms the major portion of the molecule (Table 12.1). The amino-acid sequence and length of the repeats from the different mucins varies, although they are all rich in serine, and/or threonine and proline residues. The repeat units therefore act as a scaffold for the attachment of carbohydrate side chains and result in the formation of extended molecules. The MUC1 gene

Table 12.1.    Tandem Repeat Sequences of Human Mucin Genes

| Name | Source | Amino-acid sequence | Reference |
|---|---|---|---|
| MUC1 | Mammary gland and pancreas | PPAHGVTSAPDTRPAPGSTA | Gendler et al. (1987, 1988) |
| MUC2 | Intenstine | PTTTPITTTTTVTPTPTPTGTQT | Gum et al. (1989) |
| MUC3 | Intestine | HSTPSFTSSOTTTETTS | Gum et al. (1990) |
| MUC4 | Lung | TSSASTGHATPLPVTA | Porchet et al. (1991) |
| MUC5AC | Lung | TTSTTSAP | Debailleul et al.[a] |
| MUC5B | Lung | TTVGP/S | Meerzaman et al. (1994) |
| MUC6 | Intestine | SPFSSTGPMTATSFQTTTTYPTP SHPQTTLPTHVPPFSTSLVTPST GTVITPTHAQMATSASIHSTPTG TIPPPTTLKATGSTHTAPPMTP TTSGTSQAHSSFSTAKTSTSLH SHTSSTHHPEVTPTSTTTITPNP TSTGTSTPVAHTTSATSSRLPT PFTTHSPPTGS | Toribara et al. (1993) |
| MUC7 | Salivary gland | TTAAPPTPSATTPAPPSSSAPPE | Bobek et al. (1993) |

[a] Debailleul, V., Guyonnet Duperat, V., Laine, A., Buisine, M. P., Pigny, P., Aubert, J. P. & Porchet, N. 3rd International Workshop on Carcinoma-associated Mucins, 1994.

encodes for a highly polymorphic mucin glycoprotein, which we have termed the polymorphic epithelial mucin (PEM), but which has been given a variety of other names by other laboratories, including episialin or MAM6 (Ligtenberg et al., 1990), PAS-O (Schimizu & Yamauchi, 1982) and DF3 antigen (Siddiqui et al., 1988). The tandem repeat of PEM contains 20 amino acids (Figure 12.1) and recent evidence suggests that it is the two threonine residues that flank the PDTRP motif that are glycosylated (Nishimori et al., 1994). The number of repeats in MUC1 varies from 20 to 125 in the Northern European population (Gendler et al., 1990), giving rise to the polymorphism (Figure 12.1).

The complex mucins contain cysteine-rich domains flanking the tandem repeat domain and these are likely to be involved in the formation of covalently bonded mucin aggregates after they have been secreted from the cell (Eckhardt et al., 1991; Gum et al., 1992). MUC1, however, is unique in the mucin family in that it is has a transmembrane domain, a 69 amino-acid cytoplasmic tail and lacks cysteine residues. The transmembrane domain and the cytoplasmic tail are highly conserved in the mouse homologue (Spicer et al., 1991), suggesting that they may have an important function. The tandem repeat region, however, shows conservation mainly in the serine and threonine residues. Much of the following discussion will concentrate on the MUC1 gene and its product PEM, since

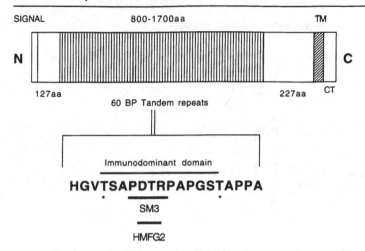

SIGNAL    800-1700aa    TM

N    C

127aa    227aa    CT

60 BP Tandem repeats

Immunodominant domain

**HGVTSAPDTRPAPGSTAPPA**
*                    *

SM3

HMFG2

\* Probable glycosylation sites

**Figure 12.1.** The structure of the MUC1 gene product, the polymorphic epithelial mucin, illustrating the tandem repeat sequence and the epitopes of monoclonal antibodies HMFG1 and SM3. TM, transmembrane; CT, cytoplasmic tail.

as an integral membrane glycoprotein it has received most attention in the investigation of immune responses.

## ■ GLYCOSYLATION OF MUCINS

The mechanisms involved in O-linked glycosylation are not as well understood as those involved in N-glycosylation. However, it is clear that, unlike N-glycosylation, the sugars are added individually and sequentially as the protein passes through the Golgi. In normal tissues, extended polyactosamine side chains, terminated with sialic acid or fucose, are linked to the protein core via GalNAc. Differences in glycosylation patterns of the same mucin-core protein are seen in different tissues, possibly as a result of different glycosyltransferases being expressed or active in different tissues.

Differences in glycosylation are also seen between normal and malignant tissues. Antibody studies have shown that carcinoma-associated carbohydrate epitopes, including O-GalNAc (Tn), sialylated Tn, O-GalNAc-Gal (T) and sialylated T, show an increased expression in carcinomas. This is clearly demonstrated for MUC1 expressed by the breast, where the breast carcinoma-associated mucin is aberrantly glycosylated and overexpressed (Burchell et al., 1987). In the normal breast, MUC1 is

(A) NORMAL MUCIN          (B) CARCINOMA ASSOCIATED MUCIN

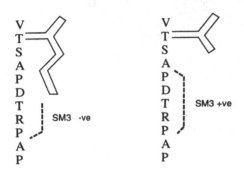

**Figure 12.2.** Glycosylation of the normal mucin (A) masks core protein epitopes such as PDTRP recognized by monoclonal antibody SM3. Aberrant glycosylation of the carcinoma-associated mucin (B) exposes PDTRP, allowing binding of SM3.

recognized by the monoclonal antibody (Mab) HMFG1, raised against the human milk fat globule. HMFG1 recognizes the epitope PDTR within the tandem repeat region (Price et al., 1990). SM3, a Mab raised against the deglycosylated milk mucin shows very little reactivity with the normal resting breast, but reacts strongly with the malignant breast. SM3 recognizes the sequence PDTRP (Burchell et al., 1989), which appears to be masked in mucin produced by normal breast epithelium, but exposed on the tumour-associated mucin, presumably due to aberrant glycosylation of the core protein (Figure 12.2). Direct analysis of sugar side chains from the milk mucin and mucin derived from a breast cancer cell line has confirmed that indeed the chains are larger and more complex in the normal mucin than in the breast cancer mucin (Hanisch et al., 1989; Hull et al., 1989). Table 12.2 summarizes results of this analysis, which indicates that premature sialylation terminates the side chains of the tumour-associated mucin.

In vitro model systems have now been developed to investigate the mechanisms underlying the aberrant glycosylation of MUC1 in breast cancer (Burchell & Taylor-Papadimitriou, 1993).

## ■ MUC1 AS A POTENTIAL TARGET MOLECULE FOR IMMUNOTHERAPY

Several features of the MUC1 gene product expressed by carcinoma cells suggest that it may have potential as an immunogen in the treat-

Table 12.2.    Major Carbohydrate Side Chains on PEM

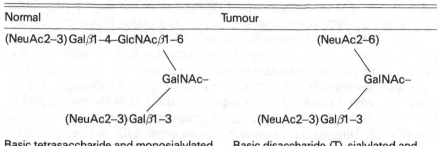

| Normal | Tumour |
|---|---|

Basic tetrasaccharide and monosialylated product. Extended and branched polylactosamine side chains, disialylated and fucosylated derivatives are also found. | Basic disaccharide (T), sialylated and disialylated products. GalNAc (Tn) and sialylated Tn.

ment of breast and other carcinomas. Firstly, MUC1 is up-regulated in breast carcinoma, as it is in the lactating breast but, significantly, it is aberrantly glycosylated in breast carcinoma resulting in the tumour-associated mucin being antigenically distinct from the normal mucin. This overexpression and aberrant glycosylation is also seen in other carcinomas including those of the colon, ovary, and pancreas. Short sugar chains, which replace the normal, long, branching carbohydrate side chains, themselves form novel epitopes with the potential to be immunogenic, and also lead to the exposure of novel immunogenic epitopes within the core protein itself. Secondly, the structure of the MUC1 gene results in these novel epitopes being repeated 25–125 times per molecule. Finally, MUC1 is normally expressed on the apical surface of epithelial cells, however, during malignancy, this apical distribution is lost and MUC1 becomes expressed over the entire surface of the tumour cell, making it more accessible to the immune system.

Although tumour-associated antigenic determinants, such as those expressed on PEM, have the potential to be recognized by some, or all of the components of the immune system, the tumours are not rejected by the host's immune system. Either the antigens are not being presented efficiently and do not evoke an immune response, or they are not being recognized by effector cells. It is not clear which components of the immune system are relevant to tumour rejection mediated by specific tumour-associated antigens. A humoral response, nonspecific cellular response involving macrophages, natural killer (NK), and lymphokine activated killer (LAK) cells, or a specific cellular response involving $CD8^+$ cytotoxic T cells and $CD4^+$ helper T cells may be involved.

A specific cellular response classically involves interaction of the T cell receptor with an antigenic peptide carried by the surface HLA molecule of the antigen presenting cell (APC), the major histocompatibility complex (MHC) class I presenting to the CD8[+] cytotoxic T cells and MHC class II to the CD4[+] helper T cells. The secretion of IL-2 is essential for the proliferation of T cells, and this requires the interaction of co-stimulatory molecules on the APC with ligands on the T cell, for example, the B7 molecule, which binds to CD28 molecules on T cells (Schwartz, 1992). Both HLA molecules and co-stimulatory molecules are found on professional APCs. Tumour cells, however, do not express B7, or in general HLA class II. Expression of HLA class I is also often lost. Tumour antigens may thus be presented in an ineffective manner by tumour cells. There is, however, increasing evidence for the immune recognition of the tumour-associated polymorphic epithelial mucin in cancer patients: PEM may be a unique molecule as data suggest that specific cellular responses do not require HLA.

## ■ IMMUNE RECOGNITION OF TUMOUR-ASSOCIATED MUCIN

### Cytotoxic T Cells

Human cytotoxic T lymphocytes (CTL) specific for the PEM molecule were first isolated from tumour-draining lymph nodes of patients with breast and pancreatic cancer by Finn and colleagues (Barnd et al., 1989; Jerome et al., 1991). CTL have also been isolated from tumour-infiltrating lymphocytes (TIL) or tumour-associated lymphocytes (TAL) infiltrating ovarian tumours that recognize MUC1-expressing ovarian tumours, but not MUC1-negative tumours (Ioannides et al., 1993). More recently, CTL have been isolated from peripheral blood lymphocytes from multiple myeloma patients (Hinoda, Third International Workshop on Carcinoma-associated Mucins, 1994).

In all cases, killing of PEM-expressing cancer cells is non-HLA restricted. Mutant cell lines T2 and CIR, which lack or express low levels of MHC class I molecules, transfected with full-length 22-repeat MUC1, were killed by CTL in cytotoxicity assays (Magarian-Blander et al. Third International Workshop on Carcinoma-associated Mucins, 1994). Although the mechanism involved is still unclear, it appears that mucin CTL epitopes are within the tandem repeat of the MUC1 molecule and therefore are repeated many times in a single molecule. It is suggested that it is the repetitive structure of the molecule that allows multiple PEM epitopes to cross link T cell receptors (TCR) of mucin-specific CTL, resulting in activation of T cells without presentation of the antigen by MHC molecules, that is, the peptide binding groove of the HLA molecule is not involved. The antibody SM3 inhibits the killing of PEM-expressing breast and ovarian cell lines, suggesting that the core protein epitopes in the vicinity of the PDTRP sequence (recognized by SM3 and selectively exposed in carcinomas) may be involved in T cell recognition. Antibodies to the TCR also inhibit cytotoxicity, whereas Mabs to MHC class I or class II molecules do not interfere with the function of the CTL. Further evidence for the involvement of the tandem repeats of the mucin molecule in unrestricted CTL killing also comes from the Finn group. MUC1 expressed by a vaccinia virus, which deletes large portions of the tandem repeats, did not induce MHC-unrestricted recognition. However, in this situation, MHC-restricted killing, dependent on the presentation of mucin peptides, was evident. A nine-amino-acid synthetic peptide (STAPPAHGV) was able to bind to HLA class I molecules (Domenech & Finn, Third International Workshop on Carcinoma-associated Mucins, 1994).

Recent data from Finn and colleagues (Magarian-Blander et al., Third International Workshop on Carcinoma-associated Mucins, 1994) has shown that mucin molecules with two tandem repeats are killed more efficiently than the full-length mucin (twenty-two repeats) when expressed by Epstein–Barr virus (EBV)-immortalized B cells. The mucin with two tandem repeats is glycosylated, but the lack of extended rigid structure is thought to allow interaction of adhesion or accessory molecules with their ligands. T2 or CIR cells (lacking MHC class I molecules) transfected with 2TR MUC1 were not recognized by CTL in cytotoxicity assays. It was suggested that MHC class I/CD8 interaction may play a role in MHC-unrestricted recognition of MUC1 by CTL, this role being more important when only a small number of repeats are present.

## Humoral Response

The therapeutic benefits of a specific antibody response are unclear, however, the knowledge that tumour antigens can evoke a tumour-specific immune response is important to evaluate the potential use of immunotherapy as a clinical treatment for cancer. Until recently no humoral responses to MUC1 were detected in cancer patients. However, Rughetti et al. (1933) recently reported a B cell immune response to the PEM molecule. EBV-immortalized B cells from tumour-draining lymph nodes from ovarian cancer patients secreted mucin-specific antibodies to PEM have now also been detected in the sera of breast, pancreatic, and colon cancer patients, using an assay based on binding to a chemically synthesized 105-amino-acid peptide (5.25 tandem repeats; Kotera et al., 1994). The frequency of antimucin responses seen in breast (8.3%), pancreatic (16.7%), and colon (10%) cancer patients is similar to that reported by others for humoral responses against other tumour proto-oncogenes or oncogene suppressor genes (for example, Crawford, Pim & Bulbrook, 1982; 9% breast cancer patients showed anti-p53 antibodies). Reactivity of MUC1 specific antibodies with the 105-residue peptide was blocked by a nine-amino-acid peptide containing the APDTRPAP motif. Most mouse Mab that are specific for mucin recognize epitopes within this immunodominant sequence.

Cancer patients with a large tumour burden are known to have high levels of circulating mucin, therefore, one explanation for the lack of antibody detection in patients sera was that MUC1-specific antibodies may form complexes with circulating mucin. A sandwich enzyme-linked immunosorbent assay (ELISA) has recently been developed by Gourevitch et al. (1995) that also allows the detection of antibodies to PEM, bound in immune complexes with circulating PEM, in at least 20% of breast and ovarian cancer patients. This humoral response to PEM may protect against disease progression (J. Hilgers & S. von Mensdorff-Pouilly, personal communication).

## ◼ MURINE MODEL SYSTEMS

The demonstration of both humoral and cytotoxic T cell responses to cancer-associated polymorphic epithelial mucin supports the idea that MUC1-based immunogens may be effective as vaccines in cancer patients. Although current evidence suggests that tumour-associated epitopes that arise from aberrant glycosylation of the PEM core protein are recognized by the immune system in cancer patients and are therefore antigenic, they fail to elicit an effective immune response against the tumour. Clearly antigen presentation is not optimal and strategies for improving this need to be developed (see Chapters 8 and 9). It is a well-known fact that carcinoma cells, which derive from epithelial cells, are particularly inefficient in antigen presentation to T cells. There may be several reasons for this, but one which has been brought into focus recently is the lack of expression of co-stimulatory molecules such as B7. Even if the tumour cells express HLA class I and can thus present peptide to cytotoxic T cells, the interaction will result in anergy if co-stimulatory signals generated by the B7/CD28 interaction do not occur (see Schwartz, 1992, for a review). Also carcinoma cells in general do not express HLA class II molecules and therefore cannot themselves activate helper T cells. In the case of the mucin, it appears that the need for HLA expression may be circumvented, however, the expression of co-stimulatory molecules is probably still necessary. A more general problem in

Table 12.3.    Possible MUCl-Based Immunogens

Cells expressing mucin
Purified mucin produced by cancer cells
Recombinant core protein
Different mucin glycoforms produced by transfected cells
Peptide or glycopeptide based on tandem repeat
Recombinant viruses (vaccinia, retroviruses)
Synthetic carbohydrates based on cancer-associated mucin side chains
Naked DNA

eliciting an efficient immune response in cancer patients is that immune responses may be suppressed, not only by exogenously administered chemotherapeutic drugs, but by the tumour itself, and this effect would almost certainly affect the response to PEM as well as to other tumour-associated antigens.

To develop protocols for improving antigen presentation, clearly animal models are required. In the case of PEM, there are also many forms of the antigen that could be used (Table 12.3) and these need to be compared for efficacy. Several models are now available and are beginning to be used to select protocols for phase I clinical trials.

### TA3-Ha Tumour Model for the Analysis of Carbohydrate Antigens

The TA3-Ha tumour is an aggressive mouse mammary tumour, which expresses high levels of a mucin, epiglycanin. Although the gene coding for the core protein of epiglycanin has not been cloned, it is clear that it is different from the mouse homologue of the MUC1 gene product. However, this mucin carries the same short carbohydrate side chains as are carried not only on PEM, but also on other tumour-associated mucins in humans. This mouse model has been used effectively to examine the efficacy of synthetic carbohydrates as immunogens. A synthetic T ($\beta$Gal1-3$\alpha$GalNAc) hapten coupled to the carrier protein keyhole limpet haemocyanin (KLH) in RIBI adjuvant (RIBI ImmunoChem Research Inc. Hamilton, Montana, USA) was successful in inhibiting tumour growth and prolonging the survival of mice bearing TA3-Ha tumours expressing the mucin epiglycanin bearing T carbohydrate epitopes (Fung et al., 1990). A humoral response and delayed-type hypersensitivity (DTH) were also reported. Disialylated OSM, which carries exclusively Tn (GAlNAc) carbohydrate side chains also provided protection against the challenge of TA3-Ha tumour cells in this murine model. The Tn antigen induced a high anti-Tn antibody response in mice, a cellular immune response (in vitro proliferation of primarily CD4$^+$ T cells) and DTH (Singhal, Fohn & Hakomori, 1991).

The studies in this murine model system have led to the start of clinical trials using synthetic carbohydrates as vaccines. Maclean and colleagues (1992) conducted phase I clinical trials in ovarian carcinoma patients with extensive metastatic disease using synthetic T-hapten coupled to KLH (T-KLH) with Detox adjuvant (RIBI ImmunoChem Research, Inc., Hamilton, Montana, USA) as an immunogen with a low dose of cyclophosphamide. They demonstrated that KLH was a suitable carrier protein and that Detox was a nontoxic adjuvant that was appropriate for the generation of high-titre anticarbohydrate antibodies in cancer patients. Trials are currently in progress using synthetic STn coupled to KLH plus Detox as an immunogen in breast, pancreatic, ovarian, and colorectal patients (Biomira, Inc., Edmonton, Alberta, Canada; Maclean et al., 1993). STn was chosen as a target structure as its expression on mucin has been shown to be a strong independent predictor of prognosis in ovarian cancer (Kobayashi, Terao & Kawashima, 1992), colorectal cancer (Itzkowitz et al., 1990), and gastric cancer (Takahasi et al., 1994; Werther et al., 1994). In primary breast cancer, however, STn expression appears to be of borderline prognostic significance, but STn positivity appears to be a marker of resistance to chemotherapy in node positive disease (Miles et al., 1994).

## Syngeneic Model Systems for MUC1 Expressing Tumours

A syngeneic mouse model has been developed in our laboratory for comparing the efficacy and toxicity of PEM-based immunogens. The human MUC1 cDNA has been transfected firstly into a mouse mammary tumour cell line, 410.4 (Lalani et al., 1991) for use in an H-2$^d$/Balb/c model system, and secondly into the RMA cell line (a Rauscher virus-induced T cell lymphoma) for use in an H-2$^b$/C57 mouse model (Graham et al., 1995). Both MUC1 transfectants express epitopes recognized by Mabs HMFG-1, HMFG-1, HMFG-2, and SM3, a similar profile to that seen in the breast cancer-associated mucin.

410.4-MUC1 transfectants showed a reduced tumour incidence compared to hygromycin-transfected controls at low inoculum. Tumours did develop in 100% of mice when sufficient cells were injected (10$^6$), although a delay in tumour growth was apparent compared to the control transfectants. Several alternative PEM-based immunogens have been tested to date using the Balb/c syngeneic model. A reduced incidence or delay in tumour growth can be achieved by: (1) immunization of mice with a low dose of transfected cells prior to tumour challenge with a higher dose (Lalani et al., 1991); (2) peptides based on the tandem repeat sequence of PEM (Ding et al., 1993); and (3) a recombinant vaccinia construct carrying the MUC1 gene (J. Lewis, H. Stauss, E.-N. Lalani & J. Taylor-Papadimitriou, unpublished observations). The expression of MUC1 by RMA transfectants also appeared to cause a delay in tumour growth and a reduced incidence at low inoculum. Moreover, cytotoxic T cell lines could be isolated from C57 mice immunized with a low dose of RMA-MUC1 ($2.5 \times 10^4$) transfectants that failed to induce tumour development. CTL specifically killed RMA-MUC1 in vitro, compared to killing of control transfectants expressing the hygromycin resistance gene only (RMA-HYGRO). Nonimmunized control mice failed to produce MUC1-specific CTL. We are currently using the model to establish the efficacy of MUC1 cDNA as an immunogen.

Syngeneic model systems have also been used by other groups to investigate the potential of vaccinia recombinants expressing tumour-associated antigens (TAA) to generate an effective immune response against tumour cells expressing the TAA. Secreted (MUC1-S) and trans-membrane (MUC1-T) forms of PEM expressed in vaccinia virus (VV) pro-vided tumour protection in immunized rats challenged with a Fischer rat fibroblast line transfected with MUC1-S or MUC1-T (Hareuveni et al., 1990). VV-MUC1-T was most effective in preventing tumour develop-ment in rats challenged with MUC1-T, where 82% of challenged mice failed to develop tumours. A similar model has also been developed in mice using a vaccinia virus (VV-MUC1) that expresses PEM with three or four tandem repeats, with the tumour-associated epitopes exposed (Acres et al., 1993). Thirty per cent of DBA mice immunized with VV-MUC1 and challenged with P815-MUC1 tumour cells failed to develop tumours. Immunized Balb/c mice showed a delay in tumour growth of 3T3-MUC1 cells. MUC1-specific antibodies were detected but did not correlate with tumour rejection. No CTL were detected.

The syngeneic models are extremely useful for comparing the efficacy of PEM-based immunogens in tumour-rejection studies and their ability to produce mucin-specific CTL, but they are limited since the human MUC1 gene is not expressed as a self antigen in mice. The mouse homo-logue of the human mucin shows only 30% homology to the human sequence in the tandem repeat domains so that the transfected tumour cell lines are in fact expressing a foreign antigen, and tolerance is not operative. To overcome the limitations of the syngeneic model, we have also developed a transgenic mouse model expressing the human MUC1 gene as a self antigen, in a tissue specific manner similar to that seen in humans (Peat et al., 1992).

## MUC1 Transgenic Mouse Model

The Tg4 transgenic mouse strain was developed using a 40 kb geno-mic DNA fragment from a cosmid clone GPEM1 from pCOS2EMBL human genomic library, and the Tg18 strain was produced from a 10.6 kb fragment of the 40 kb fragment, that contained a 1.6 kb 5'-flanking sequence and 1.9 kb 3'-flanking sequence (Figure 12.3). A homozygote strain has now been obtained (Tg18h) by breeding Tg18 heterozygotes.

The MUC1 transgenic mouse is a very appropriate system for pre-clinical testing of immunogens for toxicity studies, particularly for mon-itoring autoimmune responses. To test the efficacy of these immunogens in mice, it is, however, necessary to be able to examine their effects on tumour development. Spontaneous tumours have been produced in the

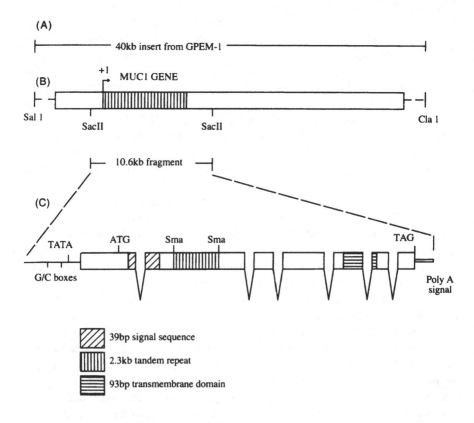

**Figure 12.3.** (A) 40-kb and (B) 10.6-kb DNA fragments from pCOS2EMBL containing the MUC1 gene, used to produce Tg4 and Tg18 transgenic mice, respectively. (C) The major features of the MUC1 gene. The diagram is not to scale.

Tg4 transgenics by cross fostering litters from the MUC1 transgenics on to BR6T female mice carrying the mouse mammary tumour virus (MMTV). The cross fostered mice were subsequently kept pregnant until tumours developed (Graham et al., 1995). Sixty per cent of mice developed spontaneous tumours: nine out of fifteen tumours were mammary tumours, 89% of which expressed both the HMFG1 and SM3 epitopes of MUC1 (Figure 12.4). The exposure of the SM3 epitope on the tumour-associated mucin indicates that aberrant glycosylation of mucin as seen in human breast cancer is also occurring in this mouse model system. Although spontaneous tumours develop slowly, they provide a more realistic model for the evaluation of therapeutic agents as each animal can be considered as an individual patient. To utilize the model to its full extent, we are currently developing transplantable tumours from the spontaneous tumours that arise.

Transplantable tumours can also be established from the MUC1 transfectants described above. Although the Tg18h transgenic mice are of H-2$^k$ haplotype and would not support tumour growth of either 410.4 (H-2$^d$) or RMA (H-2$^b$) transfectants, transgenic F1 hybrids Tg18h × C57 (H-2$^{k/b}$) and Tg18h × Balb/c (H-2$^{k/d}$) are capable of supporting growth of the transplantable MUC1-transfected cell lines, RMA and 410.4, respectively. It should also be possible to extend the transgenic mouse model by using alternative approaches to induce spontaneous tumours in the MUC1-transgenic mice. For example, by crossing the MUC1-transgenic mice with transgenic mice for an oncogene or making double transgenics by expressing an oncogene from the MUC1 (epithelial specific) promoter. In vitro the 1.6-kb 5'-flanking sequence is sufficient to produce epithelial cell-specific production of a reporter gene (Kovarik et al., 1993). These 5' sequences alone, driving the MUC1 gene are being used to produce transgenic mice to determine whether tissue specificity of expression is maintained in vivo.

# ■ CONCLUDING REMARKS

Many investigators are taking a new look at the possibility of introducing immunotherapy into the management of cancer patients. There are two main reasons for the recent optimism, namely: (1) several tumour-associated antigens have been identified and, in many cases, the genes coding for the antigens have been cloned; and (2) mechanisms involved in antigen presentation have been more clearly defined. Antigen presentation is clearly of paramount importance and is not optimal because tumours expressing novel antigens are not rejected. Mucins have come to the fore as carcinoma-associated antigens because, not only can they be overexpressed in the tumour, but the core protein can

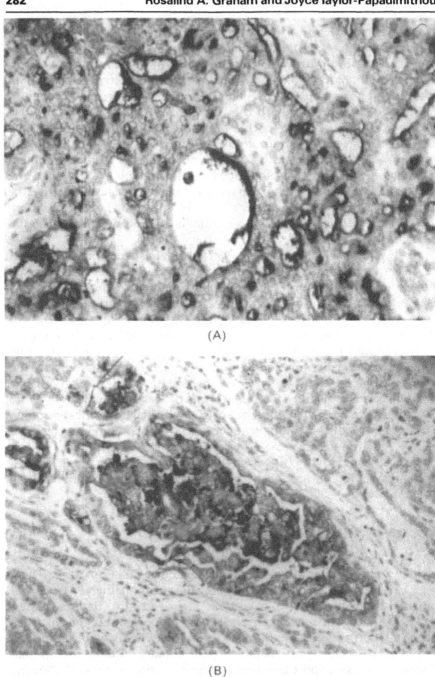

(A)

(B)

**Figure 12.4.**   Spontaneous tumours arising in cross fostered Tg4 transgenic mice expressing (A) HMFG1 epitope ( × 400) and (B) SM3 epitope ( × 250)

be aberrantly glycosylated. Indeed, the novel carbohydrate epitopes found in these complex molecules are now being tested in clinics as immunogens. It has to be noted that, while it is clear how a carbohydrate epitope can induce a B cell response, it is less clear how T cells are activated by these determinants. Nevertheless, in a mouse model some carbohydrate determinants have been shown to be extremely effective in inhibiting the growth of tumours expressing the specific epitope.

The complex mucins are extracellular and this may make them less effective for T cell activation and as targets for CTL. PEM, the product of the MUC1 gene, is a membrane glycoprotein and, as such, is an appropriate target for antibodies. The apparent lack of requirement for HLA for antigen presentation to T cells means that the antigen can also be seen by T cells as a membrane glycoprotein and not as a peptide in the groove of the HLA molecule. This unique form of presentation to and recognition by T cells is probably dependent on the repetitive structure of the molecule and suggests that the limitations normally encountered in HLA-restricted presentation are circumvented. Consequently, PEM is the focus of attention of several groups of investigators and clinical trials with PEM-based immunogens are beginning. Our own strategy has been to develop appropriate model systems in order to evaluate the various possible PEM-based immunogens, to optimize antigen presentation and to define protocols. It is 100 years after William Coley's original observation that tumours could be induced to regress by stimulating the immune system by bacterial toxins. It is hoped that immunotherapy of cancer may now begin to play some role in the management of cancer patients, and that the mucins, particularly MUC1, will be useful in the treatment or prevention of carcinomas.

# ACKNOWLEDGMENTS

We would like to acknowledge the financial support of Biomira, Inc., Edmonton, Alberta, Canada (R. Graham).

### REFERENCES

Acres R.B., Hareuveni M., Balloul J.-M. & Kieny M.-P. (1993) Vaccinia virus MUC1 immunisation of mice: immune response and protection against the growth of murine tumours bearing the MUC1 antigen. *Journal of Immunotherapy*, **14**, 136–43.

Barnd D.L., Lan M.S., Metzgar R.S. & Finn O.J. (1989) Specific, major histocompatibility complex-unrestricted recognition of tumour-associated mucins by human cytotoxic T cells. *Proceedings of the National Academy of Sciences USA*, **86**, 7159–64.

Bobek L.A., Tsai H., Biesbrock A.R. & Levine M.J. (1993) Molecular cloning, sequence, and specificity of expression of the gene encoding the low molecular weight human salivary mucin (MUC7). *Journal of Biological Chemistry*, **268**, 20563–9.

Burchell J., Gendler S.J., Taylor-Papadimitriou J. et al. (1987) Development and characterisation of breast cancer reactive monoclonal antibodies directed to the core protein of the human milk mucin. *Cancer Research*, **47**, 5476–82.

Burchell J. & Taylor-Papadimitriou J. (1993) Effect of modification of carbohydrate side chains on the reactivity of antibodies with core protein epitopes of the MUC1 gene product. *Epithelial Cell Biology*, **2**, 155–62.

Burchell J., Taylor-Papadimitriou J., Boshell M., Gendler S.J. & Duhig T. (1989) A short sequence within the amino acid tandem repeat of a cancer associated mucin, contains immunodominant epitopes. *International Journal of Cancer*, **44**, 691–6.

Crawford L.V., Pim D.C. & Bulbrook R.D. (1982) Detection of antibodies against the cellular protein p53 in sera from patients with breast cancer. *International Journal of Cancer*, **30**, 403–8.

Ding L., Lalani E.-N., Reddish M. et al. (1993) Immunogenicity of synthetic peptides related to the core protein sequence encoded by the human MUC1 gene: effect of immunization on the growth of murine mammary adenocarcinoma cells transfected with the human MUC1 gene. *Journal of Cancer Immunology and Immunotherapy*, **36**, 9–17.

Eckhardt A.E., Timpte C.S., Abernethy J.L., Zhao Y. & Hill R.L. (1991) Porcine submaxillary mucin contains a cysteine-rich domain, carboxyl-terminal domain in addition to a highly repetitive glycosylated domain. *Journal of Biological Chemistry*, **266**, 9678–86.

Fung P.Y.S., Madej M., Koganty K. & Longenecker B.M. (1990) Active specific immunotherapy of a murine mammary adenocarcinoma using a synthetic tumour-associated glycoconjugate. *Cancer Research*, **50**, 4308–14.

Gendler S.J., Burchell J.M., Duhig T. et al. (1987) Cloning of partial cDNA encoding differentiation and tumour-associated mucin glycoprotein expressed by human mammary epithelium. *Proceedings of the National Academy of Sciences USA*, **84**, 6060–4.

Gendler S.J., Lancaster C.A., Taylor-Papadimitriou J. et al. (1990) Molecular cloning and expression of the human tumour-associated polymorphic epithelial mucin. *Journal of Biological Chemistry*, **265**, 15286–93.

Gendler S.J., Taylor-Papadimitriou J., Duhig T., Rothbard J. & Burchell J. (1988) A highly immunogenic region of a human polymorphic epithelial mucin expressed by carcinomas is made up of tandem repeats. *Journal of Biological Chemistry*, **263**, 12820–3.

Gourevitch M.M., von Mensdorff-Pouilly S., Litvinov S.V., Kenemans P., van Kamp G.J., Verstraeten A.A. Hilgers J. (1995) Polymorphic epithelial mucin (MUC-1)-containing circulating immune complexes in carcinoma patients. *British Journal of Cancer*, **72**, 934–8.

Graham R.A., Stewart L.S., Peat N.P., Beverley P. & Taylor-Papadimitriou J. (1995) MUC1-based immunogens for tumour therapy: development of murine model systems. *Tumour Targeting* (in press).

Gum J.R., Byrd J.C., Hicks J.W., Toribara N.W., Lamport D.T.A. & Kim Y.S. (1989) Molecular cloning of human intestinal mucin cDNA's. *Journal of Biological Chemistry*, **264**, 6480–7.

Gum J.R., Hicks J.W., Swallow D.M. et al. (1990) Molecular cloning of cDNA's derived from a novel human intestinal mucin gene. *Biochemical and Biophysical Research Communications*, **171**, 407–15.

Gum J.R., Hicks J.W., Toribara N.W., Rothe E.M., Lagace R.E. & Kim Y.S. (1992) The human MUC1 intestinal mucin has cysteine-rich subdomains located both upstream and downstream of its central repetitive region. *Journal of Biological Chemistry*, **267**, 21375–83.

Hanisch F.G., Uhlenbruck G., Katalinic P.J., Egge H., Dabrowski J. & Dabrowski U. (1989) Structures of neutral O-linked polylactosaminoglycans on human skim milk mucins. A novel type of linearly extended poly-N-acetyl-lactosamine backbone with Galβ(1–4) GlcNAcβ(1–6) repeating units. *Journal of Biological Chemistry*, **265**, 872–83.

Hareuveni M., Gautier C., Kieny M.-P., Wreschner D., Chambon P. & Lathe R. (1990) Vaccination against tumour cells expressing breast cancer epithelial tumour antigen. *Proceedings of the National Academy of Sciences USA*, **87**, 9498–502.

Hull S.R., Bright A., Garraway K.L., Abe M., Hayes D.F. & Kufe D.W. (1989) Oligosaccharide differences in the DF3 sialomucin antigen from normal milk and the BT-20 human breast carcinoma cell line. *Cancer Communications*, **1**, 261–7.

Ioannides C.G., Fisk B., Jerome K.R., Tatsuro I., Taylor Wharton J. & Finn O. (1993) Cytotoxic T cells from ovarian malignant tumours can recognise polymorphic epithelial mucin core peptides. *Journal of Immunology*, **7**, 3693–703.

Itzkowitz S.H., Bloom E.J., Kokal W.A., Modin G., Hakomori S.-I. & Kim Y.S. (1990) Sialosyl-Tn: a novel mucin antigen associated with prognosis in colorectal cancer patients. *Cancer*, **66**, 1960–6.

Jerome K.R., Barnd D.L., Bendt K.M. et al. (1991) Cytotoxic T-lymphocytes derived from patients with breast adenocarcinoma recognize an epitope present on the protein core of a mucin molecule preferentially expressed by malignant cells. *Cancer Research*, **51**, 2908–16.

Kobayashi H., Tero T. & Kawashima Y. (1992) Serum sialyl Tn as an independent predictor of poor prognosis in patients with epithelial ovarian cancer. *Clinical Oncology*, **10**, 95–101.

Kotera Y., Fontenot J.D., Pecher G., Metzgar R.S. & Finn O.J. (1994) Humoral immunity against a tandem repeat epitope of human mucin MUC-1 in sera from breast, pancreatic and colon cancer patients. *Cancer Research*, **54**, 2856–60.

Kovarik A., Peat N., Wilson D., Gendler S.J. & Taylor-Papadimitriou J. (1993) Analysis of the tissue specific promoter of the MUC1 gene. *Journal of Biological Chemistry*, **268**, 9917–26.

Lalani E.-N., Berdichevsky F., Boshell M. et al. (1991) Expression of the gene encoding for a human mucin in mouse mammary tumour cells can affect their tumourigenicity. *Journal of Biological Chemistry*, **266**, 5420–6.

Lan M., Batra S., Qi W.-N., Metzgar R.S. & Hollingsworth M.A. (1990) Cloning and sequencing of a human pancreatic tumour mucin cDNA. *Journal of Biological Chemistry*, **265**, 15294–9.

Ligtenberg M., Vos H., Gennissen A. & Hilkens J. (1990) Episialin, a carcinoma-associated mucin, is generated by a polymorphic gene encoding splice variants with alternative amino acid termini. *Journal of Biological Chemistry*, **265**, 5573–8.

Maclean G.D., Bowen-Yacyshyn M.B., Samual J., Meikle A. et al. (1992) Active immunization of human ovarian cancer patients against a common carcinoma (Thomsen–Friedenreich) determinant using a synthetic carbohydrate antigen. *Journal of Immunotherapy*, **11**, 292–305.

Maclean G.D., Reddish M., Koganty R.R. et al. (1993) Immunization of breast cancer patients using a synthetic sialyl-Tn glycoconjugate plus detox adjuvant. *Cancer Immunology and Immunothrapy*, **36**, 215–22.

Meerzaman D., Charles P., Daskal E., Polymeropoulos M.H., Martin B.M. & Rose M.C. (1994) Cloning and analysis of cDNA encoding a major airway glycoprotein, human tracheobronchial mucin (MUC5). *Journal of Biological Chemistry*, **269**, 12932–9.

Miles D.W., Happerfield L.C., Smith P. et al. (1994) Expression of sialyl-Tn predicts the utility of adjuvant chemotherapy in node positive breast cancer. *British Journal of Cancer*, **70**, 1272–5.

Nishimori I., Perini F., Mountjoy K.P. et al. (1994) N-Acetylgalactosamine glycosylation of MUC1 tandem repeat peptides by pancreatic tumour cell extracts. *Cancer Research*, **54**, 3738–44.

Peat N., Gendler S.J., Lalani E.-N., Duhig T. & Taylor-Papadimitriou J. (1992) Tissue specific expression of a human polymorphic epithelial mucin (MUC1) in tansgenic mice. *Cancer Research*, **52**, 1954–60.

Porchet N., Van Cong N., Dufosse J. et al. (1991) Molecular cloning and chromosomal localisation of a novel human tracheo-bronchial mucin cDNA containing randomly repeated sequences of 48 base pairs. *Biochemical and Biophysical Research Communications*, **175**, 414–22.

Price M.R., Hudecz F., O'Sullivan C., Baldwin R.W., Edwards P.M. & Tendler S.J. (1990) Immunological and structural features of the protein core of human polymorphic epithelial mucin. *Molecular Immunology*, **27**, 795–802.

Rughetti A., Turchi V., Ghetti C.A. et al. (1993) Human B-cell immune response to the polymorphic epithelial mucin. *Cancer Research*, **53**, 2457–9.

Schwartz R.H. (1992) Costimulation of T lymphocytes: the role of CD28, CTLA-4 and B7/BB1 in interleukin-2 production and immunotherapy. *Cell*, **71**, 1065–8.

Shimizu M. & Yamauchi K. (1982) Isolation and characterisation of mucin-like glycoprotein in human milk fat globule membrane. *Journal of Biochemistry*, **91**, 515–9.

Siddiqui J., Abe M., Hayes D., Shani E., Yunis E. & Kufe D. (1988) Isolation and sequencing of a cDNA coding for the human DF3 breast carcinoma-associated antigen. *Proceedings of the National Academy of Sciences USA*, **85**, 2320–3.

Singhal A., Fohn M. & Hakomori S. (1991) Induction of a-N-acetylgalactosamine-O-serine/threonine (Tn) antigen-mediated cellular immune response for active specific immunotherapy in mice. *Cancer Research*, **51**, 1406–11.

Spicer A.P., Parry G., Patton S. & Gendler S.J. (1991) Molecular cloning and analysis of the mouse homologue of the tumour-associated mucin, MUC1, reveals conservation of potential O-glycosylation sites, transmembrane, and cytoplasmic domains and a loss of a minisatellite-like polymorphism. *Journal of Biological Chemistry*, **266**, 15099–109.

Takahashi I., Maehara Y., Kusumoto T., Kohnoe S., Kakeji Y., Baba H. & Sugimachi K. (1994) Combined evaluation or preoperative serum sialyl-Tn antigen and carcinoembryronic antigen levels is prognostic for gastric cancer patients. *British Journal of Cancer*, **69**, 163–6.

Toribara N.W., Roberton A.M., Ho S.B. et al. (1993) Human gastric mucin. Identification of a unique species by expression cloning. *Journal of Biological Chemistry*, **268**, 5879–85.

Werther J.L., Rivera-MacMurrary S., Bruckner H., Tatematsu M. & Itzkowitz S.H. (1994) Mucin-associated sialosyl-Tn antigen expression in gastric cancer correlates with an adverse outcome. *British Journal of Cancer*, **69**, 613–6.

# 13

## Heat Shock Protein–Peptide Complexes: Pan-valent Vaccines against Cancers and Infectious Diseases

RYUICHIRO SUTO AND PRAMOD K. SRIVASTAVA

## ■ DISCOVERY OF HEAT SHOCK PROTEIN–PEPTIDE COMPLEXES AS IMMUNOGENIC ENTITITIES

The observation that inbred mice can be immunized against syngeneic tumors forms the conceptual underpinning of the prospects of cancer immunotherapy (Gross, 1943; Prehn & Main, 1957; Klein et al., 1960; Old et al., 1962). This observation implied that tumors contained substances not present in normal tissues and that such tumor-specific substances could elicit protective immunity to cancers. We attempted to identify the tumor-specific principle responsible for eliciting this response by fractionating tumor cell lysates biochemically and testing individual fractions for their ability to protect mice specifically against live cells of the tumor used for fractionation. This approach led to identification of heat shock proteins (HSPs) as the active immunogenic principle, as it was observed that injection of apparently homogeneous HSP preparations from a given tumor to syngeneic mice or rats renders the animals resistant to that particular tumor (Srivastava & Das, 1984; Srivastava, Deheo & Old, 1986; Ullrich et al., 1986; Palladino et al., 1987; Udono & Srivastava, 1993; 1994). This finding was curious, as HSPs constitute a group of proteins that are present in all living cells of all organisms, from bacteria to mammals (Lindquist & Craig, 1988) and are by no means tumor specific. However, it was soon observed that HSPs isolated from normal tissues do not elicit immunity against any tumors tested (Udono & Srivastava, 1993, 1994). This suggested that the HSPs from normal tissues differ from their counterparts in cancers. Further pursuit of this line of enquiry has shown that the HSPs in normal tissues and cancers do not differ per se (see Srivastava & Maki, 1991); instead, HSP preparations contain a broad array of peptides tightly but noncovalently bound to the HSP molecules (Li & Srivastava, 1993, Srivastava, 1993; Udono & Srivastava, 1993). Previous workers have shown that purified preparations of the HSP grp78 can bind a broad spectrum of peptides in vitro (Flynn et al., 1991; Blond-Elguindi et al., 1993). Although it is now clear that it is the peptides rather than the HSPs that are immunogenic, the HSP-eluted peptides do not elicit immunity by themselves (H. Udono & P.K. Srivastava, unpublished). The fact of their being chaperoned by the HSP molecules is an essential prerequisite for their immunogenicity. The reason for this requirement may be imagined from recent results, which indicate that immunogenicity of HSP–peptide complexes requires the presence of functional phagocytic cells in the host (Udono et al., 1994). It is thus conceivable that the HSP–peptide complexes are taken up by the host phagocytic cells such as the macrophage, dendritic cells, or Langerhans cells and are processed such that the peptides chaperoned by the HSPs are represented by the phagocytic cells (Srivastava et al., 1994). Our preliminary results confirm this hypothesis (R. Suto & P.K. Srivastava, unpublished).

From these results and deliberations, it may be deduced that the spectrum of tumor-associated peptides is different from tumor to tumor, and is also different between tumors and normal tissues. As of now, this deduction remains to be proven through structural studies, in the case of tumor cells. As we have demonstrated that the chaperoning of antigenic peptides by HSPs is not restricted to tumor cells, but occurs in normal cells as well as in virus-infected and virally transformed cells, this problem has been approached in cells infected with the vesicular stomatitis virus. Our findings confirm the presence of presentable virus-specific peptides among the peptides eluted from HSPs purified from virus-infected cells, but not among the peptides eluted from HSPs purified from nonvirus-infected cells (R. Suto & P.K. Srivastava, unpublished).

The chaperoning of peptides by HSPs has been suggested by us to be an integral part of the phenomena of antigen presentation and priming of cytotoxic T cell response. These aspects are beyond the purview of this chapter and have been discussed at length elsewhere (Srivastava, 1993; Srivastava et al., 1994).

## ■ THE HIGH 'SPECIFIC ACTIVITY' OF HSP–PEPTIDE VACCINES

An extraordinary aspect of immunization with HSP–peptide complexes is their high 'specific activity,' that is, immunogenicity per unit quantity of immunogen. Thus, vaccination of mice with 10 $\mu$g gp96-peptide preparation from a tumor renders the mice tumor resistant. Conversion of this value into its molar equivalents is instructive: a 10 $\mu$g HSP–peptide preparation contains approximately $6 \times 10^{13}$ molecules of gp96 (as calculated from Avogadro's number of approximately $6.6 \times 10^{23}$ molecules per mole). Preliminary studies show that equimolar quantities of HSPs and peptides are present in a given preparation. Thus, approximately $6 \times 10^{13}$ molecules of peptides will be present in a 10 $\mu$g HSP–peptide preparation. Of these, one may conservatively expect 0.01% of the peptides to be the specific antigenic peptides, in the overwhelming background of self antigens (which are tolerated by the immune system). Thus, in vaccinating with a 10 $\mu$g gp96 preparation derived from a tumor, one is vaccinating with approximately $10^9$ molecules of tumor-specific antigenic peptide(s). This number is, at once, too small and quite large. Too small in that, assuming an average peptide size of 1 kDa, $10^9$ molecules to 10 pg of specific antigenic peptide, a quantity too small to be effective in vaccination by itself. On the other hand, $10^9$ specific antigenic peptides, presented efficiently to the immune system, constitute a potent stimulus as discussed eblow. We have shown recently, that effective vaccination with gp96-peptide complexes requires the participation of macrophage or other phagolytic cells (Udono, Levey & Srivastava, 1994). This requirement has been explained on the basis of the premise that macrophages bind to the HSPs through a receptor and, having bound, the peptides chaperoned by the HSP are dissociated from the HSP in an intracellular compartment, and re-presented by the macrophage in the context of its own MHC class I molecules (Srivastava et al., 1994). If one assumes that only 1% of the $10^9$ specific antigenic peptide injected is channeled productively, $10^7$ specific antigenic peptides are available. If these peptides are presented by $10^5$ macrophages, dendritic cells or other such cells, each of which presents 100 such peptides (and a much larger number of self peptides) in association with their major histocompatibility complex (MHC) class I molecules (which is sufficient for T cell stimulation), the immune system is faced with a potent stimulus. Thus, while the specific immunogenicity of HSP–peptide complexes is unusually high, the possible mechanisms for it are compatible with existing immunological dogmas. Indeed, the situation is comparable to the extremely high efficiency by which an exogenous molecule can be presented by an MHC class II molecule, if it is taken up by a B cell, which has a specific antigen receptor (antibody) for the molecule, rather than by a B cell, which does not.

# ■ UNIQUE ADVANTAGES OF HSP–PEPTIDE VACCINES FOR CANCER IMMUNOTHERAPY

## Elicitation of a CD8+ T Cell Response in Spite of Exogenous Administration

Vaccination with HSP–peptide complexes elicits a potent CD8+, MHC class I-restricted, T cell response (Blanchere et al., 1993; Udono et al., 1994; S. Janetzki, N.E. Blachere, M. Daou & P.K. Srivastava, unpublished). Most biochemically defined preparations such as proteins or peptides generally elicit antibodies or helper T cells, and not cytotoxic T cells (Raychaudhuri & Morrow 1993). Among biochemically purified, non-live cancer vaccines, HSP–peptide complexes are unique in their ability to elicit an antigen-specific cytotoxic T cell response. The reasons that uniquely permit HSP–peptide complexes to elicit a CD8+ T cell response have to do with the peculiarities of processing of HSP–peptide complexes through the host macrophage and have been discussed above (Udono et al., 1994; Srivastava et al., 1994). Parenthetically, it is interesting to note that, although vaccination with HSP–peptide complexes elicits potent immunity, vaccination with MHC–peptide complexes does not do so, at the doses tested (P.K. Srivastava, unpublished observations). This is presumably due to the fact that, although MHC molecules finally present antigenic peptides to the T cell receptors, MHC–peptide complexes presented exogenously are not able to transfer their peptides to the MHC of antigen presenting cells of the vaccinated host.

## Generation of a Memory T Cell Response

The ability to recall, or memory, is clearly an essential attribute for any vaccine. Based on a number of independent criteria, such as radiation resistance, kinetics of appearance, loss of CD45RB and expression of L-selectin lymphocyte surface antigens, the cytotoxic T cell response generated by vaccination with HSP–peptide complexes has been shown to possess characteristics of a memory response (S. Janetzki, N.E. Blachere, M. Daou & P. K. Srivastava, unpublished).

## Circumvention of the Need for Identification of T Cell Epitopes of Individual Cancers

Vaccination with HSP–peptide complexes circumvents the necessity for identification of the antigenic epitopes of cancer cells. In the case of infectious diseases, killed or attenuated bacterial or viral preparations can be used to vaccinate. Such a whole-cell vaccination approach may be impractical in the case of cancer, because cancers contain deleterious substances such as transforming DNA and immunosuppressive factors such as tumor growth factor $\beta$ (TGD-$\beta$) (Huber, Philipp & Fontana, 1992), tumor-enhancing activity (Srivastava et al., 1986; Ebert et al., 1987) etc., and clinical trials using whole cancer-cell vaccines have not proven to be particularly effective (Old & Oettgen, 1991); however, see Chapter 11 of this volume. Thus, vaccination against cancers requires one to isolate the antigenic moiety of cancer cells rather than use the whole cell approach. Unfortunately, this requirement is as prudent as it is impractical. Unlike infectious diseases, where an antigenic epitope can be identified and used for vaccination, cancers contain a wide spectrum of antigenic epitopes. Indeed, if the chemically and ultraviolet (UV)-induced cancers of experimental animals are to be any guides in this direction (Globerson & Feldman, 1964; Basombrio, 1970; Ward et al., 1989), it would appear that each cancer (and not just each type of cancer) would contain a unique set of antigens, which would be distinct for that particular cancer (see the next section for a discussion of the current enthusiasm for shared epitopes of human tumors). Thus, identification of antigenic epitopes for human cancers would prove to be a daunting, indeed impossible, task as each patient's cancer would have a distinct set of antigenic epitopes. Vaccination with HSP–peptide complexes circumvents this necessity, as HSPs are naturally complexed with the entire repertoire of antigenic epitopes generated in a cell (hence our designation of HSP–peptide complexes as pan-valent vaccines). Thus, patients can be vaccinated with HSP–peptide complexes derived from their own cancers or from cell lines derived from them, without any need for identification of the antigenic epitopes of each patient's cancer.

## Minimization of the Possibility of Generation of Escape Variants

Recently, it has become possible to identify and characterize the cancer antigenic epitopes that are recognized by cytotoxic T cells (Houghton, 1994; Coulie, Chapter 5, this volume). Vaccination with such epitopes is expected to elicit a specific antitumor immune response in cancer patients. However, in view of the profound plasticity of the genome, it is to be expected that such vaccination with a given epitope (or even a combination of a small number of different epitopes) will lead to the generation of escape variants, which will then be refractory to vaccination. This consequence is inevitable unless the immune response is directed to an epitope whose expression is essential for the malignant status of the cancer cells. This does not appear to be the case for any natural antigenic epitope so far defined nor is this to be expected. Thus, the epitope–vaccination approach, which has been so effective in the vaccination against foreign invaders, runs the risk of being self-defeating, in the case of cancer cells, for obvious reasons. In contrast to vaccination with single or multiple epitopes, vaccination with tumor-derived HSP–peptide complexes minimizes the risk of generation of immunological escape variants, because of their pan-valency, as described in the previous section. The possibility of a tumor generating variants, which will not express the entire antigenic repertoire of the original tumor, is infinitely small.

### Lack of Requirement for Adjuvants

HSP–peptide complexes elicit tumor rejection and CD8+ T cell response without the requirement of adjuvants. In view of the dearth of T cell adjuvants proven to be safe and effective for human use, this is an important advantage. It is conceivable, indeed preferable, that adjuvants that enhance the ability of HSP–peptide complexes to elicit tumor regression will be identified, but the fact that such adjuvants are not presently known, is not an impediment to the use of HSP–peptide complexes in human vaccination.

### Biochemical Purity of Vaccine Preparations

HSP–peptide complexes can be purified rapidly to apparent homogeneity and are biochemically defined preparations, free from unidentified proteins, transforming DNA and other deleterious materials. As HSP–peptide complexes will be obtained from patient's tumor samples (or cell lines derived from them), they do not contain any material to the patients have not already been exposed. These characteristics make the HSP–peptide complexes free from most potential hazards.

## ■ SHARED VERSUS UNIQUE IMMUNOGENIC ANTIGENS OF TUMORS: OF MICE AND MEN

Tumor antigens of experimental cancers have been considered historically to be antigenically distinct. Early experiments by Prehn & Main (1957), Old et al. (1962), Globerson & Feldman (1964), and Basombrio (1970) led to the definition of transplantation antigens of methylcholanthrene-induced sarcomas of inbred mice as being antigenically individually distinct, and this became the defining paradigm for cancer immunity. However, recent studies on identification of tumor epitopes recognized by cytotoxic T lymphocytes against human melanomas have begun to challenge this paradigm. So far, at least five cytotoxic T lymphocytes (CTL) epitopes have been identified and, in four of these, the CTL epitope is derived from a melanocytic differentiation antigen (see Houghton, 1994). Further, in each case, the amino-acid sequence of the melanoma CTL epitope is identical to the corresponding sequence in normal melanocytes. Thus, in contrast to the tum⁻ antigens of mutagenized tumors (Lurquin et al., 1989; Sibille et al., 1990; Szikora et al., 1990), no mutations are detected in CTL epitopes of human melanomas. These results are generating a paradigm shift in our understanding of cancer immunity. It has long been assumed that cancers would contain a repertoire of mutations, some of which will be transforming and some antigenic. The possibility that some of the transforming mutations, for example, those in rats and p53, may themselves be antigenic has also been considered (Peace et al., 1991; Yanuck et al., 1993; Disis et al., 1994; Noguchi, Chen & Old, 1994; Staus & Dahl, Chapter 7, this volume). The multimutation model of cancers also fits neatly with our understanding of the multistep nature of familial and environmentally induced cancers (see Nowell, 1988).

These assumptions regarding an inherent mutational repertoire of cancer cells are now being called into question. Firstly, the identified antigenic epitopes are not mutated, hence the ideas that cancers are recognized by the immune system because of genetic alterations stands unsubstantiated. Secondly, immunogenicity of unmutated to self antigens, particularly differentiation antigens as all known epitopes (with one exception, see van der Bruggen et al., 1991; Gaugler et al., 1994) are derived from melanocyte differentiation antigens. This observation is a reincarnation of one of the earliest speculations on the nature of tumor antigens (Old & Boyse, 1969; Boyse & Old, 1978) as differentiation antigens. The question of immune response to unaltered antigens also arises with respect to immune response to the HER2/neu oncogene product, which is not altered in tumor cells, but is overexpressed in a proportion of breast cancers (Slamon et al., 1987). Finally, the presence of unaltered CTL epitopes derived from differentiation antigens suggests that human melanomas possess shared or cross reactive immunogenic antigens. A particular tissue has only a finite set of differentiation antigens and, if genes for these antigens are not mutated in tumor cells, all tumors of a given histological origin can possess only a finite set of immunogenic antigens. Hence, the recent structural studies on CTL epitopes imply that human melanomas possess shared tumor-rejection antigens. Earlier, nonstructural studies have also suggested such cross reactivity (Darrow, Slingluff & Siegler, 1989; Hom et al., 1991; Kawakami et al., 1992).

The results of studies on specificity of antigenicity of tumors in experimental and human systems are therefore at odds with each other. Studies with tumors of mice, rats, and guinea pigs suggest that tumors are individually distinct, while studies with human tumors suggest that they are crossreactive. This divergence cannot be explained on the basis of the possibility that experimental tumors are induced by known carcinogens, while the human tumors are apparently 'spontaneous,' because spontaneous tumors of mice have also been shown to elicit individually distinct antigenicity (Vaage, 1968; Morton, Miller & Wood, 1969; Carswell et al., 1970; Koch, Zaleberg & McKenzie, 1984). In this light, it would appear that human tumors are indeed fundamentally different from experimentally induced cancers. However, closer scrutiny reveals that this distinction, which would be radical and profound, if it were to be true, is indeed only apparently so. The reasons for the discrepancy lie perhaps in the methods used to analyze individually or crossreactivity of tumors in the experimental and human systems. The methods are, of necessity, not comparable. In experimental studies, the nature of antigenicity is determined by tumor transplantation studies, while in human studies, it is measured by the presence of tumor-associated antigens, presentable by an appropriate MHC molecule to a cognate T cell receptor. The two assays, although overlapping, are almost certainly not synonymous. Indeed, when experimentally induced tumors are analysed through T cell activity, cross reactive antigens can be readily detected by cytotoxic as well as helper T cells (Rohrer et al., 1995).

The question thus shifts from the distinction between human and experimental cancers to the distinction between antigens detected by T cell assays versus those detected by tumor rejection assays. The antigens detected by the former appear to be crossreactive, while those detected by the latter appear to be unique. As tumor rejection rather than a T cell response in and of itself is the desirable endpoint in cancer vaccination, the distinction between antigens recognized by T cell assays and by tumor rejection raises questions regarding the validity of T cell assays to detect antigens of potential therapeutic significance. This concern is further highlighted of one revisits the observations of Coggin and his colleagues who have demonstrated that crossreactive tumor rejection antigens can indeed be detected even by tumor rejection assays, if one uses lower levels of tumor challenge (Coggin 1989a, 1989b). Thus, the crossreactive tumor antigens are weaker antigens with respect to tumor rejection.

These ideas have considerable bearing on the prospects of immunotherapy for human cancers. It is our belief that the current enthusiam for existence of shared tumor rejection antigens on human cancers is inconsistent with some of the most fundamental lessons learnt from immunogenicity of experimentally induced cancers. This enthusiasm derives in part from the experience with the paradigm of cellular immunity to viral antigens, where T cell response to a dominant viral epitope is sufficient to eradicate a future or ongoing infection. The viral paradigm is perhaps inapplicable to cancers because of the absence of a clearly definable dominant foreign epitope in the case of most solid cancers. We believe that immunity to cancer is directed against a large spectrum of unaltered and altered self antigens, some shared and others unique. The immunogenicity of cancers results not from the immunogenicity of one or even a small number of epitopes, but is the sum total of the immunogenicities of a large number of weakly immunogenic epitopes. As tumors arise necessarily as a consequence of random mutational events, this repertoire of epitopes is likely to be distinct for each individual cancer. If this premise turns out to be correct, immunotherapy of human cancer will once again face the challenge of developing patient-specific vaccines. As indicated in a previous section, HSP–peptide vaccines derived from autologous cancer are uniquely and powerfully suited to this challenge.

## ■ FURTHER WORK

While all the known observations on the immunogenicity of HSP–peptide complexes are in accord with our suggestions, and no observations are discordant with them, our hypothesis is clearly not yet proven. Its final validation awaits structural demonstration of association of known viral and tumor-associated antigenic epitopes and their precursors with the individual HSP molecules and elucidation of the pathway in phagocytic cells, through which the HSP–peptide complexes are taken up, processed, and the peptides re-presented by the phagocytic cells in context of its own MHC class I molecules.

While this chapter is devoted largely to the use of HSP–peptide complexes as anticancer vaccines, we would be remiss in not pointing out the applicability of HSP–peptide vaccines against infectious diseases. As HSPs chaperone the entire repertoire of peptides generated within a cell, HSP–peptide complexes isolated from virus-infected cells should be able to elicit virus-specific T cell responses, This has been indeed found to be so (Blachere et al., 1993; N.E. Blachere & P.K. Srivastava, unpublished). In this regard, it should be noted that, in contrast to HLA antigens, HSPs are nonpolymorphic and bind to antigenic peptides regardless of the HLA composition of the cells from which they are isolated. This will make it possible to vaccinate humans of any HLA composition with HSP–peptide complexes derived from virus-infected human cells of any HLA composition. Thus, with respect to vaccination against infectious diseases, HSP-based vaccines will not have to be patient specific (Suto and Srivastava, 1995).

# ACKNOWLEDGMENTS

The work described here was funded at various times by the Council of Scientific and Industrial Research, New Delhi, India (1980–3), the Cancer Research Institute, New York (1984–93), National Institutes of Health award CA44786, (1987–present), Irma T. Hirschl Foundation (1989–92), Donaldson–Atwood Foundation (1992–3), and the Martell Foundation (1991–3). R. Suto is a postdoctoral fellow of the Cancer Research Institute.

## REFERENCES

Basombrio M.A. (1970) Search for common antigenicities among 25 sarcomas induced by methylcholanthrene. *Cancer Research*, 30, 2458.

Blachere N.E., Udono H., Janetzki S. et al. (1993) Heat shock protein vaccines against cancer. *Journal of Immunotherapy*, 14, 352–6.

Blond-Elguindi S., Cwirla S.E., Dower W.J. et al. (1993) Affinity panning of a library of peptides displayed on bacteriophages reveals the binding specifity of BiP. *Cell*, 75, 717–28.

Boyse E.A. & Old L.J. (1978) Immunogenetics of differentiation in the mouse. *Harvey Lecture*, 71: 23.

Carswell E.A., Wanebo H.J., Old L.J. & Boyse E.A. (1970) Immunogenic properties of reticulum cell sarcoma SJL/J mice. *Journal of the National Cancer Institute*, 44, 1281–8.

Coggin J.H. Jr. (1989a) Shared cross protective TATA on rodent sarcomas. *Immunology Today*, 10, 76.

Coggin J.H. Jr. (1989b) Cross-reacting tumor associated transplantation antigen on primary 3-methylcholanthrene-induced BALB/c sarcomas. *Molecular Biotherapy*, 1, 223–8.

Darrow T.L., Slingluff C.L. & Siegler H.F. (1989) The role of HLA Class I antigens in recognition of melanoma cells by tumor-specific cytotoxic T lymphocytes. Evidence for shared tumor antigens. *Journal of Immunology*, 142, 3329–35.

Disis M.L., Calenoff E., E., McLaughlin G. et al. (1994) Existent T cell and antibody immunity to HER2/neu protein in patients with breast cancer. *Cancer Research*, 54, 16–20.

Ebert E.C., Roberts A.I., O'Connell S.M. et al. (1987) Characterization of an immuno-suppressive factor derived from colon cancer cells. *Journal of Immunology*, 138, 2161–8.

Flynn G.C., Pohl J., Flocco M.T. et al. (1991) Peptide-binding specifity of the molecular chaperone BiP. *Nature (London)*, 353, 726–30.

Gaugler B.B., van den Eynde B., van der Bruggen P. et al. (1994) Human MAGE-3 codes for an antigen recognized on a human melanoma by autologous cytotoxic T lymphocytes. *Journal of Experimental Medicine*, 179, 921–30.

Globerson A. & Feldman M. (1964) Antigenic specifity of benzo(a) pyrene-induced sarcomas. *Journal of the National Cancer Institute*, 32, 1229–43.

Gross L. (1943) Intradermal immunization of C3H mice against a sarcoma that originated in an animal of the same line. *Cancer Research*, 3, 326–33.

Hom S.S., Topalian S.L., Simonis T., Mancini M. & Rosenberg S.A. (1991) Common expression of melanoma tumor-associated antigens recognized by human tumor infliltrating lymphocytes: analysis by human lymphocyte antigen restriction. *Journal of Immunotherapy*, **10**, 153–64.

Houghton A.N. (1994) Cancer antigens: immune recognition of self and altered self. *Journal of Experimental Medicine*, **190**, 1–4.

Huber D., Philipp J. & Fontana A. (1992) Protease inhibitors interfere with the transforming growth factor-dependent but not the transforming growth factor-independent pathway of tumor cell-mediated immunosuppression. *Journal of Immunology*, **148**, 277–84.

Kawakami Y., Zakut R., Topalian S.L., Stotter H. & Rosenberg S.A. (1992) Shared human melanoma antigens. Recognition by tumor-infiltrating lymphocytes in HLA-A2.1-transfected melanomas. *Journal of Immunology*, **148**, 638–43.

Klein G., Sjorgen H.O., Klein E. et al. (1960) Demonstration of resistance against methylcholanthrene-induced sarcomas in the primary autochthonous host. *Cancer Research*, **20**, 1561–72.

Koch S., Zaleberg J.R. & McKenzie I.F.C. (1984) Description of a murine B lymphoma tumor-specific antigen. *Journal of Immunology*, **133**, 1070–7.

Li Z. & Srivastava P.K. (1993) Tumor rejection antigen gp96/grp94 is an ATPase: implication for protein folding and antigen presentation. *EMBP Journal*, **12**, 3134–51.

Lindquist S. & Craig E.A. (1988) The heat shock proteins. *Annual Review of Genetics*, **22**, 631–77.

Lurquin C.A., VanPel A., Mariame B. et al. (1989) Structure of the gene coding for Tum⁻ transplantation antigen P91A. A peptide encoded by the mutated exon is recognized with L$^d$ cytolytic T cells. *Cell*, **59**, 293–303.

Morton D.L., Miller, G.F. & Wood D.A. (1969) Demonstration of tumor-specific immunity against antigens unrelated to the mammary tumor virus in spontaneous mammary adenocarcinomas. *Journal of the National Cancer Institute*, **42**, 289–301.

Noguchi Y., Chen Y.T. & Old L.J. (1994) A mouse mutant p53 product recognized by CD4+ and CD8+ T cells. *Proceedings of the National Academy of Sciences USA*, **91**, 3171–5.

Nowell P.C. (1988) Molecular events in tumor development. *New England Journal of Medicine*, **319**, 575.

Old L.J. & Boyse E.A. (1969) Some aspects of normal and abnormal cell surface genetics. *Annual Review of Genetics*, **3**, 269.

Old L.J., Boyse E.A., Clarke D.A. (1962) Antigenic properties of chemically induced tumors. *Annals of the New York Academy of Sciences*, **101**, 80–106.

Old L.J. & Oettgen H. F. (1991) Cancer immunotherapy with vaccines. In V. DeVita, S. Hellman & S.A. Rosenberg (eds) *Biologic therapy of Cancer*, pp. 96–7. Philadelphia, J.B. Lippincott.

Palladino M.A., Srivastava P.K., Oettgen H.F. et al. (1987) Expression of a shared tumor-specific antigen by two chemically induced BALB/c sarcomas. *Cancer Research*, **47**, 5074–9.

Peace D.J., Chen W., Nelson H. & Cheever M.A. (1991) T cell recognition of transforming proteins encoded by mutated ras protooncogenes. *Journal of Immunology*, **146**, 2059–65.

Prehn R. & Main J.M. (1957) Immunity to methylcholanthrene-induced sarcomas. *Journal of the National Cancer Institute*, **18**, 769–78.

Raychaudhuri S. & Morrow W.J.W. (1993) Can soluble antigens induce CD8+ T cell response? A paradox revisited. *Immunology Today*, **14**, 344–8.

Rohrer J.W., Culpepper C., Barsoum A.O. & Coggin J.H. Jr. (1995) Characterization of RFM mouse T lymphocyte anti-OFA immunity in apparent tumor-free, long-term survivors of sub-lethal X-irradiation by limiting dilution T lymphocyte cloning. *Journal of Immunology*, **154**, 2266–80..

Rohrer J.W., Rohrer S.D., Barsoum A. and Coggin J.H. Jr. (1994) Differential recognition of murine tumor-associated oncofetal transplantation antigen and individually specific transplantation antigens by syngeneic cloned BALB/c and RFM mouse T cells. *Journal of Immunology*, **152**, 754–64.

Sibille C., Chomez P., Wildmann C. et al. (1990) Structure of the gene of Tum⁻ transplantation antigen P198: a point mutation generates a new antigenic peptide. *Journal of Experimental Medicine*, **172**, 35–45.

Slamon D.J., Clark G.M., Wong S.G. et al. (1987) Human breast cancer: correlation of relapse and survival with amplification of the HER-2/neu oncogene. *Science*, **235**, 177–82.

Srivastava P.K. (1993) Peptide-binding heat shock proteins in the endoplasmic reticulum: role in immune response to cancer and in antigen presentation. *Advances in Cancer Research*, **62**, 153–77.

Srivastava P.K. & Das M.R. (1984) The serologically unique cell surface antigen of Zajdela ascitis hepatoma is also its tumor-associated transplantation antigen. *International Journal of Cancer*, **33**, 417–22.

Srivastava P.K., DeLeo A.B. & Old L.J. (1986) Tumor rejection antigens of chemically induced tumors of inbred mice. *Proceedings of the National Academy of Sciences USA*, **83**, 3407–11.

Srivastava P.K. & Old L.J. (1988) Individually distinct transplantation antigen of chemically induced mouse tumors. *Immunology Today*, **9**, 78–83.

Srivastava P.K. & Maki R.G. (1991) Stress-induced proteins in immune response to cancer. *Current Topics in Microbiology and Immunology*, **167**, 109.

Srivastava P.K., Udono H., Blachere N.E. et al. (1994) Heat shock proteins transfer peptides during antigen processing and CTL priming. *Immunogenetics*, **39**, 93–8.

Suto R. & Srivastava P.K. (1995) A mechanism for specific immunogenicity of hsp-chaperoned peptides. *Science*, **269**, 1585–8.

Szikora J.P., VanPel A., Brichard V. et al. (1990) Structure of the gene of Tum⁻ transplantation antigen P35B: presence of a point mutation in the antigenic allele. *EMBO Journal*, **9**, 1041–50.

Udono H., Levey D.L. & Srivastava P.K. (1994) Cellular requirements for tumor-specific immunity elicited by heat shock proteins: tumor rejection antigen pg96 primes CD8+ T cells in vivo. *Proceedings of the National Academy of Sciences USA*, **91**, 3077–81.

Udono H. & Srivastava P.K. (1994) Comparison of tumor-specific immunogenecities of stress-induced proteins gp96, hsp90, and hsp 70, *Journal of Immunology*, **152**, 5398–403.

Udono H. & Srivastava P.K. (1993) Heat-shock protein 70-associated peptides elicit specific cancer immunity. *Journal of Experimental Medicine*, **178**, 1391–6.

Ullrich S.J., Robinson E.A., Law L.W. et al. (1986) A mouse tumor-specific transplantation antigen is a heat-shock related protein. *Proceedings of the National Academy of Sciences USA*, **83**, 3121–5.

Vaage J. (1968) Non-virus antigens in virus-induced mammary tumors. *Cancer Research*, **28**, 2477–83.

van der Bruggen P., Travsersari C., Chomez, P. et al. (1991) A gene encoding an antigen recognized by cytolytic T cells on a human melanoma. *Science*, **254**, 1643–7.

Ward P.L., Koeppen H., Hurteau T. et al. (1989) Tumor antigens defined by cloned immunological probes are highly polymorphic and are not detected on autologous normal cells. *Journal of Experimental Medicine*, 170, 217–32.

Yanuck M., Carbone D.P., Pendleton D. et al. (1993) A mutant p53 tumor suppressor protein is a target for peptide-induced CD8+ cytotoxic T cells. *Cancer Research*, 54, 3257–61.

# 14

## The Potential of Gene Transfer to Alter the Immune Response to Tumors

BERNARD A. FOX AND GARY J. NABEL

## ■ INTRODUCTION

The immune system can potentially respond to malignancies and limit their growth. In some instances, immune recognition of tumors is achieved but, often, malignancies evade such immune detection. This failure of the immune response may be due to lack of tumor immunogenicity or a tumor-induced immunosuppressive environment. One goal of gene transfer for the treatment of cancer is to manipulate the host immune response to the tumor to allow for the recognition and elimination of the malignancy. Some of the available genetic approaches focus entirely on direct immunological intervention, while alternatives include the introduction of genes that may affect cell growth. In such cases, it is also important to stimulate an efficient antitumor immune response to reduce tumor burden or eliminate metastatic foci.

This review will address the potential role of gene transfer techniques to alter the immune response to tumors. This overview will include a discussion of gene transfer methods and their advantages, limitations, and how they might be applied to target different sites. Options available to modify tumor recognition by the immune system, or bolster the insufficient or immunosuppressed antitumor immune response will also be described.

## ■ GENE TRANSFER TECHNIQUES

The introduction of novel genetic information into eukaryotic cells has been accomplished by chemical, physical and biological techniques. However, many techniques applicable to in vitro gene transfer cannot be readily applied to a clinical setting. These include approaches such as

Table 14.1. Gene Transfer Techniques Available to Deliver Vector Constructs to Target Cells

1. Naked DNA
2. DNA–ligand
3. Lipid complex/liposome mediated
4. Particle mediated
5. Viral
6. Bacterial

calcium phosphate transfection and electroporation. Fortunately, a number of gene-transfer approaches are readily transferable to clinical settings. A review of these approaches is presented below and outlined in Table 14.1.

## Naked DNA

Direct injection of 'naked' plasmid DNA into muscle and tumor has been reported (Wolff et al., 1990). This method of gene transfer is relatively inefficient with low frequency of integration into host chromosomes (Wolff et al., 1991, 1992). Some of the deficiencies inherent in this approach may also be viewed as strengths. When attempting to stimulate an immune response, inefficient expression of a target molecule may spare a majority of a tissue from destruction while fostering the rudiments of an immune response. Similarly, the transient expression of a plasmid vector, due to its episomal (nonintegrated) form tends to limit the duration of gene expression. Such limited expression may be advantageous when delivering cytokine genes or strong antigens, since extended expression, particularly of certain cytokines, may exert significant toxicity. Additionally, the failure of this plasmid to integrate reduces the potential for insertional mutagenesis. This form of gene transfer has received approval for clinical trials and may be particularly suitable as a method to perform genetic immunization for malignancy and infectious disease.

## DNA–Ligand

A number of molecular conjugates containing DNA and one or a number of other molecules, including proteins, antibodies and/or viruses, have been utilized to improve gene-transfer efficiencies. For the purpose of this review, we have combined these conjugates under the heading

DNA–ligand complexes, since a ligand for a cell membrane receptor is instrumental to this approach. During transfection, the DNA–ligand complex is internalized by target cells when the ligand interacts with its specific cell membrane receptor and induces endocytosis of the complex. This approach was first used by Wu and colleagues, who targeted asialoglycoprotein receptors on hepatic cells (Wu & Wu, 1988). Subsequently, a number of investigators have utilized DNA complexed to transferin, histones, or adenovirus (Wagner et al., 1990, 1992; Cureil et al., 1991, 1992; Chen, Stickles & Douchendt, 1994a). A disadvantage of this approach was the propensity of DNA to be incorporated into endosomes, which can degrade the complex and destroy the gene construct. Curiel and colleagues exploited the endosome-disrupting capacity of adenoviral particles to augment the escape of DNA–ligand complexes from endosomes and demonstrated increased transfection efficiency of the complex (Curiel et al., 1991, 1992b; Cotten et al., 1992). In this strategy, positively charged poly-L-lysine, complexed to inactivated virus (often linked to a specific protein), is combined with the negatively charged plasmid DNA. Poly-L-lysine links the DNA to inactivated adenovirus, which is in turn linked to a specific ligand. The resulting complex is then used to transfect target cells. Recently, Chen and co-workers targeted delivery of a plasmid to the nucleus by coupling galactosylated histones to the DNA–lysine complex (Chen et al., 1994a). Galactosylation of the histones allowed them to be endocytosed by asialoglycoprotein receptors and the nuclear localization signal sequence of the histone H1 was proposed as the mechanism responsible for augmented transfection frequencies.

## Lipid Complex-mediated Gene Transfer

Combining cationic lipid complexes with plasmid DNA vectors generates a product that can interact directly with membranes on target cells (Felgner & Rhodes, 1991). This interaction increases the efficiency of gene transfer and expression of the novel gene product compared to that observed for naked DNA alone. While efficiency of gene transfer is increased, the vectors rarely integrate and expression of the gene product is transient. The development of improved lipid formulations has increased the transfection efficiency of this approach and allowed higher absolute concentrations of DNA lipid complexes to be combined and remain in solution (San et al., 1993; Felgner et al., 1994; Nabel et al., 1994a). These properties of lipid complex-mediated gene transfer provide additional advantages over DNA alone without the drawbacks inherent to biological–viral approaches. The inherent safety of this plasmic-based approach has helped accelerate its application in clinical trials (Nabel et al., 1993; Hersh et al., 1994; Rubin et al., 1994; Vogelzang, Lestingi &

Sudakoff, 1994). It is stably delivered through catheters or by a guided needle, and could be readily applied as an adjunct to debulking surgery, where unrestrictable tumour deposits could be injected with DNA–lipid complexes.

Lipids have also been used to create unilamellar and multilamellar lipsomes. Investigators have encapsulated plasmid vectors into these structures and demonstrated increased transfection frequencies for some cells in vitro. The prospects for using liposomes to target cells in vivo will be discussed below.

## Particle-mediated Gene Transfer

This form of gene transfer was developed as a means to insert genes into plants (Klein et al., 1987). The bombardment of seeds with gold particles coated with DNA allowed the gene of interest to be carried into the seed. This approach has been successfully applied to transfect a wide range of cells in vitro and in vivo (Yang et al., 1990; Yang, 1992). While the majority of transfection can be expected to be transient, integration is possible. Cheng and colleagues have reported novel gene expression in dermis for as long as 1.5 years following particle bombardment (Cheng et al., 1993). The recent refinement of this technology into a small hand-held 'gene gun' should help expedite the application of this approach to clinical trials.

## Viral/Retroviral/Producer Cell Transfer

Murine retroviral vectors have been the most widely utilized gene transfer vehicles for clinical trials. The viral RNA backbone of these agents has been engineered such that essential structural genes encoding for capsid proteins (gag), reverse transcriptase (pol) and envelope glycoproteins (env) have been removed. These essential components to the virus life cycle are provided in trans by packaging cell lines into which these viral genes have been introduced (McLachlin et al., 1990; Hesdorffer et al., 1991). Packaging cell lines, transfected with recombinant retroviral backbone DNA, will produce infectious but replication-defective RNA retroviral vectors. These vectors provide for stable integration of proviral sequences into primary and established cells, provided the target cells are undergoing replication (Temin, 1989). The introduction of safety features into both the viral and packaging systems has increased the safety of these agents. However, recombination events and the generation of wild-type virus is still possible (Donahue et al., 1992).

Adeno-associated viruses (AAVs) and adenoviruses are two additional viral vectors that have been evaluated as vehicles for gene transfer. AAV are single-stranded DNA parvoviruses, which are not pathogenic in humans. These viruses infect and integrate into the host genome at specific regions in chromosome 19 (Muzyczka, 1992). AAV vectors may not require target-cell replication and high titers of infectious virus can be achieved increasing their potential advantages for in vivo gene transfer. Adenovirus-based vectors are currently being used for many in vivo gene-transfer applications, because they combine characteristics of high titer, infection of nondividing cells, a broad host range, and a tropism for epithelial tissue (Berkner, 1988; Graham, 1992). These vectors are double-stranded DNA viruses of approximately 35 kb. Recombinant adenovirus vectors may accommodate up to 7.5 kb of inserted DNA, increasing the potential to deliver multiple gene constructs to target cells (Graham, 1992).

**Herpes Simplex Virus**   Vectors based on defective herpes simplex viruses (HSVs) have recently been used to selectively target tumors in the brain. These vectors selectively replicate in dividing cells and exhibit direct cytotoxic activity against infected cells (Coen et al., 1989; Martuza et al., 1991). An additional advantage to HSV is its large genome, which is well suited for the development of constructs with multiple genes (Breakefield & Deluca, 1991). However, a major concern regarding these vectors is the potential destruction of normal neural tissue. Clinical application will depend on design developments or techniques which attenuate their neurotoxicity (Pakzaban, Geller & Isacson, 1994).

**Bacterial Vectors**   *Salmonella* strains, attenuated by the introduction of nonreverting mutations into gal E or aroA genes on the *Salmonella* chromosome have been effectively used to vaccinate against salmonellosis (Dougan, Hormaeche & Maskell, 1987). The vaccine is administered orally and invades the reticuloendothelial system. *Salmonella* engineered to express foreign antigens can generate protective immune responses against *Salmonella*, and both humoral and cellular immune responses to the novel antigens. This approach to gene transfer appears to be particularly well suited for the delivery of antigens presented by major histocompatibility complex (MHC) class I and class II molecules (Aggarwal et al., 1990; Flynn et al., 1990; Brett et al., 1993). Future application of this approach will most likely include the peptide tumor antigens being described for melanoma, breast, pancreatic, and ovarian tumors.

Table 14.2. Gene Transfer Options Available to Augment an Immune Response to Tumors

A. Gene transfer into tumors
  1. Cytokines
  2. Antigens (tumor specific, alloantigens, superantigens)
  3. Accessory molecules for T cell recognition/activation
  4. Suicide genes
  5. Intracellular single chain antibodies (sFv)
  6. Cytokine receptors
B. Gene transfer into T cells
  1. Cytokines
  2. Chimeric receptor genes
  3. Selectable markers/recovery–expansion–reinfusion
C. Gene transfer into antigen presenting cells, fibroblasts or muscle cells
  1. Cytokines
  2. Antigens (peptides)

## ■ MODIFICATION OF TUMOR CELLS BY GENE TRANSFER

An outline of the strategies being employed to alter the immune response to tumors is presented in Table 14.2. This section will provide some basis for these general approaches, review the experimental evidence, and comment on their future direction.

### Cytokine Gene Transfer

Cytokines can be potent mediators or modulators of an immune response. A number of cytokines have been used to modify tumor cells genetically (Table 14.3). Since components of this list will be reviewed more extensively in other chapters, we will limit our discussion of this topic to a general overview.

One advantage of cytokine gene transfer into tumour cells, particularly in a vaccine strategy, is that it provides a constant release of cytokine at the vaccine site, thereby increasing the likelihood that the desired effect will occur, whether this desired effect is on the tumor itself, on the infiltrating immune cells, or both. It appears that the future clinical application of cytokine gene transfer into tumor cell vaccines, or autologous fibroblasts combined with the vaccine, will be in combination with additional immunologically based genetic intervention. A potential short cut to bypass cytokine gene transfer into tumors is the use of slow-

Table 14.3. Cytokines Used to Augment the Immune Response to Tumors

| Cytokine | Reference |
|----------|-----------|
| IL-1 | Douvedevani et al. (1992) |
| IL-2 | Fearon et al. (1990) Gansbacher et al. (1990b) |
| IL-4 | Golumbek et al. (1991) Tepper, Coffman & Leder (1992) Tepper, Pattengale & Leder (1989) |
| IL-6 | Mullen et al. (1992) Porgador et al. (1992) |
| IL-7 | Aoki et al. (1992) Hock et al. (1991) Hock et al. (1993) Jicha, Mule & Rosenberg (1991) McBride et al. (1992) |
| IL-10 | Barth & Coppola (1994) Richter et al. (1993) Suzuki et al. (1994) |
| IL-12 | Tahara et al. (1994) |
| IFN-$\gamma$ | Gansbacher et al. (1990a) Hock et al. (1991) Watanabe et al. (1989) |
| TNF-$\alpha$ | Asher et al. (1991) Blankenstein et al. (1991) |
| G–CSF | Colombo et al. (1991) Stoppacciaro et al. (1993) |
| GM–CSF | Dranoff et al. (1993) |

release polymers or gels, which can be mixed with tumor vaccines and used to release small amounts of cytokines into the local milieu in vivo. While this approach may be safer than a gene transfer strategy, it is unclear whether this approach will provide similar therapeutic effects in vivo.

### Gene Transfer to Enhance Tumor Antigenicity

T cell recognition of antigens is generally envisioned as the T cell receptor for antigen interacting with and recognizing a small antigenic peptide presented by an MHC or human leukocyte antigen (HLA) class I or class II molecule. In order for tumors to be recognized by a cell-mediated immune response, a minimal requirement is that they express either MHC class I or class II molecules, and possesses some tumor-associated antigen(s). Numerous investigators have characterized defects in the expression of HLA/MHC molecules on both human and animal tumors, and proposed a role for this deficit in tumor progression. A decade ago, Hui and colleagues demonstrated that a tumor, which failed to express detectable levels of MHC class I and grew progressively in syngenic hosts, was rejected following transfection with a syngeneic MHC class I molecule (Hui et al., 1984). This observation, reproduced by multiple investigators, identified one mechanism that tumors use to escape the immune response and strengthened the argument for an immunological approach to cancer therapy (Tanaka et al., 1985; Wallich et al., 1985; Tanaka et al., 1986; Weber et al., 1987).

## Allogeneic MHC Gene Transfer

Tanaka and colleagues characterized the growth of tumor cells transfected with a syngenic MHC class I molecule and observed that they were less tumorgenic in allogenic animals (Tanaka et al., 1985). This result represented the first evidence that transfection of an MHC molecule, allogeneic to the tumor-bearing host, could significantly alter tumor progression. While some suggested that MHC class I expression alone was insufficient for tumor rejection, others clearly recognized the decrease in tumorigenicity following transfection with allogenic MHC class I genes (Bahler et al., 1987; Cole et al., 1987; Carlow et al., 1989; Hui et al., 1989; Ostrand-Rosenberg et al., 1990). Recently, Plautz and colleagues used direct allogenic MHC class I gene transfer to modify established tumors in mice. The introduction of allogenic MHC class I genes into progressively growing tumors led to the generation of cytotoxic T lymphocytes (CTL) reactive to the unmodified tumor and reduction of tumor growth (Plautz, 1993). Based on these studies, a phase I clinical trial was initiated to use direct allogenic HLA class I (HLA-B7) gene transfer in an effort to induce tumor regression. Five patients who did not express the HLA-B7 allele were treated without complications and recombinant HLA-B7 protein was detected in tumor biopsy tissue from all patients (Nabel et al., 1993). One patient demonstrated regression of injected nodules on two independent treatments, which was accompanied by regression at distant sites. Another patient demonstrated an increase in anti-HLA-B7 CTL precusions following gene transfer, suggesting that expression of recombinant HLA-B7 at the tumor site could sensitize precursors T cells. This observation was also consistent with previous studies, which demonstrated generation of anti-HLA-B7 CTL following direct gene transfer into arterial vessels in a porcine model (Nabel, Plautz & Nabel, 1992).

We and others have previously speculated that one potential advantage of expressing a strongly immunogenic antigen on the surface of the tumor is that it elicits a strong immune response at the tumor site. Initiation of an immune response in nature yields a series of dynamic immunological events, which can effectively immunize a competent host. While the complexity of this response is only partially appreciated, development of the appropriate cytokine cascade is thought to be essential. Thus, the elaboration of an appropriate cytokine milieu at the tumor site may induce the appropriate inflammatory response and cellular infiltrate such that the immune system recognizes both the foreign allo-antigen and the tumor cells as well. Unfortunately, some progressively growing tumors may immunosuppress or partially anergize the host's immune response. In one poorly immunogeneic murine model, direct allogeneic MHC class I gene transfer failed to halt progression of tumor growth. However, expression of the allogeneic class I molecule augmented sensitization of the antitumor immune response such that immune effector T cells could be generated by an in vitro activation process from lymph nodes draining the injected tumors (Wahl et al., 1992). Wahl and colleagues clearly demonstrated that allogeneic MHC class I gene transfer failed to halt progression of tumor growth. However, expression of the allogeneic class I molecule augmented sensitization of the antitumor immune response such that immune effector T cells could be generated by an in vitro activation process from lymph nodes draining the injected tumors (Wahl et al., 1992). Wahl and colleagues clearly demonstrated that allogeneic MHC class I gene transfer was significantly more effective at generating therapeutic T cells in this model, than gene transfer with a $\beta$-galactosidase negative control (Wahl et al., 1992, 1995). Direct gene transfer could thus possibly be used in autologous tumor vaccines with recovery of the sensitized tumor vaccine draining lymph nodes. Following activation and expansion, these tumor-sensitized T cells could be returned to the patient with a course of systemic interleukin-2 (IL-2). An alternative approach would be to generate tumor-infiltrating lymphocytes (TIL) from tumors modified by direct gene transfer. These could then be adoptively transferred back to the host together with systemic IL-2.

### Prospects for Superantigen Gene Transfer

Microbial superantigens (SAg) are a family of small peptides that can selectively activate subsets of T cells on the basis of $V_\beta$ TCR expression (Hermon et al., 1991; Johnson, Russell & Pontzer, 1991). Several investigators have already demonstrated that SAg can be potent inducers of immune responses against tumors. Newell and co-workers administered the staphylococcal SAg, SEB, to C3H mice and documented the in vivo activation of the appropriate, complimentary-reactive $V_\beta$ subsets, while nonreactive $V_\beta$ (TCR) subsets were not affected (Newell et al., 1991). When mice were administered a dose of SEB SAg at the time of tumor inoculation, there was a significant decrease in the growth of tumor. While no studies were performed to document the immunologic specificity of this reaction, these results provide a clue to the potential therapeutic effect SAg might have in the manipulation of the host's response to a vaccine or tumor challenge. Subsequently, we have demonstrated that SAg stimulation of tumor-draining lymph node (TDLN) cells can induce the differentiation of tumor-specific T cells with therapeutic activity (Shu et al., 1994). Thus the direct in vivo use of SAg may stimulate specific and/or nonspecific antitumor reactivities by triggering select $V_\beta$ T cell subsets with antitumor reactivity, or secondary to the cytokine cascade initiated by SAg activation. These potent stimulators of the immune response may offer a new approach to deal with the anergy or suppression long suspected to play a role in the failure of immunotherapy.

## Tumor Antigens

Another exciting area of immunology over the past decade has been the identification of a series of common tumor antigens. Carcinoembryonic antigen (CEA) is a well-characterized antigen associated with colon, breast, gastric, pancreatic, and nonsmall-cell lung cancer (Thompson, Grunert & Zimmerman, 1991). The cloning of the CEA gene led to the generation of a vaccinia virus vector encoding it. Administration of this recombinant viral vaccine to mice demonstrated antitumor effects against a syngeneic tumor expressing human CEA (Kantor et al., 1992). The preclinical success of this approach led investigators to test alternative strategies of generating antihuman CEA immunity without using viral vectors. Conry and colleagues recently demonstrated that direct gene transfer with a plasmid vector encoding CEA generated immune reactivity to this antigen in mice (Conry et al., 1994). These preclinical observations led to the initiation of a clinical trial of the recombinant vaccinia CEA vaccine in patients with colon cancer.

A number of tumor antigen peptides have recently been described and are likely to be the focus of future gene transfer strategies. These include peptides from melanoma, breast, ovarian, and pancreatic cancers. In each case, T cells are recognizing specific peptides presented by HLA molecules or as a repeated epitope on a protein core (Jerome et al., 1991, 1993; van der Bruggen et al., 1991; Ioannides et al., 1993a, 1993b; Slingluff et al., 1993; Storkus et al., 1993; Kawakami et al., 1994). Transfection of these genes into target cells confers susceptibility to lysis by tumor antigen-specific T cells, suggesting a role for those molecules in direct gene transfer vaccination strategies.

Proto-oncogenes can also serve as targets for the immune-mediated destruction of tumor cells. Fenton and colleagues immunized mice to mutated *Ras* and demonstrated specific protection against a subsequent challenge with tumor cells expressing the appropriate *Ras* oncogene (Fenton et al., 1993). Similarly, Carbon and colleagues immunized mice to mutant p53 protein epitopes and generated CTL, which specifically recognized and lysed syngeneic target cells expressing the appropriate mutant p53 (Carbone et al., 1994). While both examples used peptides to immunize mice, a similar strategy using plasmid vector constructs can easily be envisioned. These strategies would rely on identifying an appropriate mutated region of the gene to target with the vector construct, such that the complete proto-oncogene would not be used, thereby reducing the risk of inducing tumors in normal tissue as a result of gene transfer.

## Accessory Molecules

Previously, we described a minimal model of immune recognition, which required only T cell receptor interaction with MHC/HLA molecules presenting a TAA. In fact, there are a wide array of accessory molecules which can act to facilitate T cell recognition and activation (reviewed in Shevach, 1993).

One of the most critical accessory molecules on T cells is lymphocyte functional antigen (LFA-1). Antibody that reacts with their cell membrane determinant can inhibit essentially all activity of immune cells (Schevach, 1993). This suggests that the normal interaction of LFA-1 with its ligand ICAM-1, ICAM-2, or ICAM-3 (intracellular adhesion molecule) is an important component of a successful immune response. Many tumor cell types do not express these ligands effectively, decreasing the potential of these tumor cells to act as stimulators or targets of the immune response. This finding suggests that transfer of genes encoding this family of LFA-1 ligands may augment the generation of an antitumor immune response and be useful in the refinement of engineered tumor vaccines.

CD28 is another membrane-bound molecule important to the generation of an immune response under certain circumstances. Co-stimulatory signals provided by CD28 recognition of the B7 ligand leads to increases in cytokine production, stabilization of the message for IL-2, and maintenance of effector T cell activity (reviewed in Schwartz, 1992). Becker and colleagues recently reported that human T cells stimulated by tumor cells missing the co-stimulatory signal were anergized and secreted elevated levels of the potentially immunosuppressive cytokine, interleukin-10 (IL-10) (Becker, Czerny & Brocker, 1994). Stimulation of T cells with tumor cells transfected with B7 did not anergize the T cells and induced the secretion of significantly less IL-10. Furthermore, several animal studies have demonstrated a critical role for B7 expression by tumor cells in the generation of antitumor immune responses (Townsend & Allison, 1993; Li et al., 1994). Interestingly, Chen and colleagues have subsequently demonstrated that transfection of B7 into tumor vaccines is only effective when tumors are immunogeneic (Chen et al., 1994b). Nonetheless, results of these and other studies have stimulated investigators to engineer B7 into tumor cell vaccines. Recently, a phase I trial of B7-

transfected allogeneic melanoma cells was approved by the Recombinant DNA Advisory Committee (Sznol, 1994).

Recently, Kubin and colleagues have demonstrated that IL-12 synergizes with B7 co-stimulation of CD28 to increase proliferation and cytokine release of T cells in vitro (Kubin, Kamoun & Trinchieri, 1994). Zitvogel et al. have extended these observations to demonstrate that B7 transfection into tumor cell vaccines was further amplified by expression of interleukin-12 (IL-12) in autologous fibroblasts or tumor cells (Zitvogel et al., 1994). These interesting results provide insight into the direction that clinical trials are likely to progress.

The co-stimulatory and immune amplifying properties of accessory molecules make them likely targets for future incorporation into tumor vaccine strategies. A host of other accessory molecules have been identified and characterized. These include CD2, CD44, CD45, CD59, and OX-40 (Shevach, 1993). Future investigations will undoubtably focus on examining the effect of expressing ligands for these molecules in tumor vaccines or in combination with other genes for direct in vivo gene transfer strategies (see Chapter 8).

## Suicide Genes

The demonstration that insertion of a suicide gene into tumors combined with the subsequent administration of the appropriate prodrug could induce tumor regression and cure of animals provided an additional weapon in the gene-therapy arsenal. Moolten & Wells (1990) and Plautz, Nabel & Nabel (1991) demonstrated that transplantable murine tumors transduced with the Herpes thymidine kinase gene regressed completely following treatment with ganciclovir in vivo. Subsequently, Culver et al. (1992) demonstrated that the intratumoral transfer of retroviral producer cells producing the thymidine kinase vector resulted in transduction and eradication of experimental brain tumors in vivo following administration of ganciclovir. This approach does not need to transduce every tumor cell to be effective. Freeman et al. (1993) colleagues have documented that tumor regression can occur when only a fraction of the tumor mass expresses the gene. Recently, Mullen et al. (1994) demonstrated that some animals cured by this suicide vector-producing strategy became immune to subsequent wild-type tumor challenges. These results further support combining immunologically based intervention together with suicide-gene transfer strategies in order to increase the percentage of responding tumors and augment the generation of immune hosts. Taken together, these results have led to the initiation of clinical trials for brain and ovarian tumors (Freeman et al., 1992; Oldfield et al., 1993).

### Intracellular Single Chain Antibodies

One of the most exciting new approaches to the immunotherapy of disease is the development of intracellular single chain antibodies (sFv). Introduction of a construct encoding a recombinant sFv leads to intracellular expression of this molecule. This approach has been used to incorporate an anti-gp 120 sFv into T cells with resulting resistance to human immunodeficiency virus-1 (HIV-1)-induced syncytium formation and reduced virus production (Chen et al., 1994c). This technology has recently been applied to neutralize oncogene expression in a tumor cell line. A gene construct encoding an sFv reactive with erbB-2 was transfected into tumor cells, reducing membrane expression of the oncogene and blocking cell proliferation (Curiel, 1994). Additionally, transfection of this sFv into erbB-2 expressing tumor cells, but not control erbB-2 negative tumor cells, induced apoptosis. This novel approach to cancer gene therapy will undoubtedly be expanded and combined with both targeting and immune response-activating strategies. Future investigations need to address how generalizable is the observation that anti-erbB-2 sFv induces apoptosis in erbB-2 positive tumor cells and to what extent this approach can be translated to other oncogenes.

### Cytokine Receptors

In order for cytokines to mediate their effects on target cells directly, it is necessary for targets to exhibit an appropriate cytokine receptor. Isobe et al. (1994) recently reported that the transduction of the tumor necrosis factor-$\alpha$ (TNF-$\alpha$) receptor gene into tumor cells, which is normally negative for TNF-$\alpha$ receptor expression, conferred sensitivity to this cytokine in vitro. The result of this rather predictable experiment nonetheless demonstrates possible strategies once hurdles of vector targeting and expression are overcome.

### ■ GENE TRANSFER INTO T CELLS

Adoptive immunotherapy with TIL and IL-2 can induce regression of disseminated cancer in select patients (Rosenberg et al., 1988). It has been suggested that these T lymphocytes, which in some patients localize at the tumor site, may afford a vehicle for the delivery of therapeutic genes to the tumor (Fisher et al., 1989; Kasid et al., 1990). It may also be possible to augment, protect, or redirect the therapeutic activity of T cells using gene transfer techniques. Alternatively, labeling with a selectable marker gene, the T cells used for adoptive immunotherapy may provide a mechanism to study, recover, and subsequently expand and reinfuse T cells with antitumor activity. In this section we will review what we see as the three main avenues for gene transfer into T cells.

## Cytokines

Nishihara et al. (1988) and Miyatake et al. (1990) demonstrated the antitumor properties of a murine tumor specific T cell could be augmented by transduction. Their respective reports demonstrated that the productive integration of the interferon-$\gamma$ (IFN-$\gamma$) gene increased both in vitro cytotoxicity and therapeutic efficacy against the IFN-$\gamma$-sensitive glioma tumor cell line. Unfortunately, the difficulty in transducing primary cultures of immune T cells in the murine system has severely hampered the characterization of this approach and delineation of the appropriate cytokine strategy to employ in clinical trials. Recently, Nakamura et al. (1994) reported that TIL specific for B16 melanoma demonstrated an increased tumoricidal activity following transduction with IL-2. However, the analysis of antitumor activity in their study was limited to modified Winn-type assays, not established metastases, raising questions regarding the applicability of this approach to clinical trials.

Based on the pronounced antitumor activity of TNF in animal models, Rosenberg and colleagues have incorporated this gene into cultures of human TIL. The hypothesis of this strategy is that trafficking of engineered TIL to tumor deposits will result in localized secretion of TNF without the pronounced toxicity associated with systemic administration of this cytokine. Hwu & Rosenberg (1994) have recently reviewed the results of their TNF gene transfer studies. By modifying the TNF construct such that it bypasses the membrane-bound form, directly transcribing the smaller secreted form and coupling this to the IFN-$\gamma$-signal peptide, they report an additional fivefold increase in TNF secretion over their previous vector. TIL transduced with this improved vector are being administered to patients.

## Chimeric T Cell Receptor Genes

Immune T cells specific for tumor antigens are potent therapeutic agents in multiple animal tumor models. However, for most histologies of human cancer, it has been difficult to generate immune T cells with specificity for tumor antigen(s). The last several decades has seen the generation of antibody molecules that define numerous tumor-associated antigens. These immunological reagents have proved valuable in the diagnosis of cancer histologies but have had limited therapeutic efficacy. Kuwana et al. (1987) reported the engineering of a chimeric receptor constructed by combining the variable region of an immunoglobulin molecule, which confers immunological specificity, and the constant region of the TCR. This latter region is critical for signal transduction and activation of T cells. Subsequently, a number of investigators have extended these observations, demonstrating that T cells transduced with chimeric receptor gene constructs exhibit cytolytic activity that is redirected by the specificity of the immunoglobulin gene (Gross & Eshhar, 1992; Stancovski et al., 1993; Hwu, 1994). Refinement of this technology may allow for the insertion of appropriate chimeric receptors into CTL clones, peripheral blood lymphocytes (PBL), or hematopoietic stem cells with application to a wide variety of diseases.

## Selectable Markers/Recovery–Expansion–Reinfusion

In 1989, transduction of a murine TIL clone with the bacterial cDNA encoding resistance to the neomycin analog ($Neo^R$), G418, was reported, which afforded new avenues to investigate the trafficking, survival, and functional activities of immune T cells in vivo (Fox et al., 1989, 1990). This result demonstrated the feasibility of this approach and, together with substantial safety data, provided the Recombinant DNA Advisory Committee with sufficient evidence to perform the first clinical gene transfer protocol. Advantages of inserting genetic labels into T cells included the potential to follow cells long term because, unlike radioactive labels, the genetic marker would not decay or become diluted as cells replicated in vivo. Additionally, extremely sensitive detection of the $Neo^R$ label was possible using polymerase chain reaction (PCR). Finally, the potential to selectively recover $Neo^R$ T cells from patients following adoptive transfer of gene-marked cells opened possibilities to study functional properties of T cells associated with tumor regression.

In 1990 Rosenberg and colleagues reported on the clinical application of gene marked T cells (Rosenberg et al., 1990). Using PCR analysis, T cells marked with the $Neo^R$ gene were observed in the systemic circulation for at least 3 weeks, and as long as 2 months. In one patient, genetically labelled T cells were recovered from a tumor sample 64 days following adoptive transfer, demonstrating the capacity to recover marked cells in a clinical setting. This result verified evidence from animal models and stimulated development of methods to isolate and characterize functional activities of $Neo^R$ T cells following adoptive transfer. Recently, we reported the development of a modified limiting dilution analysis (LDA) method to analyze quantitatively and qualitatively $Neo^R$ T cells isolated following adoptive transfer (Fox et al., 1994). This methodology allowed the determination of gene-marked T cell frequency in populations of cells isolated from tissues and provided a means to extrapolate the total number of marked cells surviving in the host. Functional activities of isolated cells were also determined using this LDA approach, with both the frequency of Neo$^R$ tumor-specific CTL and cytokine gene expression being demonstrated. Application of this approach to follow and recover T cells in vivo may provide a technique to study tumor regression and to define the contributions of adoptively transferred T cells in this phenomenon.

# ■ GENE TRANSFER INTO ANTIGEN PRESENTING CELLS, FIBROBLASTS, OR MUSCLE CELLS

The same possibilities outlined for gene transfer into tumour cells may be targeted for expression in autologous antigen presenting cells (APC), fibroblasts, or muscle cells. This approach has already been used as an adjunct to tumor vaccine strategies, eliminating the requirements to isolate, culture, and modify the tumor cells themselves (Lotze et al., 1994). One can also envision the use of autologous APC transduced with appropriate tumor antigen constructs being used to vaccinate patients with malignancies. This approach may be particularly effective given the efficiency of APC function in stimulating immune responses.

Currently, these strategies are predominantly focused on in vitro manipulations of cultured cells. However, future applications are likely to focus on direct in vivo approaches to manipulate these targets. Direct gene transfer strategies that employ simple, safe, plasmid vectors, while being less efficient than their viral counterparts, may be eminently suitable for certain vaccination approaches to cancer immunotherapy. This will be particularly true for the development of tumor vaccination in an adjuvant setting, where possible risks of viral gene transfer may be unacceptable given the current state-of-the-art in gene therapy.

# ■ TARGETING GENE TRANSFER TO TUMORS IN VIVO

Table 14.4 outlines possible approaches to target gene expression at tumor sites. These approaches are subdivided under the headings physically-directed, ligand directed, and genetic.

## Physically directed

The simplest way to target gene expression at a tumor deposit is to physically apply/inject the vector construct at that location. Direct injection of a vector into a tumor deposit has been accomplished using a

## Table 14.4. Possible Approaches to Target Gene Expression at Tumor Sites

A. Physically directed
   1. Direct injection
   2. Catheter delivery
   3. Particle mediated
B. Ligand directed
   1. Antibody-targeted delivery
   2. Receptor-mediated delivery
   3. T cell-mediated delivery
C. Genetic
   1. Tumor-specific promoters
   2. Radiation-inducible promoters
   3. Drug-inducible constructs

variety of approaches ranging from lipid-complex-mediated gene transfer to injection of retroviral producer cells (Culver et al., 1992; Nabel et al., 1994b; Oldfield et al., 1993). This approach is certain to see broad application in an increasing variety of tumors over the next few years. Catheter-based delivery of vectors to tumor has been performed and is an alternative approach to deliver genes to sites not readily accessible by needle (Nabel, Plantz & Nabel, 1990; Nabel et al., 1994a). Catheter-based delivery has the unique advantage of being able to perfuse the tumor site with vector via the arterial circulation. We have used this approach to deliver vector to vascular endothelium and tumor sites (Nabel et al., 1990, 1994a).

Particle-mediated gene transfer provides an alternative method of gene transfer. Small portable 'gene gun' devices are now available to shoot particles into tumors. This will likely accelerate the introduction of this approach into the clinic.

### Ligand directed

Antibodies with specificity for cell membrane determinants have been incorporated into the liposome delivery vehicle. These immunoliposomes have increased affinity for cell types recognized by the incorporated antibody and have translated into increased transfection frequencies. Mizuno and colleagues reported a sevenfold increase in interferon production by glial cells targeted for in vitro transfection by an antibody recognizing a glioma-associated antigen (Mizuno et al., 1990). In a similar system, Holmberg et al. (1994) reported a threefold increase in transfection of glioma cells when immunoliposomes were compared to liposomes without antibody. These in vitro results have encouraged the use of this immunoliposome technology to deliver genes in vivo to sites targeted by the antibody. Significant advances in liposome technology have extended the circulating half-life of liposomes in vivo (stealth liposomes), increasing the likelihood that antibodies incorporated into their membranes may be able to target gene delivery specifically. In one study, immunoliposomes targeted to cardiac myosin heavy chain demonstrated a 16–18-fold increase in specific localization to the necrotic areas of the myocardium in rabbits with experimental infarction (Klibanov et al., 1991). These increases in tissue-specific localization have encouraged the investigation of this approach as a vehicle to target tumors in vivo. Alternatively, receptor-mediated delivery, pioneered by Wu and colleagues, offers additional strategies to target vector (Wu & Wu, 1988; Grasso & Wu, 1994). In the future it may be possible to prepare viral vectors that are engineered to express variable regions of antibody molecules or other ligands in their viral capsid. This approach may allow for systemic targeting of selected tissues or tumors.

## Genetic

Another strategy to target genetic intervention is the use of vectors with specialized promoter regions. A number of investigators have used this approach to express vector constructs preferentially in melanoma, glioma, and hepatoma cells. Recently, Vile & Hart (1993) identified promoters for tyrosinase and tyrosinase-related protein 1 that are selective for melanoma cells in vitro and in vivo. These investigators have combined this approach with direct intratumoral injection of cytokine constructs and demonstrated gene expression in vivo (Vile & Hart, 1994). In an attempt to target glioma cells, Miyao and colleagues designed constructs utilizing the promoter for the myelin basic protein gene. This approach successfully targeted these cells for expression of $\beta$-galactosidase activity (Miyao et al., 1993). Successful targeting of hepatoma cells has been accomplished by employing constructs with both the albumin enhancer element and promoter. Kuriyama and colleagues demonstrated that this construct exhibited tissue specificity in vitro and in vivo, with gene expression limited to dividing hepatocytes and hepatoma cells (Kuriyama et al., 1991).

The recent isolation of an X-ray-responsive element in the promoter of plasminogen activator provides an additional approach to target gene therapy by selective activation of gene expression (Boothman, Lee & Sahijdak, 1994). Vectors with an X-ray-responsive promoter could be used to deliver a variety of genes (see Table 14.2A) to tumor sites.

Following genetic intervention, the target tissues would be subjected to radiotherapy, selectively activating vector expression. It might be envisioned that this approach to gene radiotherapy could be applied to the wide range of radioresistant malignancies currently excluded from standard radiotherapy.

An alternative strategy to regulate novel gene expression was recently proposed by Wang and colleagues. Termed a 'gene switch' cytokine, this technology combined a mutated steroid receptor, selective for progesterone antagonists, with a transcriptional activator (Wang et al., 1994). This chimeric regulating unit was used to induce expression of gene constructs containing the specific DNA binding sites. Since the concentration of progesterone antagonists required to induce expression is lower than that needed to antagonize progesterone's effect, this gene switch might find general application in a number of approaches where regulation of gene expression is desired.

Promoters for proto-oncogenes will also be suitable enhancers for tumor-selective gene expression. Sikora and colleagues have recently proposed a number of strategies employing *c-erbB-2* promoter-controlled drug activation (Sikora et al., 1994). These approaches, which selectively target gene expression, are certain to play a significant role in the development of novel strategies to alter the immune response to tumors.

## ■ ACKNOWLEDGMENTS

We thank Drs. Walter J. Urba, Deric D. Schoof, and Kevan Roberts as well as Mr. Hong-Ming Hu, James Liu, and Erik Huntzicker for helpful discussions in the preparation of this manuscript. The excellent editorial assistance of Mary Kalez is gratefully acknowledged.

### REFERENCES

Aggarwal A., Kumar S., Jaffe R., Hone D., Gross M. & Sadoff J. (1990) Oral Salmonella: malaria circumsporozoite recombinants induce specific CD8$^+$ cytotoxic T cells. *Journal of Experimental Medicine*, **172**, 1083–90.

Aoki T., Tashiro K., Miyatake S. et al. (1992) Expression of murine interleukin 7 in a murine glioma cell line results in reduced tumorigenicity in vivo. *Proceedings of the National Academy of Sciences USA*, **89**, 3850–4.

Asher A., Mule J.J., Kasid A. et al. (1991) Murine tumor cells transduced with the gene for tumor necrosis factor-α. *Journal of Immunology*, **146**, 3227–34.

Bahler D.W., Frelinger J.G., Harwell L.W. & Lord E.M. (1987) Reduced tumorigenicity of a spontaneous mouse lung carcinoma following H-2 gene transfection. *Proceedings of the National Academy of Sciences USA*, **84**, 4562–6.

Barth R.J. Jr. & Coppola M. (1994) Lack of an immunosuppressive effect of interleukin-10 on the murine anti-tumor immune response. *Journal of Immunotherapy*, **16**, 234.

Becker J.C., Czerny C. & Brocker E. (1994) Maintenance of clonal anergy by endogenously produced IL-10. *International Immunology*, 6, 1605–12.

Berkner K.L. (1988) Development of adenovirus vectors for the expression of heterologous genes. *Biotechniques*, 6, 616–29.

Blankenstein T., Qin Z., Uberla K. et al. (1991) Tumor suppression after tumor cell-targeted tumor necrosis a gene B transfer. *Journal of Experimental Medicine*, 173, 1047–52.

Boothman D.A., Lee I.W. & Sahijdak W.M. (1994) Isolation of an X-ray-responsive element in the promoter region of tissue-type plasminogen activator: potential uses of X-ray-responsive elements for gene therapy. *Radiation Research*, 138 (Suppl.1) S68–71.

Breakefield X.O. & DeLuca N.A. (1991) Herpes simplex virus for gene delivery to neurons. *New Biologist*, 3, 203–18.

Brett S.J., Rhodes J., Liew F.Y. & Tite J.P. (1993) Comparison of antigen presentation of influenza A nucleoprotein expressed in attenuated AroA- Salmonella typhimurium with that of live virus. *Journal of Immunology*, 150, 2869–84.

Carbone D.P., Ciernick F., Wiedenfeld E., Yanuck M. & Berzofsky J.A. (1994) Development of strategies to vaccinate patients against mutations in oncopeptides. *Proceedings of the American Association of Cancer Research*, 35, 691.

Carlow D.A., Kerbel R.S. & Elliott B.E. (1989) Failure of expression of Class I mjaor histocompatibility antigens to alter tumor immunogenicity of a spontaneous murine carcinoma. *Journal of the National Cancer Institute*, 81, 759–67.

Chen L., McGowan P., Ashe S. et al. (1994b) Tumor immunogenicity determines the effect of B7 costimulation on T cell-mediated tumor immunity. *Journal of Experimental Medicine*, 179, 523–32.

Chen J., Stickles R.J. & Daichendt K.A. (1994a) Galactosylated histone-mediated gene transfer and expression. *Human Gene Therapy*, 5, 429–35.

Chen S.Y., Bagley J. & Marasco W.A. (1994c) Intracellular antibodies as a new Class of therapeutic molecules for gene therapy. *Human Gene Therapy*, 5, 595–601.

Cheng L., Ziegelhoffer P.R. & Yang N.S. (1993) In vivo promoter activity and transgene expression in mammalian somatic tissues evaluated by using particle bombardment. *Proceedings of the National Academy of Sciences USA*, 90, 4455–9.

Coen D.M., Kosz-Vnenchak M., Jacobson J.G. et al. (1989) Thymidine kinase-negative herpes simplex virus mutants establish latency in mouse trigeminal ganglia but do not reactivate. *Proceedings of the National Academy of Sciences USA*, 86, 4736–40.

Cole G.A., Cole G.A., Clements V.K., Garcia E.P. & Ostrand-Rosenberg S. (1987) Allogeneic H-2 antigen expression is insufficient for tumor rejection. *Proceedings of the National Academy of Sciences USA*, 84, 8613–7.

Colombo M.P., Ferrari G., Stoppacciaro A. et al. (1991) Granulocyte colony-stimulating factor gene suppresses tumorigenicity of a murine adenocarcinoma in vivo. *Journal of Experimental Medicine*, 173, 889–97.

Conry R.M., LoBuglio A.F., Loechel F. et al. (1994) A carcinoembryonic antigen polynucleotide vaccine has in vivo antitumor activity. *Gene Therapy*, 1, 1–7.

Cotten M., Wagner E., Zatloukal K., Phillips S., Curiel D.T. & Birnstiel M.L. (1992) High-efficiency receptor-mediated delivery of small and large (48 kilobase) gene constructs using the endosome-disruption activity of defective or chemically inactivated adenovirus particles. *Proceedings of the National Academy of Sciences USA*, 89, 6094–8.

Culver K.W., Ram Z., Wallbridge S., Ishii H., Oldfield E.H. & Blaese R.M. (1992) In vivo gene transfer with retroviral vector-producer cells for treatment of experimental brain tumors [see comments]. *Science*, 256, 1550–2.

Curiel D.T. (1994) Targeted gene delivery to accomplish gene therapy for cancer. *Journal of Immunotherapy*, 16, 235.

Curiel D.T., Agarwal S., Romer M.U. et al. (1992a) Gene transfer to respiratory epithelial cells via the receptor-mediated endocytosis pathway. *American Journal of Respiratory Cell and Molecular Biology*, 6, 247–52.

Curiel D.T., Agarwal S., Wagner E. & Cotten M. (1991) Adenovirus enhancement of transferrin-polylysine-mediated gene delivery. *Proceedings of the National Academy of Sciences USA*, 88, 8850–4.

Curiel D.T., Wagner E., Cotten M. et al. (1992b) High-efficiency gene transfer mediated by adenovirus coupled to DNA–polylysine complexes. *Human Gene Therapy*, 3, 147–54.

Donahue R.E., Kessler S.W., Bodine D. et al. (1992) Helper virus induced T cell lymphoma in nonhuman primates after retroviral mediated gene transfer. *Journal of Experimental Medicine*, 176, 1125–35.

Dougan G., Hormaeche C.E. & Maskell D.J. (1987) Live oral Salmonella vaccines: potential use of attenuated strains as carriers of heterologous antigens to the immune system. [Review]. *Parasite Immunology*, 9, 151–60.

Douvdevani A., Heleihel M., Zöller M., Segal S. & Apte R.N. (1992) Reduced tumorigenicity of fibrosarcomas which constitutively generate IL-1α either spontaneously or following IL-1a gene transfer. *International Journal of Cancer*, 51, 822–30.

Dranoff G., Jaffee E., Lazenby A. et al. (1993) Vaccination with irradiated tumor cells engineered to secrete murine granulocyte–macrophage colony-stimulating factor stimulates potent, specific and long-lasting antitumor immunity. *Proceedings of the National Academy of Sciences USA*, 90, 3539–43.

Fearon E.R., Pardoll D.M., Itaya T. et al. (1990) Interleukin-2 production by tumor cells bypasses T helper function in the generation of an antitumor response. *Cell*, 60, 397–403.

Felgner J.H., Kumar R., Sridhar C.N. et al. (1994) Enhanced gene delivery and mechanism studies with a novel series of cationic lipid formulations. *Journal of Biological Chemistry*, 269, 2550–61.

Felgner P.L. & Rhodes G. (1991) Gene therapeutics. *Nature (London)*, 349, 351–2.

Fenton R.G., Taub D.D., Kwak L.W., Smith M.R. & Longo D.L. (1993) Cytotoxic T-cell response and in vivo protection against tumor cells harboring activated ras protooncogenes [see comments]. *Journal of the National Cancer Institute*, 85, 1294–302.

Fisher B., Packard B.S., Read E.J. et al. (1989) Tumor localization of adoptively transferred indium-111 labeled tumor infiltrating lymphocytes in patients with metastatic melanoma. *Journal of Clinical Oncology*, 7, 250–61.

Flynn J.L., Weiss W.R., Norris K.A., Seifert H.S., Kumar S. & So M. (1990) Generation of a cotytoxic T-lymphocyte response using a Salmonella antigen-delivery system. *Molecular Microbiology*, 4, 2111–8.

Fox B.A., Culver K.W., Cornetta K. et al. Retroviral gene transduction of murine tumor infiltrating lymphocytes: A new approach to study trafficking in vivo. *FASEB Journal*, 3, 3496.

Fox B.A., Osterholzer J.J., Mali V. & Schomogyi M. (1994) Trafficking and survival of effector T cells in vivo. In A.E. Chang & S. Shu (eds) *Immunotherapy of cancer with sensitized T lymphocytes*, pp. 91–109. Austin, R.G. Landes Company.

Fox B.A., Spiess P.J., Kasid A. et al. (1990) In vitro and in vivo antitumor properties of a T-cell clone generated from murine tumor-infiltrating lymphocytes. *Journal of Biological Response Modifiers*, 9, 499–511.

Freeman S.M., Abboud C.N., Whartenby K.A. et al. (1993) The 'bystander effect': tumor regression when a fraction of the tumor mass is genetically modified. *Cancer Research*, **53**, 5274–83.

Freeman S.M., McCune C.S., Abboud C.N. & Abraham G.N. (1992) Treatment of ovarian cancer using HSV-TK gene-modified cells. *Human Gene Therapy*, **3**, 342–9.

Gansbacher B., Bannerji R., Daniels B., Zier K., Cronin K. & Gilboa E. (1990a) Retroviral vector-mediated gamma-interferon gene transfer into tumor cells generates potent and long lasting antitumor immunity. *Cancer Research*, **50**, 7820–25.

Gansbacher B., Zier K., Daniels B., Cronin K., Bannerji R. & Gilboa E. (1990b) Interleukin-2 gene transfer into tumor cells abrogates tumorigenicity and induces protective immunity. *Journal of Experimental Medicine*, **172**, 1217–24.

Golumbek P., Lazenby A., Levitsky H.I. et al. (1991) Treatment of established renal cancer by tumor cells engineered to secrete interleukin-4. *Science*, **254**, 713–6.

Graham F.L. & Prevec L. (1992) Adenovirus-based expression vectors and recombinant vaccines. [Review]. *Biotechnology*, **20**, 363–90.

Grasso A.W. & Wu G.Y. (1994) Therapeutic implications of delivery and expressions of foreign genes in hepatocytes. [Review]. *Advances in Pharmacology*, **28**, 169–92.

Gross G. & Eshhar Z. (1992) Endowing T cells with antibody specificity using chimeric T cell receptors. [Review]. *FASEB Journal*, **6**, 3370–8.

Herman J., Kappler J.W., Marrack P. & Pullen A.M. (1991) Superantigens: Mechanism of T-cell stimulation and role in immune responses. *Annual Review of Immunology*, **9**, 745.

Hersh E.M., Akporiaye E., Harris D., Stopeck A.T., Unger E.C. & Warneke J.A. (1994) Phase I study of immunotherapy of malignant melanoma by direct gene transfer. *Human Gene Therapy*, **5**, 1371–84.

Hesdorffer C., Markowitz D., Ward M. & Bank A. (1991) Somatic gene therapy. [Review]. *Hematology–Oncology Clinics of North America*, **5**, 423–32.

Hock H., Dorsch M., Diamantstein T. & Blankenstein T. (1991) Interleukin 7 induces CD4$^+$ T cell-dependent tumor rejection. *Journal of Experimental Medicine*, **174**, 1291–8.

Hock H., Dorsch M., Kunzendorf U., Qin Z., Diamantstein T. & Blankenstein T. (1993) Mechanisms of rejection induced by tumor cell-targeted gene transfer of interleukin 2, interleukin 4, interleukin 7, tumor necrosis factor, interferon γ. *Proceedings of the National Academy of Sciences USA*, **90**, 2774–8.

Holmberg E.G., Reuer Q.R., Geisert E.E. & Owens J.L. (1994) Delivery of plasmid DNA to glial cells using pH-sensitive immunoliposomes. *Biochemical and Biophysical Research Communications*, **201**, 888–93.

Hui K., Grosveld F. & Festenstein H. (1984) Rejection of transplantable AKR leukaemia cells following MHC DNA-mediated cell transformation. *Nature (London)*, **311**, 750–2.

Hui K.M., Sim T., Foo T.T. & Oei A.A. (1989) Tumor rejection mediated by transfection with allogeneic Class I histocompatibility gene. *Journal of Immunology*, **143**, 3835–43.

Hwu P. & Rosenberg S.A. (1994) The genetic modification of T cells for cancer therapy: an overview of laboratory and clinical trials. *Cancer Detection and Prevention*, **18**, 43–50.

Ioannides C.G., Fisk B., Jerome K.R., Irimura T., Wharton J.T. & Finn O.J. (1993a) Cytotoxic T cells from ovarian malignant tumors can recognize polymorphic epithelial mucin core peptides. *Journal of Immunology*, **151**, 3693–703.

Ioannides C.G., Fisk B., Fan D., Biddison W.E., Wharton J.T. & O'Brian C.A. (1993b) Cytotoxic T cells isolated from ovarian malignant ascites recognize a peptide derived from the HER-2/neu proto-oncogene. *Cellular Immunology*, 151, 225–34.

Isobe K., Fan Z.H., Emi N. & Nakashima I. (1994) Gene transfer of TNF receptors for treatment of cancer by TNF. *Biochemical and Biophysical Research Communications*, 202, 1538–42.

Jerome K.R., Barnd D.L., Bendt K.M. et al. Cytotoxic T-lymphocytes derived from patients with breast adenocarcinoma recognize an epitope present on the protein core of a mucin molecule preferentially expressed by malignant cells. *Cancer Research*, 51, 2908–16.

Jerome K.R., Domenech N. & Finn O.J. (1993) Tumor-specific cytotoxic T cell clones from patients with breast and pancreatic adenocarcinoma recognize EBV-immortalized B cells transfected with polymorphic epithelial mucin complementary DNA. *Journal of Immunology*, 151, 1654–62.

Jicha D.L., Mule J.J. & Rosenberg S.A. (1991) Interleukin 7 generates antitumor cytotoxic T lymphocytes against murine sarcomas with efficacy in cellular adoptive immunotherapy. *Journal of Experimental Medicine*, 174, 1511–5.

Johnson H.M., Russell J.K. & Pontzer C.H. (1991) Staphylococcal enterotoxin microbial superantigens. *FASEB Journal*, 5, 2706–12.

Kantor J., Irvine K., Abrams S., Kaufman H., DiPietro J. & Schlom J. (1992) Antitumor activity and immune responses induced by a recombinant carcinoembryonic antigen-vaccinia virus vaccine. *Journal of the National Cancer Institute*, 84, 1084–91.

Kasid A., Morecki S., Aebersold P. et al. (1990) Human gene transfer: characterization of human tumor-infiltrating lymphocytes as vehicles for retroviral-mediated gene transfer in man. *Proceedings of the National Academy of Sciences USA*, 87, 473–7.

Kawakami Y., Eliyahu S., Delgado C.H. et al. (1994) Cloning of the gene coding for a shared human melanoma antigen recognized by autologous T cells infiltrating into tumor. *Proceedings of the National Academy of Sciences USA*, 91, 3515–9.

Klein T.M., Wolf E.D., Wu R. & Sanford J.C. (1987) High-velocity microprojectiles for delivering nucleic acids into living cells. *Nature (London)*, 327, 70–3.

Klibanov A.L., Khaw B.A., Nossiff N. et al. (1991) Targeting of macromolecular carriers and liposomes by antibodies to myosin heavy chain. *American Journal of Physiology*, 261 (Suppl. 4.), 60–5.

Kubin M., Kamoun M. & Trinchieri G. (1994) Interleukin 12 synergizes with B7/CD28 interaction in inducing efficient proliferation and cytokine production of human T cells. *Journal of Experimental Medicine*, 180, 211–22.

Kuriyama S., Yoshikawa M., Ishizaka S. et al. (1991) A potential approach for gene therapy targeting hepatoma using a liver-specific promoter on a retroviral vector. *Cell Structure and Function*, 16, 503–10.

Kuwana Y., Asakura Y., Utsunomiya N. et al. (1987) Expression of chimeric receptor composed of immunoglobulin-derived V regions and T cell receptor-derived C regions. *Biochemical and Biophysical Research Communications*, 149, 960–8.

Li Y., McGowan P., Hellstrom I., Hellstrom K.E. & Chen L. (1994) Costimulation of tumor-reactive CD4⁺ and CD8⁺ T lymphocytes by B7, a natural ligand for CD28, can be used to treat established mouse melanoma. *Journal of Immunology*, 153, 421–8.

Lotze M.T., Rubin J.T., Carty S. et al. (1994) Gene therapy of cancer: a pilot study of IL-4-gene-modified fibroblasts admixed with autologous tumor to elicit an immune response. *Human Gene Therapy*, 5, 41–55.

Martuza R.L., Malick A., Markert J.M., Ruffner K.L. & Coen D.M. (1991) Experimental therapy of human glioma by means of a genetically engineered virus mutant. *Science*, 252, 854–6.

McBride W.H., Thacker J.D., Comora S. et al. (1992) Genetic modification of a murine fibrosarcoma to produce interleukin 7 stimulates host cell infiltration and tumor immunity. *Cancer Research*, 52, 3931–7.

McLachlin J.R., Cornetta K., Eglitis M.A. & Anderson W.F. (1990) Retroviral-mediated gene transfer. *Progress in Nucleic Acid Research and Molecular Biology*, 38, 91–135.

Miyao Y., Shimizu K., Moriuchi S. et al. (1993) Selective expression of foreign genes in glioma cells: use of the mouse myelin basic protein gene promoter to direct toxic gene expression. *Journal of Neuroscience Research*, 36, 472–9.

Miyatake S., Nishihara K., Kikuchi H. et al. (1990) Efficient tumor suppression by glioma-specific murine cytotoxic T lymphocytes transfected with interferon-gamma gene. *Journal of the National Cancer Institute*, 82, 217–20.

Mizuno M., Yoshida J., Sugita K. et al. (1990) Growth inhibition of glioma cells transfected with the human beta-interferon gene by liposomes coupled with a monoclonal antibody. *Cancer Research*, 50, 7826–9.

Moolten F.L. & Wells J.M. (1990) Curability of tumors bearing herpes thymidine kinase genes transferred by retroviral vectors. *Journal of the National Cancer Institute*, 82, 297–300.

Mullen C.A., Coale M., Levy A.T. et al. (1992) Fibrosarcoma cells transduced with the IL-6 gene exhibit reduced tumorigenicity, increased immunogenicity and decreased metastatic potential. *Cancer Research*, 52, 6020–4.

Mullen C.A., Coale M.M., Lowe R. & Blaese R.M. (1994) Tumors expressing the cytosine deaminase suicide gene can be eliminated in vivo with 5-fluorocytosine and induce protective immunity to wild type tumor. *Cancer Research*, 54, 1503–6.

Muzyczka N. (1992) Use of adeno-associated virus as a general transduction vector for mammalian cells. *Current Topics in Microbiology and Immunology*, 158, 97–129.

Nabel E.G., Plautz G. & Nabel G.J. (1990) Site-specific gene expression in vivo by direct gene transfer into the arterial wall. *Science*, 249, 1285–8.

Nabel E.G., Plautz G. & Nabel G.J. (1992) Transduction of a foreign histocompatibility gene into the arterial wall induces vasculitis. *Proceedings of the National Academy of Sciences USA*, 89, 5157–61.

Nabel G.J., Chang A.E., Nabel E.G. et al. (1994a) Immunotherapy for cancer by direct gene transfer into tumors. *Human Gene Therapy*, 5, 57–77.

Nabel E.G., Yang Z., Muller D. et al. (1994b) Safety and toxicity of catheter gene delivery to the pulmonary vasculature in a patient with metastatic melanoma. *Human Gene Therapy*, 5, 1089–94.

Nabel G.J., Nabel E.G., Yang Z.Y. et al. (1993) Direct gene transfer with DNA–liposome complexes in melanoma: expression, biologic activity, and lack of toxicity in humans. *Proceedings of the National Academy of Sciences USA*, 90, 11307–11.

Nakamura Y., Wakimoto H., Abe J. et al. (1994) Adoptive immunotherapy with murine tumor-specific T lymphocytes engineered to secrete interleukin-2. *Cancer Research*, 54, 5757–60.

Newell K.A., Ellenhorn J.D.I., Bruce D.S. & Bluestone J.A. (1991) In vivo T cell activation by staphylococcal enterotoxin B prevents outgrowth of a malignant tumor. *Proceedings of the National Academy of Sciences USA*, 88, 1074–8.

Nishihara K., Miyatake S., Sakata T. et al. (1988) Augmentation of tumor targeting in a line of glioma-specific mouse cytotoxic T-lymphocytes by retroviral expression of mouse gamma-interferon complementary DNA. *Cancer Research*, 48, 4730–5.

Oldfield E.H., Ram Z., Culver K.W. et al. (1993) Gene therapy for the treatment of brain tumors using intra-tumoral transduction with the thymidine kinase gene and intravenous ganciclovir. *Human Gene Therapy*, **4**, 39–69.

Ostrand-Rosenberg S., Cole G.A., Nishimura M.I. & Clements V.K. (1990) Transfection and expression of syngeneic H-2 genes does not reduce malignancy of H-2 negative teratocarcinoma cells in the autologous host. *Cellular Immunology*, **128**, 152–64.

Pakzaban P., Geller A.I. & Isacson O. (1994) Effect of exogenous nerve growth factor on neurotoxicity of and neuronal gene delivery by a herpes simplex amplicon vector in the rat brain. *Human Gene Therapy*, **5**, 987–95.

Plautz G., Nabel E.G. & Nabel G.J. (1991) Selective elimination of recombinant genes in vivo with a suicide retroviral vector. *New Biologist*, **3**, 709–15.

Plautz G.E., Yang Z.Y., Wu B., Gao X., Huang L. & Nabel G.J. (1993) Immunotherapy of malignancy by in vivo gene transfer into tumors. *Proceedings of the National Academy of Sciences USA*, **90**, 4645–9.

Porgador A., Tzehoval E., Katz A. et al. (1992) Interleukin 6 gene transfection into Lewis lung carcinoma tumor cells suppresses the malignant phenotype and confers immunotherapeutic competence against parental metastic cells. *Cancer Research*, **52**, 3679–86.

Richter G., Kruger-Krasagakes S., Hein G. et al. (1993) Interleukin 10 transfected into Chinese hamster ovary cells prevents tumor growth and macrophage infiltration. *Cancer Research*, **53**, 4134–7.

Rosenberg S.A., Aebersold P., Cornetta K. et al. (1990) Gene transfer into humans – immunotherapy of patients with advanced melanoma, using tumor-infiltrating lymphocytes modified by retroviral gene transduction. *New England Journal of Medicine*, **323**, 570–8.

Rosenberg S.A., Packard B.S., Aebersold P.M. et al. (1988) Use of tumor-infiltrating lymphocytes and interleukin-2 in the immunotherapy of patients with metastatic melanoma. A preliminary report. *New England Journal of Medicine*, **319**, 1676–80.

Rubin J., Charboneau J.W., Reading C. & Kovach J.S. (1994) Phase I study of immunotherapy of hepatic metastases of colorectal carcinoma by direct gene transfer. *Human Gene Therapy*, **5**, 1385–99.

San H., Yang Z.Y., Pompili V.J. et al. (1993) Safety and short-term toxicity of a novel cationic lipid formulation for human gene therapy. *Human Gene Therapy*, 781–8.

Schwartz R.H. (1992) Costimulation of T lymphocytes: the role of CD28, CTLA-4, and B7/BB1 in interleukin-2 production and immunotherapy. *Cell*, **71**, 1065–8.

Shevach E.M. (1993) Accessory molecules. In W.E. Paul (ed.) *Fundamental immunology*, 3rd edn, pp. 531–75. New York, Raven Press.

Shu S., Krinock R.A., Matsumura T. et al. (1994) Stimulation of tumor-draining lymph node cells with superantigenic staphylococcal toxin leads to the generation of tumor-specific effector T cells. *Journal of Immunology*, **152**, 1277–88.

Sikora K., Harris J., Hurst H. & Lemoine N. (1994) Therapeutic strategies using c-erbB-2 promoter-controlled drug activation. *Annals of the New York Academy of Sciences*, **716**, 115–24 (discussion, 124–5, 140–3).

Slingluff C.L. Jr., Cox A.L., Henderson R.A., Hunt D.F. & Engelhard V.H. (1993) Recognition of human melanoma cells by HLA-A2.1-restricted cytotoxic T lymphocytes is mediated by at least six shared peptide epitopes. *Journal of Immunology*, **150**, 2955–63.

Stancovski I., Schindler D.G., Waks T., Yarden Y., Sela M. & Eshhar Z. (1993) Targeting of T lymphocytes to Neu/HER2-expressing cells using chimeric single chain Fv receptors. *Journal of Immunology*, **151**, 6577–82.

Stoppacciaro A., Melani C., Parenza M. et al. (1993) Regression of an established tumor genetically modified to release granulocyte colony-stimulating factor requires granulocyte-T cell cooperation and T cell-produced interferon-$\gamma$. *Journal of Experimental Medicine*, **178**, 151–61.

Storkus W.J., Zeh H.J. III, Maeurer M.J., Salter R.D. & Lotze M.T. (1993) Identification of human melanoma peptides recognized by Class I restricted tumor infiltrating T lymphocytes. *Journal of Immunology*, **151**, 3719–27.

Suzuki T., Tahara H., Robbins P.D. & Lotze M.T. (1994) Discordant biologic effects of viral IL-10 and authentic IL-10 in murine tumor models. *Journal of Immunotherapy*, **16**, 245.

Sznol M. (1994) Regulatory issues: addition to appendix D of the NIH guidelines regarding human gene transfer protocol. *Human Gene Therapy*, **5**, 1182–4.

Tahara H., Zitvogel L., Storkus W.J., McKinney T.G., Robbins P.D. & Lotze M.T. (1994) Cancer gene therapy using interleukin-12 (IL-12). *Journal of Immunotherapy*, **16**, 245.

Tanaka K., Hayashi H., Hamada C., Khoury G. & Jay G. (1986) Expression of major histocompatibility complex Class I antigens as a strategy for the potentiation of immune recognition of tumor cells. *Proceedings of the National Academy of Sciences USA*, **83**, 8723–7.

Tanaka K., Isselbacher K.J., Khoury G. & Jay G. (1985) Reversal of oncogenesis by the expression of a major histocompatibility complex Class I gene. *Science*, **228**, 26–30.

Temin H.M. (1989) Retrovirus vectors: promise and reality. *Science*, **246**, 983.

Tepper R.I., Coffman R.L. & Leder P. (1992) An eosinophil-dependent mechanism for the antitumor effect of IL-4. *Science*, **257**, 548–51.

Tepper R.I., Pattengale P.K. & Leder P. (1989) Murine interleukin-4 displays potent antitumor activity in vivo. *Cell*, **57**, 503–12.

Thompson J., Grunert F. & Zimmerman W. (1991) CEA gene family: molecular biology and clinical perspectives. *Journal Clinical Laboratory Analysis*, **5**, 344–66.

Townsend S.E. & Allison J.P. (1993) Tumor rejection after direct costimulation of CD8[+] T cells by B7-transfected melanoma cells. *Science*, **259**, 368–70.

van der Bruggen P., Traversari C., Chomez P. et al. A gene encoding an antigen recognized by cytolytic T lymphocytes on a human melanoma. *Science*, **254**, 1643–7.

Vile R.G. & Hart I.R. (1993) In vitro and in vivo targeting of gene expression to melanoma cells. *Cancer Research*, **53**, 962–7.

Vile R.G. & Hart I.R. (1994) Targeting of cytokine gene expression to malignant melanoma cells using tissue specific promoter sequences. *Annals of Oncology*, **5** (Suppl. 4), 59–65.

Vogelzang N.J., Lestingi T.M. & Sudakoff G. (1994) Phase I study of immunotherapy of metastatic renal cell carcinoma by direct gene transfer into metastatic lesions. *Human Gene Therapy*, **5**, 1357–70.

Wagner E., Zatloukal K., Cotten M. et al. (1992) Coupling of adenovirus to transferrin-polysine/DNA complexes greatly enhances receptor-mediated gene delivery and expression of transfected genes. *Proceedings of the National Academy of Sciences USA*, **89**, 6099–103.

Wagner E., Zenke M., Cotten M., Beug H. & Birnstiel M.L. (1990) Transferrin–polycation conjugates as carriers for DNA uptake into cells. *Proceedings of the National Academy of Sciences USA*, **87** 3410–4.

Wahl W.L., Plautz G.E., Fox B.A., Nabel G.J., Shu S. & Chang A.E. (1992) Generation of therapeutic T lymphocytes after in vivo transfection of a tumor with a gene encoding allogenic Class I major histocompatability complex antigen. *Surgical Forum*, **XLIII**, 476–8.

Wahl W.L., Strome S.E., Nabel G.J. et al. (1995) Generation of therapeutic T lymphocytes after in vivo tumor transfection with an allogeneic Class I major histocompatibility complex gene. *Journal of Immunotherapy*, **17**, 1–11.

Wallich R., Bulbuc N., Hammerling G.J., Katzav S., Segal S. & Feldman M. (1995) Abrogation of metastatic properties of tumour cells by de novo expression of H-2K antigens following H-2 gene transfection. *Nature (London)*, **315**, 301–5.

Wang Y., O'Malley B.W. Jr., Tsai S.Y. & O'Malley B.W. (1994) A regulatory system for use in gene transfer. *Proceedings of the National Academy of Sciences USA*, **91**, 8180–4.

Watanabe Y., Kuribayashi K., Miyatake S. et al. (1989) Exogenous expression of mouse interferon gamma cDNA in mouse neuroblastoma C1300 cells results in reduced tumorigenicity by augmented anti-tumor immunity. *Proceedings of the National Academy of Sciences USA*, **86**, 9456–60.

Weber J.S., Jay G., Tanaka K. & Rosenberg S.A. (1987) Immunotherapy of a murine tumor with interleukin 2. Increased sensitivity after MHC Class I gene transfection. *Journal of Experimental Medicine*, **166**, 1716–33.

Wolff J.A., Ludtke J.J., Acsadi G., Williams P. & Jani A. (1992) Long-term persistence of plasmid DNA and foreign gene expression in mouse muscle. *Human Molecular Genetics*, **1**, 363–9.

Wolff J.A., Malone R.W., Williams P. et al. (1990) Direct gene transfer into mouse muscle in vivo. *Science*, **247**, 1465–8.

Wolff J.A., Williams P., Acasdi G., Jiao S., Jani A. & Chong W. (1991) Conditions affecting direct gene transfer into rodent muscle in vivo. *Biotechniques*, **11**, 474–85.

Wu G.Y. & Wu C.H. (1988) Evidence for targeted gene delivery to Hep G2 hepatoma cells in vitro. *Biochemistry*, **27**, 887–92.

Yang N.S. (1992) Gene transfer into mammalian somatic cells in vivo. *Critical Reviews in Biotechnology*, **12**, 335–56.

Yang N.S., Burkholder J., Roberts B., Martinell B. & McCabe D. (1990) In vivo and in vitro gene transfer to mammalian somatic cells by particle bombardment. *Proceedings of the National Academy of Sciences USA*, **87**, 9568–72.

Zitvogel L., Tahara H., Robbins P., Clark M. & Lotze M.T. (1994) B7.1 expression enhances effective OL-12 mediated antitumor immunity. *Journal of Immunotherapy*, **16**, 247.

# —15————————————————

# Applications of Antibody Gene Technology

ROBERT E. HAWKINS AND KERRY A. CHESTER

## ◼ INTRODUCTION

The last few years have seen a revolution in molecular biology that has allowed greater understanding of the mechanisms of oncogenesis. Unfortunately this greater understanding has not yet led to improved therapy. Molecular biology is now being applied to developing new antibody-based therapeutic modalities, which appear to have great potential. Antibodies are flexible binding reagents and have been investigated as tumour-targeting agents, but recent technological advances have brought many changes to the ways antibodies are made and the forms in which they can be used. Antibodies play a critical part in many approaches to targeted cancer therapy, including gene therapy, and the development of cancer vaccines. This chapter reviews the current state of antibody-guided therapy and the changes in antibody gene technology that are making these new approaches possible.

## ◼ EXPERIENCE OF ANTIBODY-TARGETED CANCER THERAPY

Since the development of monoclonal antibodies by somatic cell fusion (Köhler & Milstein, 1975) numerous antibodies to tumour selective antigens have been made. They provide useful diagnostic (for review, see Neville, 1991) and prognostic (Hawkins et al., 1989) information in the treatment of cancer, and have been tested for imaging or therapy in a variety of malignancies. In general, imaging is successful and can be better than other available techniques, although therapeutic successes have been limited (for review, see Mach, Pelegtin & Buchegger, 1991). Some of the reasons for this are shown in Table 15.1. Many of these problems are interrelated. Poor penetration, poor target specificity, and lower than

## Table 15.1. Problems Encountered in Antibody Therapy for Cancer

- Poor specificity of target antigens
- Heterogeneous expression of target antigens
- Poor penetration of solid tumours by large molecules
- Antibodies used may have suboptimal affinity
- Immunogenicity of the antibody limits long-term therapy
- Toxicity resulting from the effector arm of the antibody

optimal affinity mean that only a small fraction of the antibody reaches the tumour (usually much less than 1% injected dose) and that it frequently localizes only around the tumour vasculature. Because many antibodies have poor affinity, they remain bound for only a short time. Understanding the problems involved and applying the techniques of molecular biology to solving them should allow design and production of new molecules, which overcome at least some of these problems.

A humanized antibody has been used with good effect in the treatment of non-Hodgkin's lymphoma (Hale et al., 1988), but for common epithelial tumours, the use of human or humanized antibodies has not been reported. Indeed, the use of natural effector mechanisms is attractive both because they should have low toxicity, and because the mechanism of action is entirely different from that of radiation or cytotoxic drugs. Their use in adjuvant therapy may avoid the difficulties of tumour penetration. Encouragingly, a recent report of a randomized trial utilizing a native murine antibody as adjuvant therapy for colorectal cancer has shown a modest benefit on survival (Reithmuller et al., 1994) comparable to that obtained with chemotherapy but with less toxicity.

Antibody-guided radiation, most commonly radioiodine, has been used extensively as an alternative to harnessing natural effector mechanisms. This has the advantage that part of the problem of tumour penetration is overcome by a strong bystander effect but the low percentage of the dose received and the extensive circulation time mean that much of the radiation dose is received by other tissues, including very sensitive tissues, such as bone marrow. Even though responses (Vriesendorp et al., 1991) and, with high doses (Press et al., 1993), prolonged remission can be achieved in very radiosensitive tumours, there may be considerable toxicity.

# ■ ISSUES FOR IMPROVED ANTIBODY THERAPY

Antibody therapy is dependent on the antigens available and the characteristics of the antibodies themselves.

## Target Antigens

There are a number of classes of tumour antigens that make potential targets (Table 15.2). The main target antigens used in human trials have been over-expressed oncofetal antigens or differentiation markers. In nude mouse models, such antigens generally provide excellent targets but in humans the targeting ability is often less impressive. There may be many reasons for this, but part of the problem is the presence of the identical or cross reactive antigens in normal tissues. Even weakly cross reactive tissue may be important (Pai et al., 1991), especially if it is more accessible, as the amount bound is very dependent on the amount reaching the target (Kennel, 1991). Such cross reactivities have occasionally given rise to unexpected toxicities in human trials (Pai et al., 1991). Intensive effort has, however, revealed some tumour-specific mutant cell-surface proteins; they deserve special note both because they make ideal targets and because others may be discovered. Such markers have been encountered as a result of point mutation (for example, Her 2 in breast cancer), deletion [for example, mutant epidermal growth factor (EGF) receptors encountered in malignant gliomas] and chromosome translocation (tropomysin–tyrosine kinase fusion in colon carcinoma) (for review, see Urban & Schreiber, 1992).

Contrary to the popular view of cancer, one feature that characterizes many tumours is the increased cell death. This exposes markers not found

## Table 15.2. Target Antigens for Anticancer Monoclonal Antibodies

| | |
|---|---|
| • Unique to tumour | Immunoglobulins T cell receptors. Mutated cell-surface proteins |
| • Relative abundance in tumour | Growth factor receptors. Oncofetal antigens Dead cell markers. Altered carbohydrate groups |
| • Confined to tumour and nonessential normal tissues | Differentiation antigens |
| • Stromal targets | Endothelial activation markers. Fibroblasts activation markers |

in normal tissues, which are useful therapeutic targets if used in conjunction with effector mechanisms that have appropriate bystander effects (Epstein et al., 1988). Although certainly not ideal for eradicating *all* microscopic disease, antibodies to intracellular targets coupled to appropriate effector mechanisms may be a very effective and general approach for treatment of bulk disease. Another attractive target is the tumour vasculature, which differs from most normal blood vessels, is clearly readily accessible and is important for the continued growth of the tumour. Models demonstrate the clear potential of tumour vascular targeting (Burrows & Thorpe, 1993) and, since some novel antigens (Rettig et al., 1992) have been characterized, the way is now open for clinical trials in this area.

Advances in our understanding of carbohydrate metabolism and carbohydrate chemistry have led to the discovery that many tumours contain an abundance of altered carbohydrates (Hakomori, 1989). In some cases this involves glycolipids as well as glycoproteins, making these especially abundant targets. In addition, there is increasing evidence that such carbohydrate groups are involved as adhesion molecules and in the development of metastasis (Hoff et al., 1990). Altered carbohydrate antigen has been correlated with poor prognosis (Hakomori 1991; Itzowitz et al., 1990), so targeted therapy against such molecules is especially attractive.

## Tumour Penetration by Macromolecules

Our understanding of tumour vasculature and the penetration of macromolecules into solid tumours is incomplete but some principles are clear. Studies with various high-molecular-weight dextrans demonstrate that the tumour neovasculature is more permeable than normal blood vessels and this allows the leakage of macromolecules from the vessels (Dvorak et al., 1988; Dvorak, Nagy & Dvorak, 1991). However, once extravasated, they penetrate the tumour parenchyma slowly and inefficiently. This also applies to antibodies and must clearly be considered when designing targeting molecules.

## Binding Characteristics–Affinity and Avidity

The antibody binding to its antigen is clearly important; the specifity is one aspect but, for optimal targeting, the affinity of binding is also important. The antibody interaction with its antigen is usually described by its affinity but this is actually a composite of the kinetic 'on-rate' and 'off-rate.' These considerations are clearly complex and there is very little experimental data to define the optimal characteristics.

In addition to affinity and off-rate there are other features of binding that can be used to advantage. Natural antibodies are (at least) bivalent and use this feature to improve binding. The affinity of binding results from univalent interactions but, when binding of two or more heads occurs, this results in a much more stable interaction–known as the avidity effect. This can result in large increases in functional affinity [up to 1000-fold for an immunoglobulin G (IgG) compared to the Fab fragment of an antibody] but depends critically on the density of the target antigen in relation to the spacing of the antibody heads (Kaufman & Jain, 1992). Whole antibodies use this feature. However, by careful design it may be possible to make molecules that are small and thus penetrate well, but are avid and so bind strongly (see p. 336 below).

## Immunogenicity

Rodent antibodies are immunogenic in humans resulting in a progressively shorter half-life of injected antibody with repeated dosage. Although rare in practice, this can also result in toxic side effects such as serum sickness or anaphylaxis. Production of chimeric (Neuberger et al., 1985) or fully reshaped antibodies (Riechmann et al., 1988) allows this problem to be reduced or avoided, but rapid methods of making human antibodies directly are desirable.

## ■ ENGINEERING IMPROVED ANTIBODIES FOR THERAPY

The problems outlined above suggest that the ideal antibody fragment for therapy (Table 15.3) would be small (say < 40,000 Da), have a high affinity for and a slow off-rate from its antigen (either intrinsically or by making use of avidity effects). The molecule should be seen as human by the immune system to avoid immune responses. Nevertheless, the experience to date suggests that the amount of targeted reagent reaching the tumour will remain low in terms of the percentage injected dose per gram of tumour. This implies that the preferred effector mechanism should incorporate some amplification and should be non-toxic in the delivered form. In addition, tumour antigen heterogeneity and the difficulty of reaching all cells suggest that the effector end of the molecule should have bystander effects. The extent to which the genetic manipulation of antibodies will allow us to approach this ideal is discussed below.

## Table 15.3. The Ideal Targeting Reagent

- Small–preferably less than 40 kDa
- Bind with high affinity
- Human
- Nontoxic before bound
- Effector mechanism should amplify the amount bound
- Effector mechanism should have bystander effect

### New Methods of Making Antibodies–the Phage System

Since an antibody fragment was first expressed on the surface of bacteriophage (McCafferty et al., 1990), rapid development of this approach to making antibodies has occurred. This system has four major advantages over other existing methods for making antibodies (Table 15.4). The basic technology behind the use of phage to make antibodies is the polymerase chain reaction (PCR). Using suitable primers (Orlandi et al., 1989), PCR can be used to amplify repertoires of re-arranged V genes (Ward et al., 1989) from a variety of B cell subsets (Hawkins & Winter, 1992). Once amplified, these gene libraries can be joined together as an antibody fragment and cloned into phage expression vectors. The display of antibodies on the surface of phage means that the phage can be treated exactly as if it were an antibody, and thus selected for specificity and desired binding characteristics (Clackson et al., 1991; Hawkins, Russell & Winter, 1992). The antibody gene is selected along with the phage antibody it encodes. After the initial selection, various methods of mutagenesis can be used to improve the originally selected antibodies

## Table 15.4. Advantages in Using Phage to Make Antibodies for Therapy

- Human antibodies can be made directly
- Large numbers of antibodies can be made
- Selection for high affinity (and slow off-rate) is possible
- The antibody genes are obtained directly, allowing expression in many different forms

(Hawkins et al., 1992; Marks et al., 1992). The system can be used to make antibodies from immunized mice and, where these have been compared, they have very favourable characteristics (higher affinity and better specificity) compared to conventional monoclonal antibodies (Chester et al., 1994). They also behave well in imaging studies both in mice and humans (R.H.J. Begent, personal communication). Antibody fragments made from phage libraries thus seem destined to become the antibodies of choice.

Such antibodies may be entirely human if made from mice transgenic for the human immunoglobulin locus (Lonberg et al., 1994). However, it is possible to bypass the need for immunization completely and generate a system, which mimics, and could even improve on the immune system, entirely in vitro. By using repertoires from nonimmune humans (Marks et al., 1991), we can make and affinity mature, human antibodies to many different antigens, just as in the natural immune system (Figure 15.1). As the technology advances and the libraries become larger, the quality and number of the antibodies produced improves (Griffiths et al., 1994). It thus seems possible that the process of making useful human antibodies

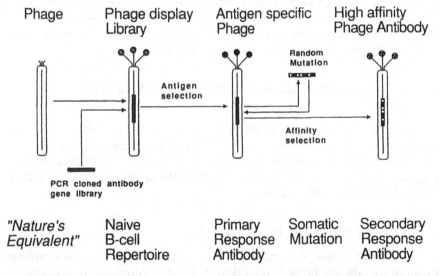

Figure 15.1  Comparison of the phage system for making antibodies from natural libraries with the immune system. The initial large repertoire of scFv fragments is equivalent to the naive B cell repertoire and, amongst this repertoire, antibodies can be found to any antigen. The affinity can subsequently be improved using methods of mutagenesis and phase selection. The use of very large libraries (Griffiths et al., 1994) allows antibodies equivalent to secondary immune responses to be isolated directly. Mutagenesis and selection could then be used to produce even higher affinity antibodies (Hawkins et al., 1993).

may eventually be done from a 'single-pot' library (Winter et al., 1994). As polyclonal antisera have been shown to be more effective than monoclonal antibodies in the treatment of recurrent Hodgkin's disease with radio-labelled antiferritin antibodies (Vriesdorp et al., 1991), it may be that the use of monoclonal cocktails will improve on single antibodies. Indeed, it may be expected that, in view of tumour antigen heterogeneity, the use of multiple antibodies to multiple antigens will be more effective still, so the ability to generate large numbers of highly specific high-affinity human antibodies may bring further benefits for therapy.

As suggested above, specificity, affinity, and off-rate are important features of an antibody. Recent evidence suggests that, in an animal models, the use of higher affinity antibodies leads to improved anti-tumour activity and improved survival (Schlom et al., 1992). The use of the bacteriophage system allows the initial selection of antibody by affinity (Chester et al., 1994) and also allows the improvement of existing antibodies (Hawkins et al., 1992) even to very high affinities (Hawkins et al., 1993a).

The final advantage of the phage system is that it permits the selection of antibodies as cloned DNA, which can very easily be expressed in an ever-increasing number of ways. This facilitates the attachment of many novel effector mechanisms and even the direct use of in vivo gene expression to deliver the therapeutic antibody.

## New Molecules for Antibody-targeted Cancer Therapy

Genetic manipulation allows the production of an endless variety of antibody-derived molecules. The basic types are shown in Figure 15.2. The ideal therapeutic agent does not exist but developments of new reagents that fulfil at least some of the criteria for an ideal molecule (Table 15.3) have been reported.

### Improving Tumour Penetration

Two approaches that have been investigated to improve tumour penetration are antibody–interleukin-2 (IL-2) conjugates, which appear to increase the local vascular permeability (LeBerthon et al., 1991) or the use of small antibody fragments. It has been shown that scFv versions of antibodies [molecular weight (MW) = 27,000] permeate deep into the tumour after 30 minutes, whereas it takes 24 hours or more for a whole IgG molecule (MW 150,000) to achieve comparable penetration (Yokata et al., 1992). Even then, the penetration of IgG at distances greater than 50 $\mu$m from the blood vessel is less than that for an scFv. These are

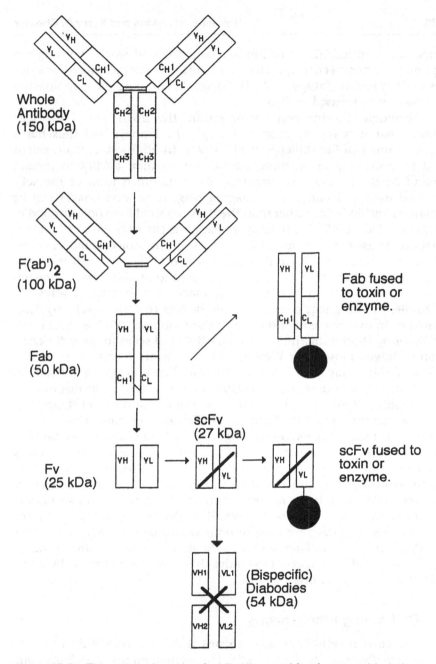

**Figure 15.2** The various formats of antibodies used for therapy with their molecular weight. The size is important for tumour penetration and is also an important determinant of the circulating half-life. The Fab and scFv can also be produced as bispecific antibodies. Diabodies (Holliger et al., 1993) may be expressed as bispecific fragments without further manipulation. These fragments can be produced in eukaryotic cells or bacteria.

important considerations for tumour targeting and when choosing the optimal effector mechanism. The use of antibody engineering to produce an scF–IL2 fusion (Savage et al., 1993) would combine these approaches but has yet to be used in vivo.

Although allowing better penetration, the small size of the scFv means that it is rapidly cleared through the kidneys and thus has a short serum half-life (Milenic et al., 1991). In addition, it is univalent and so must rely on intrinsic affinity rather than avidity to remain bound in the tumour. Nevertheless, an unmodified form of the scFv may be used as a convenient imaging reagent because images can be obtained within hours rather than the days required for whole antibodies (Colcher et al., 1990). For therapy, radiation is the only effector function that can be used without increasing the size of the molecule but the short blood half-life means that only a low fraction of the dose will reach the tumour. However, scFvs are being engineered to modify these characteristics. Bivalent scFv molecules can be made in a number of ways, for example, by using tags of amphipathic helices that are covalently associated or in dynamic equilibrium with the monomer (Pack & Plückthun, 1992) or by shortening the single chain linker of scFvs to force dimerization (Holliger, Prospero & Winter, 1993). Such molecules overcome the loss of avidity, may have longer circulation time and yet are still able to penetrate the tumour well. Small bispecific antibodies can be made either as diabodies (Holliger et al., 1993) or by the use of different dimerizing tags, which preferentially form heterodimers (Kostelny, Cole & Tso, 1992). Antibody dimers comprising two different antibodies binding two different molecules in the same tumour would simultaneously increase both avidity and specificity. If the two antibodies are not covalently associated but dimerize with appropriate affinity, it may even be possible to build up larger molecules within the tumour from small ones in the circulation. Because the small molecules penetrate well, the amount reaching deep into the tumour would be relatively large. Once a critical concentration has been reached, dimerization to form a bivalent molecules would be expected to render the binding more stable by virtue of the functional avidity.

### Cell-killing Mechanisms

The current cell-killing mechanisms that have been linked to antibodies are illustrated in Figure 15.3a. The relative merits of each are compared in Table 15.5. The effector mechanisms that will probably benefit most from the ability to engineer antibodies are the use of natural immunological mechanisms of cell killing and the antibody-directed enzyme prodrug therapy (ADEPT) approach. Radiation has been used

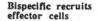

Radiation     **Toxin**     **Enzyme**

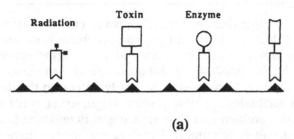

**(a)**

## (i)   Virus targeting

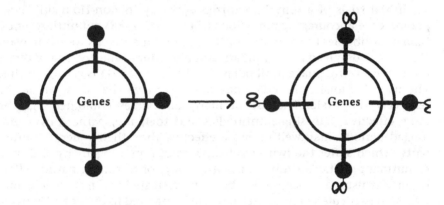

Wild Type Virus      Recombinant virus incorporates scFv
fusion to allow binding to target cell

## (ii)   Targeting delivery of plasmid DNA

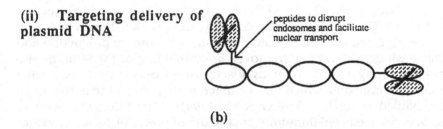

**(b)**

**Figure 15.3** Current and future methods of antibody-guided therapy. (a) In addition to native antibodies, a number of methods of antibody-mediated cell destruction are currently used. The relative merits of each are compared in Table 15.5. (b) In the future, antibodies are increasingly likely to find a role in gene therapy. The availability of antibody genes facilitate a number of novel uses, including the targeting of gene delivery using viruses. If the efficiency can be improved, the direct targeting of plasmid DNA delivery holds promise and we may speculate on the form of the eventual complex. Gene therapy has the potential advantage over protein therapy that many molecules of the therapeutic protein can then be produced locally. This may include therapeutic antibody fragments.

extensively and new isotopes that may have improved characteristics are being investigated (Waldmann,1991) but the basic problem is to target a sufficient dose to the tumour without systemic toxicity – improved antibody design may make this possible for radiation sensitive tumours, but for others large improvements are needed. Similarly, although the development of toxins is facilitated by new protein engineering constructs (Rybak et al., 1992) the problems of tumour antigen heterogeneity and tumour penetration to all cells remain. For drug conjugates there is a further problem of directing sufficient drug to the target. This may be improved by the use of more potent drugs.

Initial trials of a fully humanized antibody in non-Hodgkin's lymphoma gave encouraging remissions (Hale et al., 1988) but until recently human antibodies to common epithelial tumour antigens were not available. The widespread use of humanization (Carter et al., 1992a) and direct production using phage antibodies (Marks et al., 1991) is changing this. The use of human antibodies has the advantage that they should be relatively non-toxic. The use of many antibodies combined may be more effective than single antibodies and their use, perhaps over prolonged periods, may well be more effective than their rodent counterparts, which suffer the twin disadvantages of immunogenicity and poor recruitment of effector functions. Other ways of recruiting natural effector mechanisms are increasingly being investigated and may be advantageous. In particular, various methods are being used to direct and activate T cells using antibodies. These include the use of bispecific antibodies to recruit effector cells (Staerz, Kanagawa & Bevan, 1985). Such molecules have been used with apparent good effect in the treatment of malignant glioma (Nitta et al., 1990) and the new methods of producing bispecific antibodies (Carter et al., 1992b; Kostelny, Cole & Tao, 1992; Holliger et al., 1993), based on genetic manipulation, will simplify production and enable widespread testing. Improved understanding of the immune system is allowing optimal methods of activating T cells to be devised using bispecific antibodies, which may be much more powerful than the use of unmodified antibodies (Renner et al., 1994). Other interesting ways to harness cell-mediated immunity are the use of powerful T cell activators, such as superantigens, linked to antibodies (Dohelstein et al., 1991), or linking cytokines such as IL-2 to antibodies (Savage et al., 1993; Sabzevari et al., 1994). Such natural mechanisms may be used alone, in combination with systemic cytokines and perhaps with adoptive immunotherapy (Rosenberg 1992) to further stimulate the antitumour response.

Of the artificial effector mechanisms, the ADEPT system (Bagshawe, 1989) is attractive. In this approach an antibody is used to target an enzyme to the tumour and retain it there while the conjugate clears from the circulation. At this stage a nontoxic prodrug is given, which is activated by the enzyme to produce a cytotoxic drug at the tumour site. This system has the attraction that it includes an element of amplification and that the final cytotoxic molecule is small, allowing diffusion throughout the tumour. Thus, it is unnecessary to reach all the cells and activation of the prodrug in the vicinity of the tumour may be sufficient. The obvious drawbacks are the need to develop appropriate drugs/antibody–enzyme combinations (for review, see Senter et al., 1993) and the difficulty of obtaining optimal timing of prodrug delivery. The enzyme must be stable, not be present in the circulation and yet not be recognized as foreign by the human immune system. Such reagents have been tested but the ideal approach has not yet been found. The expression of human $\beta$-glucuronidase as an antibody fusion (Bosslet et al., 1992) is the only report of an entirely human construct. Appropriate drugs are not yet widely available, but preliminary tests with epirubicin glucuronide as the prodrug appear promising (Haisma et al., 1992) and nitrogen mustard glucuronides (Wang et al., 1992) are further possibilities. To develop smaller reagents with better ability to penetrate tumour deposits, fusions based on the scFv fragment and small monomeric enzymes can be made (Gosborn et al., 1993) and this approach seems attractive.

# ■ IDIOTYPIC VACCINATION

Methods of developing cancer vaccines and gene therapy are developing rapidly. The idiotypic immunoglobulin on B-cell lymphomas is an attractive target (Stevenson & Stevenson, 1975) but the vaccine must be made for each patient. Based on advances in antibody gene technology and gene therapy, it is possible to overcome the technical difficulties in making these vaccines for patient-specific treatment. This may represent a paradigm for vaccination against other specific target antigens when they are identified. A number of features make B-cell lymphoma a particularly attractive prospect for immunotherapy. First this is the most common type of tumour in immunosuppressed people, second a true tumour specific antigen is present on its surface (the idiotypic immunoglobulin) (Stevenson & Stevenson, 1975), third the tumour cells express good levels of major histocompatibility complex (MHC) class I and fourth they can be good antigen presenting cells (Stevenson & Hawkins, 1994). Furthermore, successes have been achieved with a variety of immunotherapeutic approaches including anti-idiotype monoclonal antibodies (Miller et al., 1982) and interferon therapy. Although there are many other therapies for malignant lymphoma disseminated, low-grade tumours are very rarely (if ever) cured and there is little evidence that current treatment prolongs survival.

Antiidiotype monoclonal antibody therapy has been tested and an overall response rate of 68% obtained. This may in part be attributed to direct cross-linking of surface immunoglobulin leading to apoptosis (Vuist, Levy & Maloney, 1994). Active immunotherapy through idiotypic vaccination has the attraction over monoclonal antibody therapy that escape from a polyclonal B and T cell response will be harder and that persisting immunity may be able to control residual dormant tumour should it subsequently become active. Pioneering work by Levy to test this approach has shown that, in advanced disease, vaccination was unsuccessful, but in earlier stage disease it is promising with immunological responses and tumour regressions being obtained (Kwak et al., 1992). The method used is very time consuming.

The use of advances in antibody gene technology allows the rapid identification and isolation of the genes comprising the tumour idiotype by PCR amplification and sequencing (Hawkins et al., 1994). Following identification of the genes, there are many possible methods for making a vaccine but again new techniques may provide the optimal solution (Tang, DeVit & Johnston, 1992). Direct inoculation of plasmid into muscles gives rise to surprisingly high levels of cell transfection and expression can persist for many months (Wolff et al., 1990). Using plasmid vaccination potentially bypasses the need for recombinant protein production (Hawkins et al., 1993b). Potentially this approach has additional advantages. As the antigen should also be presented on MHC class I molecules, it may be a good method of generating cytotoxic T cell responses and this has been demonstrated for several foreign proteins (Ulmer et al., 1993) but has yet to be demonstrated for a tumour antigen in a syngeneic host. Plasmid vaccination has yet to be tested in people but a phase I clinical trial is set to start in the near future. This approach is simple and allows logical extension by the inclusion of adjuvant molecules to enhance the immune response. This may be a very powerful means of generating of immunity to any cancer specific antigen (Urban Schreiber, 1992).

# ■ GENE THERAPY

Cancer gene therapy is a major area and cross fertilization with developments in antibody gene technology are also occurring. These give rise to new ways of using antibodies, which are particularly convenient if antibodies are available as cloned genetic material as from phage libraries (see pp. 332 above). These newer applications of antibodies, which take advantage of the manipulation of antibody genes, are illustrated in Figure 15.3b.

## Cell Targeting

Adoptive immunotherapy using lymphokine activated killer cells (LAK) or tumour-infiltrating lymphocytes (TILS) has had some success in tumours where there is some evidence of host immune response (Rosenberg, 1992). For other tumours, adoptive immunotherapy seems unlikely to be successful. Novel approaches to solving this problem have been developed by Eshhar (Eshhar et al., 1993; Hwu et al., 1993) and it may prove possible to develop T cell-based therapies targeted to tumours by monoclonal antibodies displayed on their surface (Hwu et al., 1993). Improvements allow more efficient cell activation (Eshhar et al., 1993) but it remains to be seen how such cells will behave in vivo.

## Using Genes to Deliver Antibodies

One of the drawbacks of protein therapy of all types is the difficulty and cost of making and testing large quantities of the therapeutic molecule. The rapid progress with methods of bacterial expression (Carter et al., 1992b; Skerra and Plückthun, 1988) alleviate this problem but, certainly, from a practical point of view, the use of gene transfer as a means of producing antibodies is attractive. The permanent production of proteins required for corrective gene therapy requires stable integration of genes and is perhaps best achieved using integrating viruses (for example, retroviruses or adeno-associated virus). However, for therapy with antibodies or any of the derivatives mentioned above, short-term production is all that is required. Certainly a number of possible constructs have been expressed in non-B cells and could be delivered with suitable vectors (Primus et al., 1993; Dorai et al., 1994). Adenoviruses are being evaluated for delivery of therapeutic proteins and are flexible vectors for gene transfer, which allow the incorporation of relatively large amounts of foreign DNA (Lemarchand et al., 1992) and can give high level expression for at least 70 days (Engelhardt et al., 1994). If this is not sufficient, it may be possible to develop methods in which the gene transfer complex is non-immunogenic and thus the treatment is repeatable. Such methods for in vivo gene transfer include liposomes, protein-coupled DNA or even direct injection of DNA (for review, see Felgner & Rhodes, 1991). Currently these are rather inefficient but, by incorporating the relevant parts of viral coat proteins into the DNA–protein complex, the efficiency of DNA entry into the cell is improved (Wagner et al., 1992). Further improvements to these approaches may make repeated therapy possible and enable efficient in vivo production of any therapeutic proteins including antibodies.

Entirely novel ways of using antibodies are also possible as in the use
of intracellular antibodies (Biocca et al., 1990). If directed at appropriate
targets (Biocca et al., 1994; Deshane et al., 1994), these may be able to
inhibit tumour growth in highly selective ways. However, there is the
considerable hurdle of very high efficiency (targeted) gene delivery to
be overcome before therapeutic benefits can be expected from such
approaches.

## Using Antibodies to Deliver Genes

Direct expression of an appropriate toxin within the tumour itself is
perhaps an ideal. For this, targeted delivery of genetic information is
needed. One approach is the use of antibodies to target the genes.
Antibodies can be used to target liposomes (Leonetti et al., 1990), viruses
(Roux, Jeanteur & Piechaczyk, 1989) or even directly to target DNA for
gene delivery to specific tissues (Trubetsky et al., 1992). The size of such
particles means that access to tumour tissues is severely limited. Here, if
safe replication-competent viral vectors can be developed, viruses would
have the decisive advantage that one infected cell will produce not only
many molecules of the therapeutic agent but also many progeny viruses,
which can infect more cells by local spread. In this regard the report of
stable incorporation of a functional antibody into the envelope protein of
a retrovirus is exciting (Russell, Hawkins & Winter, 1993). If the viral
infection can be directed by the antibody, then it would allow targeted
DNA delivery. Even without this feature the antibody would retain the
virus on antigen positive cells. Thus some degree of targeting will be
achievable and should be valuable in terms of both safety and efficacy.
Certainly there are problems of efficient gene transfer and problems of
immunogenicity, but, in time, if these can be overcome or circumvented,
then such recombinant viruses could provide an efficient means of reaching large tumour deposits.

## ■ CONCLUSION

Molecular biology is a rapidly changing antibody-targeted therapy.
First, new targets are being discovered. Second, it has led to the development of new methods of making antibodies, which should be superior to
the cell-based methods. Third, the antibodies can be expressed in many
forms with many different effector molecules. The most important
advances are likely to be from the use of small fragments, from improved
methods of recruiting natural effector mechanisms and from targeting
enzymes to activate prodrugs. Indeed, these methods may be especially
effective if used together. The ADEPT system should be very effective but

the problem of drug resistance in a small proportion of the tumour will be an ever-present problem. Nevertheless, at the very least, we can expect to reduce drug toxicity by such an approach. By contrast, the strength of natural mechanisms of immune surveillance is their low toxicity and entirely different mode of action. The use of true human antibodies or true human bispecific antibodies may allow prolonged therapy. This may be augmented by stimulation of T cell immunity either with cytokines, by (antibody-targeted) adoptive immunotherapy or by using immunization with tumour-specific antigens to stimulate the immune system. Such combined approaches should be very effective at directing the immune system to eradicate or suppress residual disease. Finally, gene therapy techniques for the treatment of cancer are making rapid progress. Antibodies may either be used to target appropriate genes or the appropriate vectors may be used to allow in vivo production of antibody-based molecules.

With the plethora of new techniques available that allow the production of new therapeutic molecules involving the use of antibodies, it is certain that all possible permutations cannot be tested. Perhaps the main need now is to apply our knowledge of the principles involved to design suitable molecules and test them in appropriate clinical settings.

## REFERENCES

Bagshawe K.D. (1989) Towards generating cytotoxic agents at cancer sites. *British Journal of Cancer*, 60, 275–81.
Biocca S., Neuberger M.S. & Cattaneo A. (1990) Expression and targeting of intracellular antibodies in mammalian cells. *EMBO Journal*, 9, 101–8.
Biocca S., Pierandrei-Amaldi P., Campioni N. & Cattaneo A. (1994) Intracellular immunization with cytosolic recombinant antibodies. *Bio/Technology*, 12, 396–400.
Bosslet K., Czech J., Lorenz P., Sedlacek H.H., Schuermann M. & Seeman G. (1992) Molecular and functional characterisation of a fusion protein suited for tumour specific prodrug activation. *British Journal of Cancer*, 65, 234–8.
Burrows F.J. & Thorpe P.E. (1993) Eradication of large solid tumors in mice with an immunotoxin directed against tumor vasculature. *Proceedings of the National Academy of Sciences USA*, 90, 8996–9000.
Carter P., Kelley R.F., Rodrigues M.L. et al. (1992b) High level Escherichia coli expression and production of bivalent humanized antibody fragment. *Bio/Technology*, 10, 163–7.
Carter P., Presa L., Gorman C.M. et al. (1992a) Humanisation of an anti-p185[HER2] antibody for human cancer therapy. *Proceedings of the National Academy of Sciences USA*, 89, 4285–9.
Chester K. A., Begent R.H.J., Robson L. et al. (1994) Phage libraries for generation of clinically useful antibodies. *Lancet*, 343, 455–6.
Clackson T., Hoogenboom H.R., Griffiths A.D. & Winter G. (1991) Making antibody fragments using phage display libraries. *Nature (London)*, 352, 624–8.

Colcher D., Bird R., Roseli M. et al. (1990) In vivo tumor targeting of a recombinant single-chain antigen binding protein. *Journal of the National Cancer Institute*, **82**, 1191–7.

Deshane J., Loechel F., Conry R.M., Siegel G.P., King C.R. & Curiel D.T. (1994) Intracellular single-chain antibody directed against erbB2 down-regulates cell surface erbB2 and exhibits selective anti-proliferative effect in erbB2 overexpressing cancer cell lines. *Gene Therapy*, **1**, 332–37.

Dohlestein M., Hedlund G., Åkerblom E., Lando P.A. & Kalland T. (1991) Monoclonal antibody-targeted superantigens: a different class of anti-tumor agents. *Proceedings of the National Academy of Sciences USA*, **88**, 9287–91.

Dorai H., McCartney J.E., Hudziak R. M. et al. (1994) Mammalian cell expression of single-chain Fv (sFv) antibody proteins and their C-terminal fusions with interleukin-2 and other effector domains. *Bio/Technology*, **12**, 890–7.

Dvorak H.F., Nagy J. A. & Dvorak A.M. (1991) Structure of solid tumors and their vasculature: implications for therapy with monoclonal antibodies. *Cancer Cells*, **3**, 77–85.

Dvorak H.F., Nagy J.A., Dvorak J.T. & Dvorak A.M. (1988) Identification and characterization of the blood vessels of solid tumors that are leaky to circulating macromolecules. *American Journal of Pathology*, **133**, 95–109.

Engelhardt J.F., Ye X., Doranz B. & Wilson J.M. (1994) Ablation of E2A in recombinant adenoviruses improves transgene persistence and decreases inflammatory response in mouse liver. *Proceedings of the National Academy of Sciences USA*, **91**, 6196–200.

Epstein A.L., Chen F. M. & Taylor C.R. (1988) A novel method for the detection of necrotic lesions in human cancers. *Cancer Research*, **48**, 5842–8.

Eshhar Z., Waks T., Gross G. & Schindler D.G. (1993) Specific activation and targeting of cytotoxic lymphocytes through chimeric single chains consisting of antibody-binding domains and the gamma or zeta subunits of the immunoglobulin and T-cell receptors. *Proceedings of the National Academy of Sciences USA*, **90**, 720–724.

Felgner P. L. & Rhodes G. (1991) Gene therapeutics. *Nature (London)*, **349**, 351–2.

Gosborn S.C., Svensson H.P., Kerr D.E., Somerville J.E., Senter P.D. & Fell H.P. (1993) Genetic construction, expression and characterisation of a single chain anti-carcinoma antibody fused to β-lactamase. *Cancer Research*, **52**, 2123–7.

Grifiths A.D., Williams S.C., Hartley O. et al. (1994) Isolation of high affinity human antibodies directly from large synthetic repertoires. *EMBO Journal*, **13**, 3245–60.

Hale G., Clark M. R., Marcus R. et al. (1988) Remission induction in non-Hodgkin lymphoma with reshaped monoclonal antibody CAMPATH-1H. *Lancet*, **ii**, 1394–9.

Haisma H.J., Boven E., van Muijen M., de Jong J., van der Vijgh W.J.F. & Pinedo H.M. (1992) A monoclonal antibody-β-glucuronidase conjugate as activator of the prodrug epirubicin-glucoronide for specific treatment of cancer. *British Journal of Cancer*, **66**, 474–8.

Hakomori S. (1989) Aberrant glycosylation in tumors and tumor-associated carbohydrate antigens. *Advances in Cancer Research*, **52**, 257–331.

Hakomori S. (1991) Possible functions of tumor-associated carbohydrate antigens. *Current Opinions in Immunology*, **3**, 646–53.

Hawkins R.E., Roberts K., Wiltshaw E., Mundy J., Fryatt I.J. & McCready V.R. (1989) The prognostic significance of the half-life of serum CA125 in patients responding to chemotherapy for epithelial ovarian carcinoma. *British Journal of Obstetrics and Gynaecology*, **96**, 1395–9.

Hawkins R.E., Russell S.J. & Winter G. (1992) Selection of phage antibodies by binding affinity: mimicking affinity maturation. *Journal of Molecular Biology*, **226**, 889–96.

Hawkins R.E., Russell S.J., Baier M. & Winter G. (1993a) The contribution of contact and non-contact residues of antibody in the affinity of binding to antigen: the interaction of mutant D1.3 antibodies with lysozyme. *Journal of Molecular Biology*, **234**, 958–64.

Hawkins R.E. & Winter G. (1992) Cell selection strategies for making antibodies from variable gene libraries: tapping the memory pool. *European Journal of Immunology*, **22**, 867–70.

Hawkins R.E., Winter G., Hamblin T.J., Stevenson F.K. & Russell S.J. (1993b) A genetic approach to anti-idiotype immunisation. *Journal of Immunotherapy*, **14**, 273–8.

Hawkins R.E., Zhu D., Ovecka M., Winter G., Hamblin T.J. & Stevenson F.K. (1994) Idiotypic vaccination against B-cell lymphoma: rescue of variable region gene sequences from biopsy material for assembly as single chain Fv 'personal' vaccines. *Blood*, **83**, 3279–88.

Hoff S.D., Irimura T., Matsushita Y., Ota D.M., Cleary K.R. & Hakomori S. (1990) Metastatic potential of colon carcinoma: expression of ABO/Lewis-related antigens. *Archives of Surgery*, **125**, 206–9.

Holliger P., Prospero T. & Winter G. (1993) Diabodies: small bivalent and bispecific antibody fragments. *Proceedings of the National Academy of Sciences USA*, **90**, 6444–8.

Hwu P., Shafer G.E., Treisman J. et al. (1993) Lysis of ovarian cancer cells by human lymphocytes redirected with a chimeric gene composed of an antibody variable region and the Fc gamma receptor. *Journal of Experimental Medicine*, **178**, 361–6.

Itzkowitz S.H., Bloom E.J., Kokai W.A., Modin G., Hakomori S. & Kim Y.S. (1990) Sialosyl-Tn: a novel mucin antigen associated with prognosis in colorectal cancer patients. *Cancer*, **66**, 1960–6.

Kaufman E.N. & Jain R.K. (1992) Effect of bivalent interaction upon apparent antibody affinity: experimental confirmation of theory using fluorescence photobleaching and implications for antibody binding assays. *Cancer Research*, **52**, 4157–67.

Kennel S.J. (1991) Effects of target antigen competition on distribution of monoclonal antibody to solid tumors. *Cancer Research*, **52**, 1284–90.

Köhler G. & Milstein C. (1975) Continuous cultures of fused cells secreting antibody of predefined specificity. *Nature (London)*, **256**, 495–7.

Kostelny S.A., Cole M.S. & Tso J.Y. (1992) Formation of a bispecific antibody by use of lecine zippers. *Journal of Immunology*, **148**, 1547–53.

Kwak L.W., Campbell M.J., Czerwinski D.K., Hart S., Miller R.A. & Levy R. (1992) Induction of immune responses in patients with B-cell lymphoma against the surface-immunoglobulin idiotype expressed by their tumors. *New England Journal of Medicine*, **327**, 517–22.

LeBerthon B., Khawai L.A., Alaudin M. et al. (1991) Enhanced tumor uptake of macromolecules induced by a novel vasoactive interleukin 2 immunoconjugate. *Cancer Research*, **51**, 2694–8.

Lemarchand P., Jaffe H.A., Danel C. et al. (1992) Adenovirus-mediated transfer of a recombinant human α-antitrypsin cDNA to human endothelial cells. *Proceedings of the National Academy of Sciences USA*, **89**, 6482–6.

Leonetti J-P., Machy P., Degols G., Lebleu B. & Laserman L. (1990) Antibody-targeted liposomes containing oligodeoxyribonucleotides complementary to viral RNA selectively inhibit viral replication. *Proceedings of the National Academy of Sciences USA*, **87**, 2448–51.

Lonberg N., Taylor L.D., Harding F.A. et al. (1994) Antigen-specific human antibodies from mice comprising four distinct genetic modifications. *Nature (London)*, **368**, 856–9.

Mach J-P., Pelegrin A. & Buchegger F. (1991) Imaging and therapy with monoclonal antibodies in non-haematopoietic tumors. *Current Opinion on Immunology*, 3, 685–93.

Marks J.D., Griffiths A.D., Malmqvist M., Clackson T.P., Bye J.M. & Winter G. (1992) By-passing immunisation: improving the affinity of a human antibody by chain shuffling. *Bio/Technology*, 10, 779–83.

Marks J.D., Hoogenboom H.R., Bonnert T.P., MacCafferty J., Griffiths A.D. & Winter G. (1991) By-passing immunization: human antibodies from V-gene libraries displayed on bacteriophage. *Journal of Molecular Biology*, 222, 581–97.

McCafferty J., Griffiths A.D., Winter G. & Chiswell D.J. (1990) Phage antibodies: filamentous phage displaying antibody variable domains. *Nature (London)*, 348, 553–4.

Milenic D.E., Yokota T., Filpula D.R. et al. (1991) Construction, binding properties, metabolism, and tumor targeting of a single-chain Fv derived from the pancarcinoma monoclonal antibody CC49. *Cancer Research*, 51, 6363–71.

Miller R.A., Maloney D.G., Warnke R. & Levy R. (1982) Treatment of B-cell lymphoma with monoclonal anti-idiotype antibody. *New England Journal of Medicine*, 306, 517–22.

Neuberger M.S., Williams G.T., Mitchell E.B., Jouhal S.S., Flanagan J.G. & Rabbitts T.H. (1985) A hapten-specific chimaeric IgE with human physiological effector function. *Nature (London)*, 314, 268–70.

Neville A.M. (1991) Detection of tumor antigens with monoclonal antibodies: immunopathology and immunodiagnosis. *Current Opionion in Immunology*, 3, 674–8.

Nitta T., Sato K., Yagita H., Okumura K. & Ishii S. (1990) Preliminary trial of specific targeting therapy against malignant glioma. *Lancet*, 335, 368–71.

Orlandi R., Güssow D.H., Jones P.T. & Winter G. (1989) Cloning immunoglobulin variable domains for expression by the polymerase chain reaction. *Proceedings of the National Academy of Sciences USA*, 86, 3833–7.

Pai L.H., Bookman M.A., Ozols R.F. et al. (1991) Clinical evaluation of intraperitoneal pseudomonas exotoxin immunoconjugate OVB3-PE in patients with ovarian cancer. *Journal of Clinical Oncology*, 9, 2095–103.

Pack P. & Plückthun A. (1992) Miniantibodies: use of amphipathic helics to produce functional, flexibly linked dimeric Fv fragments with high avidity in Escherichia coli. *Biochemistry*, 31, 1575–84.

Press O.W., Eary J.F., Appelbaum F.R. et al. (1993) Radiolabeled-antibody therapy of B-cell lymphoma with autologous bone marrow support. *New England Journal of Medicine*, 329, 1219–24.

Primus F.J., Finch M.D., Masci A.M., Schlom J. & Kashmiri S.V.S. (1993) Self-reactive antibody expression by human carcinoma cells engineered with monoclonal antibody genes. *Cancer Research*, 53, 3355–61.

Reithmuller G., Schneider-Gadicke E., Schlimok G. et al. (1994) Randomised trial of monoclonal antibody for adjuvant therapy of resected Duke's C colorectal carcinoma. *Lancet*, 343, 1177–83.

Renner C., Jung W., Sahin U. et al. (1994) Cure of xenografted human tumours by bispecific monoclonal antibodies and human T-cells. *Science*, 264, 833–5.

Rettig W.J., Garin-Chesa P., Healey J.H., Su S.L., Jaffe E.A. & Old L.J. (1992) Identification of endosialin, a cell glycoprotein of vascular endothelial cells in human cancer. *Proceedings of the National Academy of Sciences USA*, 89, 10832–6.

Riechmann L., Clark M., Waldmann H. & Winter G. (1988) Reshaping human antibodies for therapy. *Nature (London)*, 332, 323–7.

Rosenburg S.A. (1992) The immunotherapy and gene therapy of cancer. *Journal of Clinical Oncology*, 10, 180–99.

Roux P., Jeanteur P. & Piechaczyk, M. (1989) A versatile and potentially general approach to the targeting of specific cell types by retroviruses: application to the infection of human cells by means of major histocompatibility complex class I and class II antigens by mouse ecotropic murine leukaemia virus derived viruses. *Proceedings of the National Academy of Sciences USA*, **86**, 9079–83.

Russell S.J., Hawkins R.E. & Winter G. (1993) Retroviral vectors displaying functional antibody fragments. *Nucleic Acids Research*, **21**, 1081–5.

Rybak S.M., Hoogenboom H.R., Meade H.M., Raus J.C.M., Schwartz D. & Youle R.J. (1992) Humanization of immunotoxins. *Proceedings of the National Academy of Sciences USA*, **89**, 3165–9.

Sabzevari H., Gillies S.D., Mueller B.M., Pancock J.D. & Reisfeld R.A. (1994) A recombinant antibody–interleukin 2 fusion protein suppresses growth of hepatic human neuroblastoma metastates in severe combined immunodeficiency mice. *Proceedings of the National Academy of Sciences USA*, **91**, 9626–30.

Savage P., So A., Spooner R.A. & Epenetos A.A. (1993) A recombinant single chain antibody interleukin-2 fusion protein. *British Journal of Cancer*, **67**, 304–10.

Schlom J., Eggensperger D., Colcher D. et al. (1992) Therapeutic advantage of high-affinity anticarcinoma radioimmunoconjugates. *Cancer Research*, **52**, 1067–72.

Senter P.D., Wallace P.M., Svensson H.P. et al. (1993) Generation of cytotoxic agents by targeted enzymes. *Bioconjugate Chemistry*, **4**, 3–9.

Skerra A. & Plückthun A. (1988) Assembly of a functional immunoglobulin Fv fragment in Eschericha coli. *Science*, **240**, 1038–41.

Staerz U.D., Kanagawa O. & Bevan M.J. (1985) Hybrid antibodies can target sites for attack by T-cells. *Nature (London)*, **314**, 628–31.

Stevenson F.K. & Hawkins R.E. (1994) Molecular vaccines against cancer. *The Immunologist*, **2**, 16–19.

Stevenson G.T. & Stevenson F.K. (1975) Antibody to molecularly-defined antigen confined to a tumour cell surface. *Nature (London)*, **254**, 714–716.

Tang D-C., DeVit M. & Johnson S.A. (1992) Genetic immunization is a simple method for eliciting an immune response. *Nature (London)*, **356**, 152–5.

Trubetsky V.S., Torchilin V.P., Kennel S.J. & Huang L. (1992) Use of N-terminal modified poly(l-lysine)-antibody conjugate as a carrier for targeted gene delivery in mouse lung endothelial cells. *Bioconjugate Chemistry*, **3**, 323–7.

Ulmer J.B., Donnelly J.J., Parker S.E. et al. (1993) Heterologous protection against influenza by injection of DNA encoding a viral protein. *Science*, **259**, 1745–9.

Urban J.L. & Schreiber H. (1992) Tumor antigens. *Annual Review of Immunology*, **10**, 617–44.

Vriesendorp H.M., Herpst J.M., Germack M.A. et al. (1991) Phase I–II studies of yttrium-labelled antiferritin treatment for end-stage Hodgkin's disease, including radiation therapy oncology group 87-01. *Journal of Clinical Oncology*, **9**, 918–28.

Vuist W.M.J., Levy R. & Maloney D.G. (1994) Lymphoma regression induced by monoclonal anti-idiotypic antibodies correlates with their ability to induce Ig signal transduction and is not prevented by tumour expression of high levels of Bcl-2 protein. *Blood*, **83**, 899–906.

Wagner E., Zatlouski K., Cotton M. et al. (1992) Coupling of adenovirus to transferrin-polysine/DNA complexes greatly enhances receptor-mediated gene delivery and expression of transfected genes. *Proceedings of the National Academy of Sciences USA*, **89**, 6099–103.

Waldmann T.A. (1991) Monoclonal antibodies in diagnosis and therapy. *Science*, **252**, 1657–62.

Wang S-M., Chern J-W., Yeh M-W., Ng J.C., Tung E. & Roffler S.R. (1992) Specific activation of glucuronide prodrugs by antibody-targeted enzyme conjugates for cancer therapy. *Cancer Research*, **52**, 4484–91.

Ward E.S., Güssow D., Griffiths A.D., Jones P.T. & Winter G. (189) Binding activities of a repertoire of single immunoglobulin variable domains secreted from Escherichia coli. *Nature (London)*, **344**, 544–6.

Winter G., Griffith A.D., Hawkins R.E. & Hoogenboom H.R. (1994) Making antibodies by phage display technology. *Annual Review of Immunology*, **12**, 433–55.

Wolff J.A., Malone R.W., Williams P. et al. (1990) Direct gene transfer into mouse muscle in vivo. *Science*, 247, 1465–8.

Yokata T., Milenic D.E., Whitlow M. & Schlom J. (1992) Rapid tumor penetration of a single-chain Fv and comparison with other immunoglobulin forms. *Cancer Research*, **52**, 3402–8.

# Index

ABC (ATP-binding cassette) superfamily
    of transmembrane transporters, 52
accessory molecules, 310–11
acute lymphoblastic leukemia (ALL), 169
acute myeloblastic leukemia (AML), 169
acute myeloid leukemia (AML), 210
adenoviruses (Ads), 135–6
ADEPT system, 338, 342
adoptive immunotherapy, 18
allogeneic cell vaccines, 253–7
allogeneic MHC gene transfer, 307–8
antibody, 30
    basic types, 334
    cell-killing mechanisms, 336–9
    engineering, 331–9
    gene delivery, 342
    gene technology, 327–48
    gene therapy, 341–2
    immunogenicity, 331
    intracellular, 342
    phage system, 332–4
    tumor penetration, 334–6
antibody binding characteristics, affinity
    and avidity, 330–1
antibody-dependent cellular cytotoxicity
    (ADCC), 18, 20
antibody-dependent complement-
    mediated lysis, 18
antibody-guided radiation, 328
antibody-targeted cancer therapy, 327–8
antibody therapy, 329–31
    antiidiotype monoclonal, 340
    problems encountered in, 328
anti-CD2, 194
anti-CD3, 194
antigen, see tumor antigens
antigen presentation, 39–68, 129–30
    by MHC, 185
    by MHC class I molecules, 70–1
    in malignancy, 55–60
antigen presenting cells (APC), 14–16,
    47, 57, 59, 171, 172, 187, 191, 274
    gene transfer, 315
antigen processing, 39–68, 129–30

defective, in tumor cells, 83
in malignancy, 55–60
MHC class I pathway for, 49–53
MHC class II pathway for, 53–5
antigen receptors, MHC molecules as,
    41–9
antigen recognition, 128–9
antigen-specific unresponsiveness, 189–
    91
antigenicity, 7–9, 22–6
    enhancement of, 306
antiidiotypic antibody vaccines, 245
archaebacterium, 50

B cells/lymphocytes, 39, 40
B7, 186–8, 195, 311
B7-1, 187–9, 192
B7-2, 187–9, 192
B7-CD28 interaction, 191–2
bacterial DETOX-coupled lysate vaccine,
    249–52
BAGE gene, 105, 154
BCG, 243, 248, 254
Burkitt lymphoma, 76

calnexin, 53
carbohydrate
    antigen analysis, 277–8
    chemistry, 330
    metabolism, 330
carcinoembryonic antigen (CEA), 309
CD2, 311
CD3, 53
CD4, 171
CD4$^+$ T cells/lymphocytes, 2, 41, 57–8,
    86, 106, 109, 171, 187, 208
    in antitumor response, 59–60
    presentation of tumor-associated
        antigens to, 57–8
CD4$^+$ T helper cells, 14, 16, 21, 59, 107,
    274